Gathering Medicines

∴

Gathering Medicines

∵

NATION AND KNOWLEDGE IN
CHINA'S MOUNTAIN SOUTH

Judith Farquhar
and Lili Lai

THE UNIVERSITY OF CHICAGO PRESS
CHICAGO AND LONDON

The University of Chicago Press, Chicago 60637
The University of Chicago Press, Ltd., London
© 2021 by The University of Chicago
Published 2021
Printed in the United States of America

30 29 28 27 26 25 24 23 22 21   1 2 3 4 5

ISBN-13: 978-0-226-76351-4 (cloth)
ISBN-13: 978-0-226-76365-1 (paper)
ISBN-13: 978-0-226-76379-8 (e-book)
DOI: https://doi.org/10.7208/chicago/9780226763798.001.0001

Library of Congress Cataloging-in-Publication Data

Names: Farquhar, Judith, author. | Lai, Lili, author.
Title: Gathering medicines : nation and knowledge in China's
Mountain South / Judith Farquhar and Lili Lai.
Description: Chicago : University of Chicago Press, 2021. |
Includes bibliographical references and index.
Identifiers: LCCN 2020038864 | ISBN 9780226763514 (cloth) |
ISBN 9780226763651 (paperback) | ISBN 9780226763798 (e-book)
Subjects: LCSH: Medicine, Chinese—China, Southeast. |
Medicinal plants—China, Southeast. | Healers—China,
Southeast. | Zhuang (Chinese people)—Medicine. |
Yao (Southeast Asian people)—Medicine.
Classification: LCC R603.S8 F37 2021 | DDC 610—dc23
LC record available at https://lccn.loc.gov/2020038864

Contents

.

Preface

In July of 2011, research for this book took us to Jinxiu, in the Guangxi Zhuang Self-Governing Region. Jinxiu town is the administrative center for a Yao nationality self-governing county. Located outside this booming county town, at the intersection of two regional roads with a lot of truck traffic, sits a hospital of Yao nationality medicine (*Yaoyi Yiyuan* 瑶医医院) with forty inpatient beds, four or five outpatient clinics, and a diverse staff of several dozen medical professionals. Some of these doctors and nurses are Yao, some are members of the Han majority, and a few belong to other nationality groups. But the medical care they deliver there is marked as particularly Yao.

Lili had been to this hospital before our first visit together, and one of our project's local researchers, Yang Jian, was employed there as well, training in Yao medicine with senior resident Dr. Goldstamp Huang.[1] On this occasion, we were welcomed as old friends, then, and enthusiastically (re)introduced to the work of the hospital over a period of several days. This short but informative visit was rather typical of our itinerant field research on minority nationality medical systems in China's mountain south. Invited by leaders at the State Administration of Traditional Chinese Medicine (SATCM) in Beijing, in 2010, to bring an anthropological component to a new national initiative to "develop the nationality medicines" of (ideally) all fifty-five registered minorities, Lili invited Judith as field research partner and co-author. The SATCM then helped us to recruit research associates for seven medically various nationality groups, expecting them to help us *in situ* with local languages, contacts, experienced insights, and logistics. Yang Jian was at the time a newly appointed resident in the Yao Hospital, and she is recognized as a member of the Han majority. But she was working hard to learn the particularities of Yao medicine, and in the course of several visits we were fortunate to be able to join her in Jinxiu-area wards and clinics. She sent us many insightful field notes over the years of our multi-sited research.

Toward the end of the second day of our 2011 visit, Hospital Director

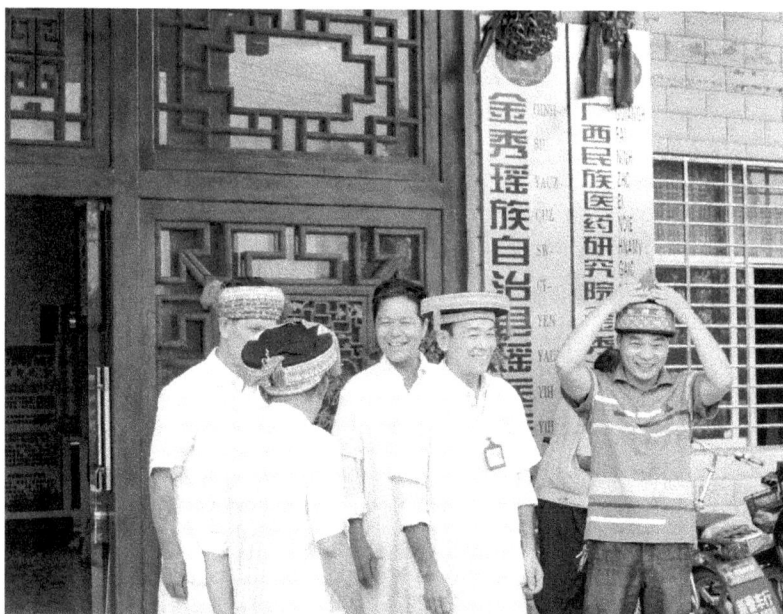

Figure 1. Staff at a Yao nationality hospital prepare to pose for a group photograph.

Liang (whose nationality is Han, but who has a father-in-law who is a famous Yao medicine doctor in private practice) and several of the Yao doctors decided we'd better take a group photo in front of the building's wide main door. As our small group of visitors, senior staff, and a research assistant began to gather in front of numerous identifying signs at the entrance, one of the white-coated doctors said, "Wait, we have to get our hats!" All of the medical staff, including the logistics manager (who was also our omnicompetent driver during this visit), laughing as they went, rushed back inside to get their Yao-style hats and put them on for the picture.

The hats were elaborately folded of red and black cloth and embroidered with colorful thread, showing different styles indicative of particular Yao subgroups. Everyone was either able to grab their own proper hat or borrow one from a colleague. Han nationality staff were not shy about wearing Yao hats. And for some of the pictures we took, our friends loaned us—foreigners that we are—Yao hats to wear.

Everyone thought it was imperative to pose for these pictures in the proper nationality headgear and at the same time found the hasty scramble to locate their fancy hats from clinic offices fairly hilarious. So did we, but as outsiders we were in a better position to laugh at the "ethnicity" embodied in this medical institution than our white-coated medical hosts were. Indeed, they were laughing not at their hospital's nationality character, but rather at the silly need to remember to assume a nationality sign for show, as we all assembled a snapshot directed toward a world outside Jinxiu, beyond the Great Yao Mountains enfolding this place, and even far from Guangxi province.

This was not the only occasion on which we asked ourselves, how essential is the "nationality" character of this medicine?[2] Did it matter that Director Liang, who is of the majority Han nationality, has his own Yao hat and wears it for ritual appearances? What does it mean that 90 percent of the many staff portraits displayed in the hospital's lobby include some form of Yao or other nationality hat in the picture? How often do these cosmopolitan medical people wear their hats, and for what occasions? We had seen already that older Yao women quite often wear their beautifully folded hats every day, all day, as a matter of propriety. Was it, perhaps, the conservative (and possibly gendered) propriety of hat wearing that was making the medical staff laugh as they dug out their Yao hats?

Whatever the nature of the joke we all shared that day in July, it was nevertheless clear to us during our stay in Jinxiu and in the Great Yao Mountains that nationality is no joke there. Our lighthearted hat play took place in full awareness that there were seriously ill patients in the hospital building behind us (perhaps looking out the window as we played). We all knew that some of these inpatients had traveled a long way to consult Yao doctors, desperate for effective therapy after experiencing painful disappointments with both biomedicine and traditional Chinese medicine (TCM). It was, thus, important to everyone (or at least most of us) that the services offered there are Yao nationality medicine (not traditional Chinese medicine, not Western medicine). Here, as in many other places in China's mountainous south, locality, nationality, natural medicines, and grassroots knowledge are drawn together into a multidimensional and highly valued form of expert life.

The Yao Hospital is a modern facility offering an array of medical services, some of them biomedical and some understood as traditional Chinese medicine (TCM). This kind of combination is required to be in place by county and prefectural health department and Ministry of Public Health regulations. The specialty of the hospital, however, is Yao therapeutics using local medicines from the nearby mountains. One sign of this Yao character is the large wooden soaking tubs furnished in alcoves for every room in the wards. We noted these tubs on our first tour of the fully occupied wards, and during this visit we learned more about the typically Yao therapeutic method of taking daily baths in a warm herbal soup, the mixture of medicines being customized to the particular chronic pathologies of the patient.[3]

The day of our group photo, we had visited the two-room *materia medica* research archive that had been assembled by two senior doctors tasked with

Yao medicine research. The walls were lined with more than one hundred portraits of "classic Yao medicinals of the Great Yao Mountains and commonly used drugs in Yao medicine," and there were dried samples in glass jars and pressed between stacked sheets of archival paper. Our senior clinician guide paged through his collections, lovingly pointing out the botanical and pharmaceutical characteristics of each plant. His reverence before these archive samples suggested to us that the plants themselves were more Yao than any official nomenclature could indicate, embodying better than any doctor or nurse the nature of Yao medicine.

In a subsequent visit, we got to know the most senior and famous of the attending practitioners of Yao medicine, Dr. Goldstamp Huang, a little better. On a day when he saw, in his outpatient clinic, six visitors from Beijing who had driven all night to have a Yao medicine consultation, Dr. Huang also personally prepared a very special herbal plaster for the severe skin lesion of a lymphoma patient. This hospital patient had undergone several bouts of chemotherapy without improvement. But Dr. Huang hunted up (first in the forests and then in a Jinxiu herb market) a rare herb called "seven leaf stem" (*qiye yizhihua* 七叶一支花) and ground it into a paste personally, in the hope that this cancer patient's fate might change with Yao medicine.[4]

We two anthropologists were far from being the first who had traveled long distances to appreciate Yao nationality medicine. This became obvious to us on our first day in Jinxiu town, when we had lunch with the director of the county health department, seeking her approval for our research. This skilled administrator had no concerns about the ethnicity-conscious attentions of anthropologists.[5] Learning that we were interested in the development of Yao nationality medicine, she warmly advised us to walk down the street after lunch to investigate an herbal medicines street market. She said, "If you want to understand Yao medicine, go talk to those street market herbalists."

One of our doctor hosts from the Yao Hospital accompanied us down the street after lunch. He was as curious as we were to learn what forest products were on sale today. The string of booths stretching along the riverside street contained the collections of a number of licensed natural drugs vendors, with some sellers also spreading out their (possibly unlicensed) wares on the side of the road. Every dealer in locally sourced drugs had posted a detailed sign listing the illnesses that could be reached with their own particular and traditionally Yao "secret formulas" (*mifang* 秘方) and "magical techniques" (*miji* 秘技). A few of them were performing treatments in their booths using Yao forms of needling. One of these, an elderly woman wearing a Yao hat, was pricking the hands of a small child. The little girl, folded in her father's arms, was crying only a little. At the time we found it interesting that the head of the health department should send visiting investigators from Beijing to see medical treatments taking place so clearly outside the formal sector of the public health system.

Later that afternoon we visited the Museum of the Yao Nationality, where we saw well-researched exhibits about the worldwide Yao diaspora; the cultural, linguistic, historical, and geographic differences among Yao subgroups; the "customs and habits" (风俗习惯) of Yao people in the Great Yao Mountains; and lots of displays of dance, food, and costume (including hats, of course) typical of Yao nationality culture.[6]

The "culturing" of life in the Great Yao Mountains visible in the museum was matched by small- and larger-scale cultural commodification efforts that we kept encountering. Walking in Jinxiu town, we noticed a medicinal wine store, where we sat for a while with its cook/proprietor, who had produced herbal rice wine in her own kitchen and packaged it in beautifully labeled bottles: "Yao Family Yang Booster" and "Old Wine from the Yao Mountains." She gave us samples. Later, we met and enjoyed interviewing a housewife retired from the county government who had a thriving mail-order business in Yao medicinal wines; she encouraged her granddaughter to model Yao costume for our cameras.[7] And our friends in the hospital pharmacy proudly pointed out their seven herbal mixtures for Yao medicinal baths, assuring us that these collections of dried herbs in their attractive metal packages are being shipped "even to the United States" from Jinxiu, the homeland of Yao medicine.[8]

There is no missing the sense of belonging to a nationality in Jinxiu, and it is tempting to see Yao nationality culture as inseparable from life in the Great Yao Mountains of northern Guangxi. But Yao culture and healing, like the diasporic ethnic Yao population, have gone global. In 2013 we were able to preview—on a video screen in the entranceway of the Jinxiu Yao Hospital—a glossy documentary made for China Central Television about the mystical Yao mountains and the magic of Yao nationality medicine. It was a little eerie for us to see our new and old friends from the town and hospital wearing "native costume" (always including Yao hats) instead of the everyday clothes in which we recognized them, stirring vats of black beetle wine, and participating in Daoist rituals in the firelit dark. The narration emphasized the mysteriousness of it all and made our sophisticated medical friends look a lot more wild than they are in daily life. But we suppose that few in Jinxiu really objected to the mystique generated by these kinds of widely mediated representations. After all, the mediated magic of culture is good for business.[9]

Perhaps the film brought more medical tourists, like Dr. Huang's six Beijing patients in 2012, to the Yao Hospital in Jinxiu and to the affiliated Yao

Wellness Spa then being planned by Director Liang. There is, further, a Yao medicine hospital far to the north in Beijing, specializing in cancer treatments. This institution was founded by a leader from a group of Yao who migrated from the south to northeastern China a couple of generations ago, but this family still claims roots in the "magic" of Guangxi's Great Yao Mountains, and they purchase and collect specialty herbs from the high forests around Jinxiu for use in the Beijing hospital.[10] Nationality medicine modernizers in Guangxi's capital, Nanning, where Zhuang nationality medicine is more common and more highly developed than the Yao medicine based in the northern part of the province, have internationalized China's southern local medicines through their publication programs. And they have pressured Yao medicine experts to standardize nomenclatures of drugs and diseases so that medical education and certification in this minority nationality specialty can be advanced and repopulated with freshly trained experts.[11]

In the chapters that follow, we describe aspects of the rich and complex, and not only local, gatherings of minority nationality medicine, as we found them growing and changing in China's southern mountains. The Jinxiu notes above should give readers a sense of the depth of knowledge and the breadth of the networks on which we were able to draw as we traveled through southern nationality areas collaborating with medical people, public health cadres, our trained research associates, writers and scholars, other anthropologists, and each other.[12] Lili and Judith were very much a part of the minority medicines development project that had been inaugurated in Beijing a few years before we began our travels. Often, we two were incorporated in field survey teams from health departments and research centers, as when we traveled in a van through western Yunnan with six or seven researchers and a cinematographer from the Yunnan Academy of TCM (see chapter 5). Sometimes we relied on local buses, three-wheeled motorcycles, or the practical arrangements of one of our research associates to get to the clinic or farmhouse of an interesting interviewee, as tended to be the case in Lisu country.[13] And we two outsiders to southern mountain life gratefully accepted instruction (not to mention the gift of many a textbook) from medical experts whose work was being supported and recognized by the SATCM and other parts of the Ministry of Public Health. There is no doubt that everywhere we went we were perceived as representatives of the state, with its developmental, regulatory, and knowledge-producing agenda. Yet almost everyone we met warmly welcomed us, often seeing us as partners in the common task of gaining more recognition for minority knowledge and practice.

Along the way, we adopted a few medical muses: healers and activists whose deep understanding of medicines and long lives of service to their communities kept our curiosity very much alive. One such muse is a Yao medicine practitioner with a drug-stuffed stall in the Shuijie (Water Street) Herbal Medicines Market in Nanning. We called her "Granny Waterstreet" and visited her both in her market stall and at her apartment in Nanning. She is Yao, as is attested by her vendor's license on prominent display in the market; two of her daughters, also licensed as Yao herbalists, practice in the market, and all three of these minority women, hailing from an area rather far north of Nanning, perform treatments in their stalls as well as selling herbal medicines. We asked where the family gets all these medicines, and Granny Waterstreet told us about her long life of itinerant drug collecting as an herbalist traveling throughout the southern mountains. She was also trained as a barefoot doctor, and for her Nanning clients she consults on a wide variety of disorders. She probably spent time on that market street by the river back in Jinxiu, selling rare herbs and advising on "secret formulas." Nowadays she still travels back to the Great Yao Mountains, where family members continue to gather medicines and process them to be transported to her urban practice in Nanning.

Our friend and fellow researcher Fang Meijian grew close to Granny Waterstreet and her family. We recall one visit with Meijian to the apartment, where our shared Granny unpacked a complete Yao nationality costume and encouraged our young friend to model it for us. Feeling a bit self-conscious, as a young person of a different nationality (Meijian is Zhuang), she wrapped herself in Granny's hand-embroidered skirt and blouse and belt and put on a spare hat. (Granny Waterstreet told us she never takes off her own Yao hat except at night.) We duly took pictures—and later discussed with Meijian the sense of possible inappropriateness we all felt when she was modeling somebody else's heritage and memory for foreigner cameras.

By that time we were all well aware of how much experience, labor, and learning had been devoted in Granny Waterstreet's life—but not only hers—to being Yao and mobilizing the powers of the Great Yao Mountains for healing. Our doctor and nurse friends at the Yao Hospital probably know her and her children, they respect the kind of knowledge she has amassed in her travels, and they remain dependent in many ways on folk herbalists like her who are active in the informal sector. Even the hats that marked the hospital staff as Yao for a snapshot were probably handmade, like Granny Waterstreet's, by mothers and grandmothers, and therefore full of personal meaning. These medical men, as they scrambled to get their hats on for an anthropologist's photograph, were enjoying the moment with us. But

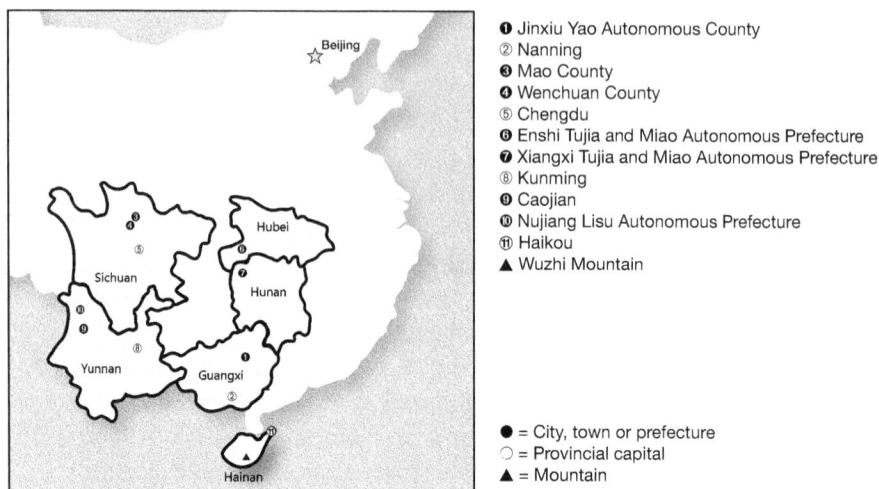

Figure 2. Chinese provinces where research was conducted, showing research sites most frequently mentioned. Map courtesy of Jenny Addison.

perhaps they could laugh at unnecessary cultural symbolism (while engaging it) because they knew how substantial, effective, and creative the Yao medicines in which they specialized, and with which they lived daily, can be. *Gathering Medicines* invites you to witness the myriad powerful things offered up to knowledge and practice by a minority nationality medicines movement in contemporary China.

Introduction

I dream of a new age of curiosity. We have the technical means for it; the desire is there; the things to be known are infinite; the people who can employ themselves at this task exist. Why do we suffer? From too little: from channels that are too narrow, skimpy, quasi-monopolistic, insufficient. There is no point in adopting a protectionist attitude, to prevent "bad" information from invading and suffocating the "good." Rather, we must multiply the paths and the possibilities of comings and goings.
MICHEL FOUCAULT, "The Masked Philosopher"

Minority nationality medicine: Is that a thing? Answering this skeptical but interesting question will be a main task for the rest of this book. Our starting point on the journey is an anthropological insistence on a pluralistic universe, one in which medicine has a history and geography expressing profound differences in bodies, tools, and concepts. There are a great many "minority nationalities" in China, and there are even more forms of bodily suffering and styles of healing—possibly these things to be known are infinite. But the emergence in contemporary China of not just one but many minority medicines is a development worth tracking and a form of life deserving recognition.

Certainly there is a standard term for minority nationality medicines: *shaoshu minzu yiyao* (少数民族医药). The concept is recognized immediately by our Chinese-speaking and China-dwelling friends. When we say we have been doing research on the "development of minority nationality medicines," these acquaintances nod sagely and respond with kind words: "how interesting," "good for you!," or "wow, that's cool!" Perhaps these cosmopolitan Chinese friends are just being polite, but there is no doubt that they recognize what we are researching and have no trouble acknowledging the interest of the subject of minority nationality medicines. Some of those we talk with express a larger curiosity. They want to know how a nationality medicine might differ from the "Chinese medicine" and "Western medi-

cine" services available in their cities, and they enjoy our slide shows stuffed
with images from specialty clinics in county hospitals and showing the work
of elderly herbalists in mountainside farmhouses.

With this topic, and with the Masked Philosopher, we are dreaming of
a new age of curiosity, one in which the local knowledges of those persons
and places perceived as remote from all centers could multiply the paths
and the possibilities of all our worldly comings and goings. There is nothing
new or unique about this undertaking. In many respects this book is anthropology as usual: comparative, relativistic, locally attuned, and appreciative
of the everyday and the down-to-earth. We sometimes think of ourselves, in
company with other anthropologists and theorists, as following the traces
of some nomad sciences, attentive to ontological differences among those
who reside in China's peripheries, and rescuing epistemological heterogeneity from "quasi-monopolistic" impositions of information thought to be
"good" by agents of modern states.[1] Still, it must be admitted that this exploration of emergent kinds of medicine is taking place in a nation committed to medical pluralism and multiculturalism. Thus this project must
not only be microscopic about cultural life and knowledge but also attend
to more large-scale and even global processes. Minority forms of life and
healing never subsist untouched by the biopolitics advanced by modern
nation-states. These cultural forms both are creatures of the majority agenda
pursued by state agents and also exert pressures on government institutions
from below and outside all formal state apparatuses. Government practices and market forces, development programs and international politics,
science policies and public health agendas play through and configure the
down-to-earth practices we present in this book. Our preference has been
to let these macroscopic formations reveal their powers—and the limits to
them—in their contemporary national Chinese mode of existence, alongside the mundane work and concerns of our nationality medicine interlocutors, even as the stories told herein multiply and fold together the things to
be known in China's mountain south.

In this introduction, then, we will begin the work of answering the question "Is that a thing?" by reporting on minority nationality medicines as a
local development, as a medical and epistemological phenomenon, and as
a health care institution. Catching contemporary nationality medicine in
the act of becoming something important in China and the world, we es-
chew definitional abstractions in favor of historically located descriptions.
The stories that fill these pages, like those already seen in the preface, show
us many forms of knowledge, modes of action, styles of cultural belonging,
active nonhuman interlocutors, and constructive social labor. They reflect
our experience as researchers, and they acknowledge the work of the wise

and generous healers, historians, farmers, state agents, trekking herbalists, health activists, and cooking mothers and grandmothers among whom we gathered minority nationality medicines. Judith and Lili were transformed by this research. We hope the encounters gathered in this book will be transforming for readers as well.

"MINORITY NATIONALITY MEDICINE"

Like any emergent social assemblage in a vast modern nation-state like China, minority nationality medicine is complicated. All concepts evoked by even the standard term noted here need to be interrogated. We must ask not only "what is a 'nationality' [*minzu* 民族]"—now, in China, and in salient histories—but also what does it mean to be part of an officially recognized minority population in a strongly unified country like China? There is a large, diverse, and careful historical literature on the nationality question in modern China, but in our view it has not quieted on-the-ground uncertainties about nationality belonging and the nature of the multicultural nation. We will return to *minzu* in this introduction, but most of the time we let the translated term "nationality" play through the stories gathered in the five chapters, where it usually refers to one of China's officially registered national minorities.

"Medicine," too, raises historical questions: here the term usually used in Chinese is *yiyao* (医药), literally "medicine and pharmacy," but as will be seen in (at least) chapters 2 and 5 below, many in China think that "medicine" is quite different from "pharmacy." And even the English word and global concept of "medicine" evokes immediately an ambiguity between "medicine" as drugs and remedies and "medicine" as a profession, clinical institutions, various branches of knowledge, and so forth. There is even some evidence that a modern concept of medicine, in which diseases with known causes are found in individual bodies and targeted with surgical and chemical technologies, was rather a novelty in parts of China as recently as the first decades of the People's Republic (founded in 1949). The concept of medicine itself, what it is and what it is not, needed to be taught in primary care public health training programs, and in some respects it is still being argued about. We see the legacy of a global conceptual technology transfer— the spread of medicine as a modern form of knowledge and power—still alive in today's small-scale struggles and resistances about who and what can be deemed "medical" and thus serve as a legitimate element in a national public health apparatus.

So one preliminary response to the "Is that a thing?" question would be no, "it" is not. Minority nationality medicine in today's China, however often it is spoken of with a single term, is not one stable bounded entity with a secure place in history or geography. The localized medical systems of China's more populous nationalities (e.g., Tibetan, Mongolian, Uyghur) are quite different, ideologically and technically, from the nationality medical systems that we saw being gathered in the south and southwest. In a philosophical language, this social complex, minority nationality medicine, is not a being but a process of becoming. Hence the title of this book: *Gathering Medicines* investigates an active and diverse process of drawing (many!) things together to craft a useful coherence—actually, a series of them. The work of gathering occupies the center of attention in this book, as we try to catch broad social things in the act of becoming recognizable, useful, and even, at times, coherent. People, like the medical and cultural activists of whom we often speak below, deliberately gather diverse elements into an assemblage called Yao medicine, or Zhuang medicine, or Achang medicine. But scattered things—plants, markets, road networks, health schools, honeybees, chronically ill patients, and so on—with their own complex histories and trajectories also spontaneously gather into mixtures that can surprise activists, health department functionaries, and anthropologists alike. Such mixtures and assemblages may come to earn the name of minority nationality medicine and be recognized as new modes of existence that work well as knowing practice. Because it is medicine and expertise that are at issue in this process, an anthropology of this emergence turns naturally to curiosity about knowledge.

AN ANTHROPOLOGY OF KNOWLEDGE

Knowledge comes in many forms, only a few of which can be put in a mental bucket and carried home. (This image recalls Karl Popper's lampooning, in his critique of commonsense knowledge, of "bucket theories of mind.")[2] In the course of our research, for example, everywhere we went to inquire about local or nationality medicines, we were told that the true healers, the wise local experts, all climbed mountains to gather medicines (*shangshan caiyao* 上山采药). This practice of finding, collecting, and naming the useful parts of wild plants (but not only plants), this way of learning from the life of the high forests, was always presented as the *sine qua non* that grounded the authority, efficacy, and superior wisdom of these herbalist gatherers. Impressed with their very specialized and practical knowledge, we quickly began to see our anthropological project as a form of gathering medicines (and indeed, we often had to go uphill to do our work). The "medicines" we gathered, like the many natural drugs that healers found in the high forests they frequented, came in many varieties. In alphabetical order, here are the seven nationality groups on whose medical development processes we focused: Achang, Li, Lisu, Qiang, Tujia, Yao, Zhuang.

But we realized that only some of what anthropologists gather is representable as formal knowledge that can be taken away, "written up," and transmitted as "information."[3] Embodied skill, canny perceptiveness, or even a fated relationship to inherited understanding was more important to users of local medicines than formal training and published facts were. Indeed, knowledge *of* the local (natural drugs, forests, common diseases, and much more) *is* local in its very nature. Shared traditional lore can be an intimate agent along with the body and person of the knower, she who draws near to things. Wishing to relativize knowledge, and to work (at times) beyond the reach of China's official medical institutions, we had to consider how to do an anthropology of emergent and diverse medical knowledges — in the plural — in China's ethnic south. And we had to constantly reconsider what could be discovered, and what would be transformed, in the process.[4]

Insofar as this study is an anthropology of knowledge, then, we have been required to reflect on what we mean by that term, especially now that we have been (re)educated in particular styles of knowing in the course of nationality medicine fieldwork.[5] As anthropologists and pragmatists, we have long preferred to attend to knowing as a practice (rather than to knowledge as a domain or an object).[6] Since the 1980s, much thinking in the human sciences has advanced a practice approach to the study of knowledge formations, in what might be called a postepistemological orientation. Foucault's archaeologies, science and technology studies, the anthropological turn to practice, feminist epistemology, a philosophical return to the pragmatists, challenges to all universal foundations, and a general queering of theory have supplemented the long-standing materialism and relativism of social and cultural anthropology. All these intellectual developments have issued an open invitation to more and richer empirical exploration. We have been encouraged to ask, again and again, *how* do "minority nationality" medical people, climbing remote mountains and gathering unknown drugs, *know*?

In a recent discussion aimed at a critical sociology and philosophy of science readership, we developed a way of thinking about knowing practice, a way of seeing it afresh, that is indebted to the Confucian ethical tradition.[7] Our favorite source, the third- or fourth-century BCE text called "The Great Learning," with extreme economy lists the different kinds of action that can help a true lord bring order and peace to the world. At the core of the text is a practice of knowing, an approach to knowledge (that ancient word *zhi* 知) that has occasioned hundreds of years of commentaries. The key sentence is: "knowledge arises from the action of drawing near to things" (*gewu zhi zhi* 格物致知).[8] This seems so simple and obvious, presenting a kind of empiricism, and even a charter for fieldwork! Yet for "The Great Learning," knowledge attained in this active way is not a mass of cognitive *representations* of things—gathered up in Popper's bucket, as it were. Rather, it is advice for ethical rulers, showing how the true human (*zhenren* 真人) can be a foundation of effective governance, which is to say, ethical action (or at least exemplary nonaction) in a given world. Therefore, to attain to knowledge is at the same time to live a good life, to come to embody the good, and to do it well. These ethical positions are patently obvious in "The Great Learning" itself, and they were elaborated in influential Chinese commentaries over two millennia. At the same time, knowledge was deobjectified: like "minority nationality medicines," knowledge, for those steeped in the Confucian (non)epistemological tradition, is not exactly a freestanding thing or (heaven forbid!) object.[9] Knowledge for the authors of "The Great Learning" and other Confucian works on knowledge seems to have been a kind of ethical becoming, a cultivation, a mode of governance, and a knowing practice. Seen in this way, medicine presents itself as a preeminent domain for lordly practice, but this is an ethics that arises from premises very different from those founding modern bioethics.

Is East Asia's ancient advice on rulership connected in any way to modern medical and epistemological pluralism?[10] We think there are many reasons to span these millennia in thought. Much of the theory that has become canonical in modern traditional Chinese medicine (TCM) is derived from ancient texts like the *Yellow Emperor's Inner Canon* and expressed in a classical language, especially that of rulership. "The liver rules dispersion of *qi*, the heart rules blood": statements like these are key principles organizing TCM, and they have occasioned much interpretation in classrooms and synthetic works. The mode of action referenced by the word "rules" (*zhu* 主) is far from self-evident for moderns, so understanding how organ systems work in relation to body substances, as in these examples, requires an experienced grasp of a great many physiological regularities. If a medical expert is to effectively influence pathophysiological processes toward better health, he must have a feel for the kind of action that is rulership, both that of the body's key agencies and that of the wise healer.

Ruling in the twenty-first century is quite a different thing than it was thought to be in the Warring States or Han periods (both prior to 221 CE). But medicine is still intimately linked to sovereign power. In China, medical care provided directly or indirectly by the socialist state has long included, alongside modern biomedical services, the official clinical, research, and educational institutions of traditional Chinese medicine. TCM as it has been institutionalized in China can thus be thought of as a statist medicine—indeed as the first statist traditional medicine in the world, given that the institutional modernization of Chinese medicine began in the twentieth century well before the social sciences and the World Health Organization had acknowledged the importance of "traditional medicines."[11] Volker Scheid has traced the expansion and slowly growing dominance of "currents of tradition" originating in the Yangtze River delta region.[12] These schools of thought and styles of practice incorporated local visions of medicine and the body during the Qing and Republican periods when China was becoming a modern nation-state, and they gradually achieved a kind of intellectual hegemony in an extremely diverse field. This was a complexly braided process of co-construction of medical authority and regime legitimacy. The TCM Scheid shows as emerging into leadership over several hundred years officially became a state medicine in the mid-1950s, being advanced at that time with a great deal of nationalist (and implicitly Han-dominant) language.[13]

But it is hard to read this recent history as an example of imperial or colonizing domination over "the folk" by a totalitarian state. The oft-presumed relation of domination and resistance between "the common people" and "the state apparatus" in the domain of knowledge production—which is what concerns us here—does not begin to account for all the relations of power involved in modern medical rulership and the management of suffering bodies. A language of state elites dominating victimized or silenced subalterns from above might work for some situations of medical pluralism (even, perhaps, in the United States where there is one hegemonic medical system). But the relation between vernacular healing and official medical knowledge in China is more complex. Minority medicines, we will show, are as much generated by locally instituted powers, in interesting novel forms, as they are regulated and limited by a modern state apparatus.

We have been speaking here of "nomad" medical knowledge, taking the term from Gilles Deleuze and Félix Guattari, who compare but do not radically contrast two kinds of knowledge, "nomad (or 'vague') science" and "royal (or 'state') science."[14] These authors are thinking more about indigenous lore than medicine, it would seem, but they do hit upon some descriptions that are rather neatly suited to modern Chinese medical pluralism. A nomad science is itinerant and vagabond, variable, laden with singularities, taking the form of passages and flows. It has a supplementary relationship with royal science, which is committed to rendering expertise stable, sedentary, predictable. Royal science has a public voice, a written history, a claim on collective resources. It trades in representations and classifications, while nomad science exists as events, oral lore, solutions to ever-new problems. It is tempting to see the "old herbal doctors" (*lao caoyi* 老草医) of whom we often heard—who were renowned for traveling through the subtropical forests of China's mountainous south, valorized for their embodied knowledge of natural herbals, known as familiars of wild powers—as heroic Deleuzian nomads resisting all commerce with the state and other instituted authorities. But that would not be quite right. There can be no pure (free) nomadism, just as there can be no pure (totalitarian) royal science. In speaking of the power relations between royal or state science and nomad or "vague" science, for example, Deleuze and Guattari invoke an image of a single field of interaction and an actively shifting borderline:

> What we have, rather, are two formally different conceptions of science, and, ontologically, a single field of interaction in which royal science is perpetually appropriating the contents of vague or nomad science, and nomad science is perpetually releasing the contents of royal science. At the limit, all that counts is the constantly moving borderline.[15]

We will show throughout this study that state institutions, ever in formation and ever vulnerable to decline of their powers, must grapple with and perpetually appropriate the call of the wild or the charm of the nomadic. Citizens and patients want to benefit from the "natural" forcefulness of "traditional" medicines, and therefore official public health authorities must find ways to claim that they too, like the nomads they often stigmatize, know how to deploy wild powers. Whatever Deleuze and Guattari mean by nomad science "releasing the contents" of royal science, we can attest to the attraction, confessed by even the most rigorous systematizers of statist medicine, toward the powers of wild plants and the wisdom of illiterate healers, and to the intrinsic interest of technologies for controlling ghosts and magical parasites. Perhaps these state functionaries, some of whom we speak with in the following chapters, feel that the "content" of what they know is "released" in practice only when well-trained experts succeed in recovering some of the powers of the forest for clinical application, working from a settled base in licensed centers of medicine. "At the limit, all that counts is the constantly moving borderline": If we take "the borderline" to be a wide zone of interaction between various agencies, all making their own claims, this is a useful formula for understanding encounters between state agenda and popular expertise.[16]

MEDICAL EMERGENCES

The *things* addressed by modern medicine, and constituted within it, have been central to the dominant understanding of modernity itself. Bodies (discrete, individual, suffering, with organs); diseases (ontological, biologi-

cal, found in bodies); techniques (diagnostic, surgical, invasive or manipu-
lative); and drugs (chemical, systemic, with effects and side effects). These
things developed early in the history of modern medicine and were drawn
together in a profession and a system of institutions that enjoy undeniable
authority throughout the world. Medicine has given us moderns a master-
ful account of the fundamental reality in which we live: an effective set of
bodies, disorders, techniques, and drugs the truth of which cannot be de-
nied.

At the same time, modern medicine has given us taken-for-granted objects that influence not only how and with what materials we are able to
think *anything*, even far beyond the clinic and the sickbed, but even how we
perceive, or not, the natural necessities that constrain us. In the social sciences we divide individual from society, in philosophy and science we distinguish word from world and cause from effect, in religion and aesthetics we
sort out the spiritual from the material. The history of medicine has shown
that none of these master dualisms took such a radically relational and differential form before clinical medicine made its most successful claims to
represent and intervene in a newly "objective" real world.[17]

But hegemonic accounts of what is "simply natural" are never completely
effective. The discovery of state-sanctioned medical pluralism in anthropological and global public health research, especially in the 1970s, destabi-
lized moderns' taken-for-granted acceptance of biomedical authority and,
we like to think, even challenged the naturalness of social categories like
"the individual" and explanatory notions like etiological "cause." China
played a role in altering the very nature of the things that had come into
existence for and in biomedicine, generating globally circulated information
about herb-gathering barefoot doctors and acupuncture-assisted surgeries.
This is a history of non-Western science that has only now begun to be told,
but it is an important background for the more recent knowledge formations we examine in this book.[18]

Medicine of the globalized modernist sort is certainly important and recognizable in China's contemporary public health system, including in TCM
hospitals and nationality areas. Though many researchers (we among them)
have shown that there are stubborn conceptual and ontological differences
between "Western medicine" and "Chinese medicine,"[19] which differences
are not easy to reconcile in contemporary hybrid clinical practices, certain modern things still powerfully influence what is known by East Asian
medicines.[20] It is widely presumed in TCM, for example, that medicine addresses disease (rather than, for example, routine health and wellness), that
pathology works inside skin-bounded human bodies, and that mechanistic
interactions between the organs of an anatomical body account for symp-

toms and other bodily experiences. At times, philosophers reading the two-thousand-year archive of medicine in Chinese use a nonmodernist Chinese language to undermine these presumptions, but most TCM workers seem to hold that the most ethical and even most truthful way forward for their field is to adopt the material world to which biomedicine refers in its standardized discourse and globalized practice.

In our readings below of nationality medicine discourse, and of local healing practices that mostly go untheorized, we have often highlighted the epistemological and ethical gestures through which nationality medicine practitioners orient their work to the officially dominant system of biomedical and integrative services. All practitioners of medicine in China work in full awareness of therapeutic plurality, at least of the kind that juxtaposes the institutionalized health services of biomedicine and TCM.[21] Doctors of the new minority nationality specialties were always ready to answer our "what's the difference?" questions, though they were not always good at articulating precisely what is local and particular about their approaches to medicine and pharmacy.

To the end of understanding what happens when medicine pluralizes in today's world, then, we developed our own approach to nationality medical things. In chapter 1, we witness institution building at its foundations and in its relation to official and unofficial (or "wild") authority. We emphasize there that instituting is a process of structuration rather than a fixed order of superior powers (a royal science?) that constrains more nomadic forms of experience. In chapter 2, "Knowledge," we consider the epistemological specificity of some nationality medicines that stand in contrast to other systems. Here we delve especially deeply into the gathered expertise of Zhuang nationality medicine, showing how it addresses bodies and their disorders in ways that truly differ from the approaches of TCM. In chapter 3 we look for forms of bodily life that tend to go unseen by the modern medical gaze, arguing that any anthropology of "the body" must expect to find pluralities of bodily practice and experience that run very deep. Chapter 4, "Plants," proposes a southern mountain nature within which local medical experts find their effectiveness and make a healing place. The chapter explores some unique intimacies with the natural world and with its powerful things, which are expressed in the lives of herbalists. And in chapter 5, "Encounters," we present some nationality medicine forms of sociality, including encounters of healers with "medicine proper." The aim of this last chapter is to open *Gathering Medicines* to the marvelous excess, which we found in our research travels, over and beyond any "narrow, skimpy, quasi-monopolistic, insufficient" form of the anthropological imagination.[22] If there are fifty-five nationality medicines now emergent in China, we'd like to think that there are at least as many nameless nomad worlds engaged by a very diverse scatter of local healers. Some of these men and women we were privileged to meet and interview.

From the beginning of our research project, we concerned ourselves with the social processes that could be witnessed as minority nationality medicines came into some kind of recognized existence. Led by our own previous training and research experience, we perceived the operation of a historical model that made this new nationality manifestation of modern medicine unique. With Lili formally trained at the Beijing University of Chinese Medicine and continuing research on TCM in graduate school, and Judith in previous projects having sought out a rich literature recounting the development and establishment of TCM in China, we were able to perceive a certain historical vision of knowledge and the nation at work in nationality medical activism. This model had a name in the form of a set of state-articulated policy directives that guided research and institution-building: *salvage, sort, synthesize, elevate* (*fajue* 发掘, *zhengli* 整理, *zongjie* 总结, *tigao* 提高). These directives were adopted for developing nationality medicines in the early 2000s because Chinese medicine, or TCM—assembled in the 1950s and 1960s and then reassembled and vastly expanded in the 1980s— had itself been "salvaged and sorted, synthesized and elevated."

The effort to establish a second official medical system, TCM, in the early years of the People's Republic of China was an explicitly nationalist and socialist project asserted by a globally embattled Maoist state. Sean Hsiang-lin Lei's important study of struggles over modernization between biomedical interests and an emergent "national medicine" (*guoyi* 国医) profession demonstrates that the roots of modern epistemological and technical work on TCM run rather deep. He shows that an ambitious collective *sorting* of the therapeutic heritage of Chinese medicine was mounted in the 1930s in response to strong attacks from new alliances of biomedical doctors.[23] David Lampton explains the growth, twenty years later, of official support for a modernizing "Chinese medicine" (*zhongyi* 中医) as an unavoidable government approach to achieving universal health care provision in a vast country with very scarce biomedical resources.[24] And once central government recognition was accorded to Chinese medicine as a health care resource with Ministry of Public Health support in the mid-1950s,[25] it was possible for TCM professionals and intellectual leaders to undertake the work of not only salvaging and sorting, but also synthesizing and elevating Chinese medicine to the status of a state-supported science. Two decades later, well into the "Reform and Opening Up" period, central government support was made available for the development of ethnically marked medicines (see chapter 2 for a more detailed history). With state guidance, it has been widely accepted among nationality medicine and public health actors that it is through these four kinds of action—salvaging, sorting, synthesizing, and elevating—that nationality medicines will of necessity have to be built. This is, thus, an approach to collective practice that has become "modular," in Benedict Anderson's sense.[26] It was no wonder that, as we began our work, everything we read about the nationality medicine movement deployed these four terms. Regardless of what these words have come to mean in recent practice, their continuing currency suggests that many people learned how to advance the cause of local medical interests by living through and reflecting on the example of a mid-twentieth-century nationalist, clinical, historically rich, and thoroughly official TCM.

What historical processes of development, in today's China, are denoted by the terms salvage, sort, synthesize, and elevate? The fact that the process of assembly should begin with *salvaging* (*fajue* 发掘) tells us much about how the plurality of folk medicines and cultures was conceived by the Beijing leadership, even as early as the modernizing 1930s. A salvaging process does not presume a blank slate on the ground and among the people, nor does it imagine any need for *ex nihilo* invention. Rather a salvage operation works with the scattered healing resources, the drugs and the techniques, that are locally ready-to-hand, known to folk healers, and known by the people to be effective. For ethnic groups that have no deeply rooted written heritage, these elements needed to be sought in such long-standing locations as the embodied knowledge and skills of recognized healers, in the notes and records of collecting herbalists, and scattered through county gazetteers with their stories of local worthies, miracle cures, herb markets, and place names. For both TCM and the developers of minority nationality medicines, to salvage often meant to travel around conducting social and natural scientific surveys, interviewing and even working alongside healers, and then filing a full report upward to the health departments of the prefecture, province, or national government.[27]

It was the unsystematic yet empirically fascinating results of this kind of salvage process that would then be subject to *sorting* (*zhengli* 整理) in the hands of various kinds of experts (historians, clinicians, educators, SATCM researchers). In the history of TCM, one hallmark of the official sorting of the medicine that had been "inherited from the laboring masses' several-thousand-year history of battling against disease" was an act of discriminating: "preserving the essence and discarding the dross."[28] These phrases were part of the nationalist rhetoric framing the medical works that issued from the vast traditional medicine construction project of the 1950s and 1960s. For the minority medicines, too, essential elements needed to be distinguished from dross. What this meant in practice was that medical practices would be *secularized* and *individualized*. Wild forms of therapy were mostly (but not entirely) made to conform to a modern medical object world and a conventionally embodied individual-in-society model.[29] The shaman, for example, while acknowledged to have healing powers in some individual cases, was not to be included in any textbooks or certifying exams. And Daoists like Wonderfont Zhao, introduced in chapter 1, were sorted as two kinds of practitioners, one aspect of him wearing the white coat of a medical man and another continuing to work on cosmic order as a diviner and ritualist.

The term *zhengli* is sometimes used to speak of an editing project, as well; and in practice it has been clear that one of the first and most important products of a sorting process is textbooks. Editing curricular materials for schools of minority medicine that did not yet exist, researchers in most cases saw their collective aim as reproducing expertise through training a younger generation of officially certified doctors. They had to consider what kind of knowledge could (sooner or later) be incorporated into licensing and certifying examinations that would allow newly trained nationality doctors to participate in a well-regulated science-based public health system. The detailed tables of contents from medical texts (on which we draw in part; see chapters 2 and 3) reflect an expert *sorting* of dispersed but very complex kinds of local knowledge.[30] Any given healer's mind and practice was unlikely to have been as orderly as these compulsively structured chapters and sections. But perhaps some of the scattered experts we met admired the results of the sorting process?[31]

The third step in the social construction of a minority medicine is *synthesizing (zongjie* 总结).[32] The already-existing concepts and objects that gather into a new mode of medical treatment, even after they are sorted into useful groupings, as in a table of contents and well-edited textbooks, are widely perceived as existing as a fragmentary scatter. If this thing-under-construction is to be a modern medicine, its substance must cohere into a structured whole, a corpus (*tixi* 体系) that can incorporate standard procedures and express deep ordering principles. We saw this epistemological demand at work in the aspirations and survey research of Institute Director Ma (discussed in chapters 2 and 5), as he tried to extract medical theory from Achang nationality herbalists. He was convinced that these excellent doctors, practicing a particular form of medicine that Director Ma and his team were salvaging and sorting as Achang nationality medicine, were withholding from him the deep synthetic principles that informed their practice. At the very least, he hoped that they would work with him to represent their knowledge and techniques as a *medical system*, comparable with both TCM and "Western medicine." His orientation on the problem and task of synthesizing, or finding the theory, the underlying coherence, was not his alone. He had developed these attitudes in conversation with national leaders of the minority nationality medicine movement: *zongjie* synthesizing has been a crucial step in the emergence of China's nationality medicines.

And finally, the fourth part of this recognized medical development process was elevating (*tigao* 提高). This term like the previous three refers back to the history of modern TCM. Elevating in that field has tended to mean scientizing. A very large proportion of the research funds commanded by the various institutions of TCM, over the decades, has been devoted to laboratory research and clinical trials aimed at confirming, explaining, and refining the efficacies of Chinese medical therapeutics.[33] Very few minority nationality medical initiatives have had the resources to devote to any similar scientizing process, but we did meet Zhuang medicine researchers in Nanning, attached to the Zhuang medical school and hospital, who were exploring phytochemical research on locally known natural drugs.

There is another sense to *tigao*-elevating as well, we think. Commercialization and globalization through the establishment of high-profile institutions (like the Yao Hospital in Beijing mentioned in the preface) and the expansion of a web presence are perceived by many we know as forms of *elevation* of a local specialty into a medical service available to the whole world. As noted, for example, Yao nationality herbalists have elevated their expertise by giving it a global presence with their online enterprises selling herbal baths and wines.

These four kinds of activity are not temporally distinct stages or discrete phases of a unidirectional historical development. All such modes of assembly operate in tandem, as activists try to construct, from scattered fragments, a corpus of medicine that can serve the people, be viable in a changing market for therapeutic services, and achieve legitimate authority in a region and, eventually perhaps, the nation and the world. As many unique forms of nationality medicine emerge in China after the millennium, nothing institutional or authoritative can be taken for granted. We met no activists who felt they could rest on their laurels. The work of salvaging must go on even as resources are sought to support some elevating research; synthesizing is a concern even before lists of practices and pharmaceuticals are sorted into some useful order.

In many cases the work of salvaging and sorting, synthesizing and elevating, has successfully constructed institutions and discourses recognizable as that relatively novel thing, a minority nationality medicine. (We are thinking especially of Zhuang, Qiang, Tujia, and Yao projects, among the groups encountered in this book.) These new formations meet the modern definition of medicine (as noted above, medicine proper involves diseases, discrete bodies with organs, drugs, etc.), and they are not the same as "traditional Chinese (Han nationality) medicine" or "Western (bio)medicine." Nor are they identical among themselves, given that different southern nationalities differently emphasize things like *gu* parasites (蛊), *sha* disorders (痧), and needling-tweaking techniques (*zhentiao* 针挑). Not to mention the many local characteristics of nationality *materia medica*. Nationality activists boasting more successful developments can now claim bricks-and-mortar institutions and ongoing institutional building projects (see chapter 1). They have risen to the occasion of sorting and synthesizing bodies of knowledge keyed to responsible clinical practices (see chapter 2). Though we never found cleanly distinct nationality or ethnic bodies as we traveled through different medical worlds, locally preferred therapeutic body manipulations nevertheless offered much to challenge our conventional assumptions about how humans can be embodied (see chapter 3). We have found, further, that experts in nationality medicine are deeply respectful of the powers of the plant world and of the forest's fragile actors (see chapter 4). Above all, we were impressed that activist representatives of even the most "elevated" and "systematic" nationality medicines we studied had a deep respect for healing "on the ground." In an effort to capture these complex relationships, chapter 5 reports some encounters between medical and anthropological rationalizers and the nomad scientists of various wild healing worlds.[34]

Perhaps the emergent nationality medical systems are not long for this world, given the vicissitudes of Beijing's nationality policy and health care financing, and the uneven successes of local cultural activism. There is a complex popular and professional demand for more responsive and modernized biomedical services throughout China. But it is not just "the folk" or cultural conservatives who seek out the nomad sciences of nationality medicine when they are facing stubborn bodily disorders. Indeed, the "royal" medicines of an increasingly plural public health system—those that are recognized, certified, institutionalized—are widely distrusted by rural and urban, minority and Han consumers. Many patients with chronic illness, and their families, do not talk of finding "world-class medicine," like that advertised by American academic medical centers, but rather simply want to find a good doctor. Perhaps only a few care whether that personal virtue, that fated "fit" between healer and sufferer, has anything to do with nationality. Thus the salvaging and sorting initiative that has assembled minority medicines in some places has not been entirely successful for every group, as for example among the Lisu people of Yunnan, where there is not (yet) any collectively recognizable style of practice that could be called "Lisu medicine."

Indeed, among the seven groups on whom we focused our inquiries, we found the Lisu group's medical expertise to be the most scattered. Very few of these rural healers admitted to sharing any part of their work with other Lisu medical workers, and most of them were working as generalist village doctors. At the other end of a certain historical continuum, which we began to see between medicines that were more scattered and those that were more gathered, were the Zhuang medicine (ZM) professionals in and around the Guangxi Zhuang Self-Governing Region's capital, Nanning. These historians, clinicians, administrators, and teachers of medicine shared a great deal of specialized Zhuang medicine knowledge and technique, as will become especially evident in chapter 2.[35] ZM development projects had benefited, rather unusually from the early 1980s, from the salvaging and sorting efforts of a few visionary leaders.

Others among the seven groups studied here had wise and effective leadership as well, though they began the process of instituting medicine a bit later than ZM and faced some different challenges. Here we are thinking of the Qiang group in Sichuan, which really began to expand only with post-2008 earthquake recovery funding from Beijing, much of it markedly aimed at Qiang nationality institutions. In addition, the stories of Yao medical work we have offered in the preface reflect the rather hyperactive development work of several local leaders in Jinxiu, but it appears that in that area of northern Guangxi nationality medicine lagged a bit behind the Yao heritage and culture work of the 1990s.[36] In the case of Tujia medicine, a specialty belonging to a large group that is found in both Hunan and Hubei provinces, leading researchers were indebted to the insights of a few inspired clinicians for the local knowledge they collected. But even these luminaries practiced in small specialty clinics housed in TCM and biomedical general hospitals. Only the Zhuang, among our group, could boast a medical school, several hospitals, a museum and research center, and a nationally prominent publication program. This all seems to be evidence that Zhuang medicine was well on its way to becoming a statist therapeutics, except for the fact that the nomad expertise of healers like Wonderfont Zhao still commanded such respect.

More similar to the nonorganized Lisu healers than to the Zhuang, Qiang, Yao, and Tujia experts were the two other groups we studied: the Li of Hainan Island, whose local *materia medica* have been studied and published, but for whom thus far there are few recognized Li nationality healers; and the Achang group, where the expertise of two families of healers was being salvaged and sorted by researchers from the Yunnan Academy of TCM. Indeed, it was partly owing to the call of the central government for the development of minority nationality medicines that the work of Lisu, Li, and

Achang healers could come to our attention at all. And our anthropological gaze and persistent questions about history and practice undoubtedly had some small impact on the claims to fame and official recognition made by emergent medical systems. Our outsiders' efforts to gather minority medicines, in other words, were one of many (trans)national practices that converged with local medical development projects to bolster and recognize the still uncertain reality of minority nationality medicines.

NATIONALITY HATS

The preface to this study reports a moment of explicit construction of nationality. Recall the scene: before posing for a group photograph that would become part of the anthropologists' archive, and possibly a news item for the Yao Medicine Hospital, medical staff dug out their embroidered red and black Yao hats and put them on for the picture. Hats were swapped and loaned for various poses, and nonminorities like Lili and Judith were cheerfully invited to borrow a Yao hat.

One reason this costume play seemed just a little ridiculous to all of us (even if it also seemed somehow necessary) was that it was taking place deep in the heart of a Yao nationality self-governing county, in the famously "cultural" Great Yao Mountains, and we were posing in front of the elaborate signage of an explicitly Yao medical institution. Moreover, most of the people we had met in this Yao heartland were members of one or another Yao subgroup. Why would a "mere symbol" of Yao identity such as a Yao hat need to be superimposed on this well-established and substantive Yao-ness? Was this little performance just an empty show, a tableau aimed back at the mediated gaze of the metropole and the world?[37]

This was not the only encounter we had with modern Chinese nationality that made us think twice about the practical significance—shallow or deep—of nationality. One kind of answer to our standard question about a person's nationality became rather predictable: "I'm Zhuang. Actually, I only realized it in middle school, when I registered as Zhuang because of certain advantages [e.g., added points on the national college entrance exam]. My mother is half Zhuang, even though my father is Han. My sister, though, didn't bother." This sort of thing is thought of in minority areas as instrumental or tactical nationality membership, and nobody is shocked or surprised by it.

Working in the domain of nationality medicine, though, reminded us that registered identities are not simple or obvious anywhere; they are certainly not "natural." This might especially be the case where particular medicines are being developed for particular populations. When local drugs, traditions, and diseases are being addressed, nationality identities might be naturalized or even racialized (though we saw little evidence of such essentialisms). Most often we saw a rather flexible mode of nationality identification. This was exemplified by Brilliance Zhang in Hubei province. Dr. Zhang was known as a developer of both Tujia and Miao medicine. He operated a hospital clinic that advertised both types. He had published on nationality medicine, and he was quite helpful to us in explaining the differences and similarities between Tujia and Miao medicines and TCM (tacitly recognized in these parts as Han). We found it interesting that he claimed an authoritative position on several nationality forms of knowledge, not really bothering to make an issue of his own nationality identity (which we recall as Miao, though for our project he was supposed to represent Tujia medicine).

But historical ethnic contrasts, and their related tensions, can run deep. We had a fascinating talk, for example, with an Achang nationality activist, whom we met staffing a county-level office of legal affairs. This well-educated cadre, Evertrue Zhou, said that his spell in the army had opened his eyes to the benefits of being identified as a minority. As a county official, he was working to improve educational opportunities for Achang youth, hoping that the bad old days of his compatriots hiding their minority status while being stigmatized anyway would not return. He felt strongly that the Achang *as* Achang had been important in the history of the county and that their nationality contribution should be remembered and valued.[38] For him, nationality status and recognition were a central project, one he was undertaking in the county offices on behalf of his Achang friends and relatives.[39]

These examples could be multiplied, but they still would not converge on a single modern Chinese understanding of ethnicity or nationality.[40] There is a national ethnic affairs commission in Beijing that continues to issue and revise national policies governing the media presentations and knowledge production activities affiliated with the national minorities. The English language names of some long-standing nationalities universities and institutes, for example, have recently changed to feature the thoroughly Chinese term *minzu* (nationality, 民族); Central Minzu University in Beijing is an example. This change reflects discomfort with the rather foreign denotations of the usual English terms "nationality" and "ethnic." *Minzu* may confuse outsiders, but at least it refers to a uniquely Chinese concept and historically known thing. As national law changes, the functional significance of *minzu* changes as well: the implications of various arrangements targeting the nationalities—from specialized universities to clinics in nationality self-governing counties—need to be rethought in relation to regulations governing the Han majority. Waivers of the family planning policy enjoyed by some *minzu*, for example, are less consequential now that regulations have loosened for everyone. And self-governing *minzu* polities enjoy sometimes more and sometimes less autonomy, particularly on the fraught question of religious development.

There are fifty-five officially recognized minority nationalities (*shaoshu minzu* 少数民族) in today's China, and there have been since 1979 (most were registered much earlier, in the 1950s). Thomas Mullaney has provided a history of the 1950s state project of salvaging and sorting the nationalities of China at a time when a Stalinist model for defining nations was influential, but not ultimately successful, at least in ethnically diverse Yunnan province. To qualify as a nationality under the Stalinist definition, the "four commonalities" of language, territory, mode of production, and cultural psychology were (at first) required.[41] Few southern groups could meet these criteria, and in a fascinating struggle among experts of various kinds, the work teams tasked with naming and delimiting a workable number of Chinese nationalities developed "a plastic definition of ethnicity." Even then, in the first years of the People's Republic, researchers "were attempting to engineer a measure of commensurability between local concepts of ethnic identity and those promulgated by the emerging social scientific state."[42] We see this plasticity in play still, especially when we attend to local approaches to identity and belonging rather than to social science hairsplitting and classificatory arbitrariness. As noted above, we also were able to witness the preferences and interventions of the state-supported social scientists as we accompanied survey researchers into minority areas and assisted their work. The ongoing project of defining minority nationality medicine and filling its categories with material life, at many social scales, is more interesting to us than any politics of ethnicity at the national level. This process, which we sometimes think of as institution-ing (see chapter 1), becomes truly visible only in relation to its unofficial, relatively untamed or nomad other, local healing and embodied expertise.

When one attends to the contemporary life of national culture and politics in the People's Republic of China, minority nationality medicine is an obvious *thing*, a policy arena in the act of becoming a significant matter of concern for the state. "Minority nationalities," however, are not new issues anywhere. In modern states, ever in formation and tirelessly reasserting biopolitical sovereignty, ethnic groups are not just primordially existing objects of a "natural" official interest. Rather, the modern nationalities as such are *creatures* of the modern state, as Thomas Mullaney's study of nationality formation in Yunnan in the 1950s has amply shown.[43] On the other hand, in a place like China, neither the nation with its peoples and cultures nor the sovereign state with its political concerns for hegemonic control of territories and productive forces is new. Laura Hostetler, for example, has studied the

Qing imperium's representation of the diverse nations under governance in Chinese spheres before the twentieth century, showing that "ethnography and cartography" involving non-Han groups were matters of imperial concern long before the revolutions that started China's "short twentieth century" of state building.[44] As such, the nationalities have been grandfathered in as targets of state power/knowledge. Wang Hui, tracking Russian nationalism alongside the twentieth-century rise of the Chinese nation-state, similarly reminds us that the semiautonomous "internal" nationalities were a concern for government in China well before Joseph Stalin legislated a nationality theory that became "modular" for nation-building in the socialist world.[45] And Partha Chatterjee, in an extended critique of nationalism theories, points out that not all nationalist movements have served the interests of singular groups, though in China Han chauvinism has not gone unnoticed and multicultural harmony is far from guaranteed.[46] The PRC was founded as a "multicultural unity," and though this image of a single nation with an irreducibly diverse population has had its vicissitudes—for example, during the later Maoist period the global solidarity of workers was more emphasized than the friendship of ethnically marked peoples—the nationalities have been made to contribute to, rather than undermine, national unity.

The appearance of a state-led minority nationality medicines initiative in the early 1980s, with significant new funding from the Ministry of Public Health appearing in the early 2000s, is not particularly surprising, then, in the context of the history of the modern Chinese nation. Even apart from the early Reform era shift, in the early 1980s, away from direct health care provision by the central government at little or no charge—this was a policy change that saw local medical institutions scrambling to find private sources of revenue and anxious to create market niches for specialist care—a "liberal" public health policy imperative emerged as a further refinement of the overall national development agenda. In China's case, liberal reform, sometimes referred to as "Getting on Track with the World" (*zouxiang shijie* 走向世界), involved a vast reorganization project for state resources. Not only huge industrial plants but also medical and educational institutions were asked to market their work in a neoliberal "socialism with Chinese characteristics." Many forms of socialist nurturance and care were exchanged for the debatable freedoms and mercies of national and global market competition. But at least in the eyes of Asian socialists, legitimate modern sovereignty requires, first, paternalistic care for the people in the form of medical services (or at least universal health insurance) that reach the perceived needs of all kinds of citizens. And second—and we think this is more important for explaining the appearance of minority nationality medicines—the national politics of the Reform Era include an acknowledgment from the central government that "the people" are irreducibly cultural; China's citizens have long been bearers of local languages, local knowledge, local values, and local needs. In other words, biopowers allied with the modern state need to be microscopic and productive, seek to wrap around the particular subjects who are interpellated and configured as Chinese citizens, and enable rather than constrict the culturally diverse lives of the people.

One task of the centralized leadership, then, is to generate reliable and responsible knowledge about salient social worlds within China's borders. Culture in modern nations cries out to be known and recognized,[47] which is one reason why Lili and Judith were often introduced to local experts in nationalities cultures, whether or not these "culture experts" knew anything about medicine. At the same time, direct state provision of health services has always been supplemented by care from those who are far from expert in modern biomedicine but who have much experience in treating afflictions where they occur. "Folk medicine" (*minjian yiyao* 民间医药) experts (the healing grannies, the traveling herbalists) tend to be denounced as charlatans by the modern biomedical profession, but as we will show here, even elite health care consumers and some medical professionals in China suspect that "wild" and "folk" therapies have special powers. In the shifting relationships between the "royal science" of Western medicine and the "nomad sciences" of minority healing traditions, then, the powers of folk therapeutics must be acknowledged even as they are partly coopted by official institutions.[48]

Henceforth in these pages the term nationality will be used to refer to social formations that are marked as belonging to some minority, and not always just one. In this we follow ordinary Chinese usage in which anything labeled as *minzu* is expected to have a minority nationality character, however vaguely conceived. Nationality names in common usage, and "nationality" as a generic term, make a claim of sorts, but this claim is not usually about personal identity, or communitarian belonging, or even resistance to Han majority domination. These semiotic habits thus set Chinese nationality apart from most of the ethnic nationalisms studied in the anthropology and sociology literature. The referents of this historically resonant modifier, in China, seem at present to have much to do with senses of local culture and nationality character.

LOCALITY AND PLACE

In the course of itinerant field research, as we traced connections through far-reaching networks, we began to refer to things appearing to have a nationality character as nothing more (or less) than *local*. Finding the "minority nationality" character of many expressions hard to discern, yet noting rich stores of particular knowledges that were still unrecognized by any state-authorized medicine (such as traditional Chinese medicine [TCM] or bio-medicine), at times we felt we were truly at the grassroots, "among the folk." Yet local medicines and pharmaceutical knowledge do not form a stable body of lore and craft that preexists visits from health and anthropology re-searchers, waiting to be discovered as nationality medicine, or even as local folk traditions. Everywhere we went we witnessed the ongoing work of as-sembly that was producing a thing, a "system" of medicine that was only sometimes called by a nationality name.[49]

Indeed, some of our more canny collaborators from research institutes and health departments chose to introduce us to "culture experts" (*wenhua ren* 文化人) who were specialists in local characteristics (*bendi tese* 本地特色). We could not always agree with these experts' uses of the culture con-cept, but we were impressed with their senses of place.[50] We recall one long car trip in Zhuang country where a very talkative culture expert sitting in the front seat lectured us about the history of every place name in this part of Guangxi (Judith was following along on a printed map, and was impressed with the comprehensiveness of his speculations). In retrospect, it does not matter to us that the historical background he reported, full of sage-kings and local worthies, battles and intrigues, seemed to be mostly philological guesswork. The more salient point was that he was filling the map of his home territory with cultural meaning and local history, and that he often taught this information to schoolchildren and tourists as well as to visiting researchers. This Zhuang expert was quite sincere about the culture he was gathering.[51] A historical and personal orientation to place, through more than names, was more important to him than the fine points of an "objec-tive" history would have been.

Similarly, a culture expert we met among the Achang group in Yunnan proudly showed us the hand-carved wooden saddles made by a few elderly local craftspeople. This embattled nationality group, long discriminated against (they said) by the much larger Bai community surrounding them, was doing deliberate culture-work. They wanted to show us how these saddles evoked a nearly forgotten Achang history of horse-craft and mili-tary service to premodern Chinese empires. In both cases we were witness-ing local place-making at work, even as these particular efforts were flying a contemporary banner of minority nationality.

We were not the only researchers who wondered about the relation be-tween nationality medicines and local cultures. The most senior national leader of the minority nationality medicine movement is Zhu Guoben, re-tired vice-director of the SATCM in Beijing. Zhu is a prolific scholar and experienced fieldworker who has written authoritatively on the medical systems of the nation's registered minorities.[52] In a keynote address at a 2012 conference in Sichuan, where many experts in Qiang medicine had gathered to assess the progress of their recent development work, Professor Zhu challenged a certain nationality idea among these minority medicine activists. Pointing out that the "Qiang medicine" practiced in Mao County where the meeting was being held was not much like the "Qiang medicine" being developed in a region closer to the Tibetan plateau (the latter significantly incorporating elements from Tibetan medicine), he asked whether the object of our investigations should be "local medicines" rather than "nationality medicines." Of course, any such shift in perspective would still require collective efforts to fill the notion of the local with meaningful and differential content. And Professor Zhu admitted to us in a later conversation in Beijing, when we asked about this question of the local, that "nationality" is a rubric that cannot be abandoned. But he, more than anyone perhaps, is aware of the social labor that goes into developing this thing, minority nationality medicine. And we think he was wise to remind his colleagues that locality might yield a more nuanced understanding of the social and scientific phenomena in question.

So let's reconsider local phenomena: We discovered during a visit to Nanning (Guangxi) that senior leaders of the nationality medicine movement in that city had a professional relationship with Wonderfont Zhao, the "instituting" Zhuang medicine practitioner who figures prominently in chapter 1. Dr. Zhao proudly showed us a draft of the preface for his forthcoming textbook that had been written and annotated by Huang Hanru, an eminent historian. We were suitably impressed. Perhaps Zhu Guoben wasn't thinking about Zhuang medicine when he made his comments on the local in Sichuan and Beijing, but for us no one illustrates better than Dr. Zhao does the intimate connection of nationality and locality.[53]

Wonderfont Zhao is the very model of a modern nationality doctor, and as we show in a reading of his business card (chapter 1), he wears many Zhuang nationality hats. But as we talked with him over the course of a long afternoon, it was not Zhuang-ness that he wanted us to see in his life and work. It was local depth and substance. He wanted us to know immediately, for example, that he was a thirteenth-generation Daoist master, all his ordained forebears having provided ritual services in the same region of southern Guangxi. His own family's home place, Settled Peace township, was a few hours' drive distant, but he traveled there often to collect the herbs native to the place for use in his practice. His former "Zhuang Medicine Academy" students were scattered over the nearby countryside as village doctors, and he told us they climbed mountains and gathered herbs—as did he—to help him maintain a rich but idiosyncratic pharmacy. The county seat in which his practice was located is known throughout the south, moreover, as the site of a large periodic natural drugs market; one of the textbooks Wonderfont has authored is an insider's guide to that market. When we asked for a look at his case records or pharmacy notes, he fetched instead a notebook that held a long prose poem written by his father (who had been a local schoolteacher as well as a Daoist), in his father's hand. The text was a paean to the beauties of the enchanted landscape of Settled Peace, and Wonderfont was anxious for us to appreciate the elegance of his father's writing. As we probed his Zhuang medicine habits, we learned that he emphasized the use of local herbs in conjunction with ritual and divination, and we pointed out that he did not seem to subscribe to all the key elements of Zhuang medicine that we had been learning about in Nanning, a long bus ride away. In retrospect, it seems incredible that we were able to learn so much about Wonderfont Zhao's placement in a particular world, rooted in many years, even many generations, of healing, teaching, and self-cultivation. Nationality seems a shallow label for such a profoundly local life; but Wonderfont was happy to assume the officially recognized nationality name, Zhuang. Moreover, his practice shows better than many that a sense of local place is constantly under construction, being asserted as a positive value for the life of families and other collaborating groups.

"Local" worlds are not naturally occurring totalities resting on firm social and cultural foundations. Dr. Zhao knew better than anyone how much ongoing labor was required to produce and propagate the situated knowledges for which he was famous.[54] At least in a heavily mediated and well-integrated globalizing country like China, the local and all its specific characteristics are always under construction, always being gathered. They are also, very often, thrown up as a contrast, even a form of resistance, to the national and the global.

There is a more radical and historically resonant way of thinking about locality and place. We are reminded of a statement Judith noticed posted in an aboriginal arts store in Sydney, Australia. The sentiment is credited to Ivan Namirrkki in 2003: "We didn't create this culture recently. It lies in the ground, it lies in the earth, but we are bringing it out." Here, discovery and invention, salvaging and sorting, are combined in one profoundly committed and deeply felt process. We will see in the chapters of this book that culture work and medical development rely on a concept of local natures. At the same time, they actualize particular worlds in physiologies, in plants, in tools.[55] And all these things—bodies, botany, techniques—fill local worlds with a specific lived and taken-for-granted character.[56] When in chapter 4 we turn to the shared life of plants and people, the notion of locality will emerge as both richer and more contingent than any concept of state-mandated ethnicity or therapeutic universality. We will show in what follows that global and national medicine, ethnic or otherwise, really touches down and achieves efficacy only in *places*. Sometimes these places take the names of nationalities.

A TRAVELING ANTHROPOLOGY

We confess immediately that the topic of minority nationality medicines in China is too large for us. Many of our Chinese friends who hear about our research think we might be investigating the very rich archives and institutions of Tibetan medicine, Uyghur medicine, or Mongolian medicine. These three minority nationalities (they are so classified in China) in China's north and west by now have developed rich histories of institutionalization in the fields of medicine and pharmacy. Since the early 1980s these groups have received considerable government and international support for "salvaging and sorting" local healing practices and traditional literatures. It is important to these development processes that all three of these groups have medical writings in their own classical languages.[57]

Rather than focus on these quite established traditional medicine projects, however, we turned our attentions to some less well-known groups who were, when we started our work in 2010, still actively engaged in laying the foundations of one or another nationality medicine. Our encounters during field research with a diverse collection of nationality activists, public health researchers, healers, and herbalists, identified (closely or remotely) with seven differently situated nationality groups, all in the mountainous southern parts of China, were extremely rewarding. Embarking on a project of tracing several kinds of health and medicine development, we sought out people and communities who we hoped would surprise us, teach us something we didn't already know, express with their personal stories and everyday work something specific to the place where we found them. Our research aim was, then, to catch development in the act.[58] We aimed to gather the scattered medical and social realities that are coming into view and contributing to the assembly of this thing called minority nationality medicine in China.

In keeping with this desire for encountering the unexpected, and this intention of gathering evidence of emergent medicines, our field research was highly mobile. In our work with seven nationality and local groups, we traveled through six provinces, circling around and within nationality institutions and traveling through minority nationality self-governing counties and prefectures. We worked with government representatives (usually county and township health department staff), medical staff in formal clinics, and a few regionally important scholars. The associates we met in these settings, perhaps presuming that we were especially after wild knowledge or nomad sciences,[59] conscientiously introduced us to healers and herbalists practicing well outside of the formal public health system. Many experts we met in this way gave us glimpses of worlds of nomad healing that would never be recognized by any modernizing and standardizing scientific system, and we were sometimes amazed by the willingness with which herbalists and other healers shared their personal histories and trade secrets, often on very short acquaintance. As we traveled, though we did not stay long anywhere, our local friendships grew deeper, and we returned several times to many of our multiple sites of research.[60]

Gathering Medicines, then, is an ethnographic study of a far from classic field. Our work obligations in Beijing and Chicago, and funding limitations as well, made it impossible for either of us to stay in one community, in classic anthropological fashion, for a year or more. The deeply rooted cultural life of any single isolated and unique village society eluded our traveling participant-observation. And the collective life that we were able to take part in came to us through relatively short encounters, like those we narrate throughout the book. Traveling, as we so often were, with state-supported researchers—most of whom were, like us, also outsiders in the nationality areas we visited—we began to take these committed and skilled itinerant investigators themselves as our most immediate "field." With them, we took up different points of view (not just a "state gaze") on the work of nationality activists, trying to get a sense of the dimensions and features of new medical formations as they became publicly recognized things.

Because our initial approach to many field sites was facilitated by the State Administration of Traditional Chinese Medicine (SATCM), we anthropologists were quite properly perceived as state representatives in this process. We have no doubt that many healers we spoke with did not want to be "seen by the state," nor did they see any need to satisfy anthropological curiosity, coming as it did from another world. Many were careful not to tell us too much.[61] But as we often explained to our local research hosts, we were not interested in collecting secret knowledge, and in the writing of this book we do not pretend to "ethnographically" understand the intimate social relations and deep historical memories of any one people who have lived together in a small place for most of their lives.

Nevertheless, this itinerant method allowed us to triangulate minority nationality medicine, that heterogeneous and creative formation-in-becoming, through its changing relations with other modes of knowledge and practice. We attended to the points of view of researchers with the

State Administration of TCM; listened to those of ordinary people seeking more adequate medical care or building a career in public health; shared the visions of activists arguing that Yao or Zhuang or Tujia existence is grounded in a particular embodiment and a special relationship to natural powers; and kept in mind the perspectives of the cultural anthropology in which we two authors had both been trained. The encounters through which minority medicines drew attention to themselves and established working relationships with wider worlds (including our own) became especially interesting to us. Sometimes a "local culture" was at issue. But more often we felt that our far from singular terrain of research, minority nationality medicines, was a network of relations more or less in the act of gathering itself, becoming a thing.

METHODOLOGY, COLLABORATION

We have already made frequent reference to our practical (and sometimes impractical) methods of undertaking field research together, and our concrete activities as fieldworkers will be continuously evident in the stories that follow in all five chapters. If there is a quality that sets our approach to social research in China apart from ethnography as usual (if there is such a thing), however, it is our commitment to many kinds of collaboration. Our own long-standing friendship and sharing of inspirations from many fields, and our efforts to write together truly and well, form the foundation of this book. We decided early on to adopt one anthropological-authorial voice, even while striving to recover in translation the many voices of a diverse collection of interlocutors in south and southwestern China. Many of the interviews we conducted were recorded and transcribed, often by members of our assisting group (about whom, see below). This practice enabled both of us to devote close attention to the particular ways local authorities on minority medicines spoke of their lives and views. But the opportunities we had during our research travels to visit medical lives in person and witness the work of healers in their homes and clinics were a precious form of collaboration as well.

The two of us have different field research skills: Lili is much better than Judith at comprehending local dialects in the south, thanks to her history of living and studying in several parts of China. And she is an indomitable interviewer, tirelessly pursuing every interesting comment that is dropped and happy to diverge from our back-of-the-hand short list of topics of interest. Judith is especially disciplined about keeping notes and maintaining a useful photo archive, and she notices significant local practices that Lili can overlook or take for granted. Just by virtue of being noticeably a stranger in nationality areas, moreover, Judith by her presence sometimes elicited explanations of and rationalizations for local practices that would otherwise go unstated or presumed.

As for the writing of this book, and the several articles that have appeared before it, we have completely relied on each other, from the times when the most basic structures of the arguments were decided upon to the final wording of every description and interpretation. We have been immensely lucky to be in a position to work closely together, at the University of Chicago Center in Beijing, in writing a book of this size and ambition. It all belongs to both of us.

But other collaborations beyond Lili and Judith's are just as important. It is methodologically significant, for example, that our starting point was in a central government agency, the State Administration of Traditional Chinese Medicine (SATCM). Lili has long-standing ties to a few leaders of the SATCM in Beijing, and in 2010 she was invited to add an anthropology component to an ambitious series of surveys planned by the agency. She was then able to invite Judith to join this nascent minority nationality medicines project, and no one at the SATCM—as far as we know—objected to having a foreigner involved.

Though at first we were not sure how our style of work would articulate with the aims and practices of this government agency, we considered this research to be an extraordinary opportunity that was not to be missed. Aware from our previous research of the salvaging and sorting process though which TCM had developed, and learning from Lili's colleagues that there was a relatively recent policy turn toward encouraging minority medicines, we jumped at this chance. At the very least, we reasoned, we would be able to address some classic questions in medical anthropology. Not only could we catch the state-led process of salvaging and sorting folk medicines in the act of bringing indigenous knowledges out from the earth where they (presumably) lay, we could say much about what happens when a national medical system pluralizes (again).

Working with a research unit of the SATCM in Beijing, we selected nationality groups that offered—we were told—good conditions for anthropological research, and we began to establish local connections in five provinces. Because we two could make only relatively short trips to research sites in Hubei, Sichuan, Guangxi, Yunnan, and Hainan, we decided to recruit and train a few research associates (one per site, at a minimum) who could connect us to interesting local experts and keep an eye on developments involving nationality medicine during times when we were absent. In seven groups, this model of collaboration worked well, though in different ways for different sites. We designed a series of three five-day workshops—

in Yunnan, Beijing, and Hainan—and working together, in these workshops our group crafted anthropological methods suitable to an itinerant and episodic fieldwork process.

Because we all had so much fun during these training conferences in Beijing, Yunnan, and Hainan between 2011 and 2014, experimenting with ethnographic methods and fitting them to the large task facing us, we want to name and recognize the group who first agreed to be part of the project: Working in Sichuan, Zhang Jing brought her ethnobotanical expertise to bear on our work, and Zhang Dan gave us the benefit of her knowledge of Qiang religion and mythology. In Nanning, Luo Jie was an important interlocutor on Zhuang medicine thanks to her academic specialty in the history of medicine, and Fang Meijian, with Wei Qian, proved to be an indomitable fieldworker over a long period of time. The research staff of the Yunnan Academy of TCM, especially Ma Kejian, Lu Yuhui, Zhao Jingyun, and Yang Yuqi, graciously added our methods and agenda to their ongoing research on Achang and Lisu medicine. In Yao country, Yang Jian was a thoughtful observer working as a medical resident at the Jinxiu Yao Hospital. Dai Shuiping shared her ethnopharmacological Hainan Island with us with great sensitivity both to plants and to people. And experts on Tujia medicine Yang Fuming in Enshi, Hubei, and (later) Tian Huayong and Hou Qinian in Xiangxi, Hunan, generously took us on research road trips through the beautiful mountains of that region.

Some of the results of our group's collaborative research were published together as a series of papers, authored by individuals and collaborating groups, in a special issue of the *Guangxi Minzu University Journal*.[62] Though Lili and Judith made their last long field trip in 2014, Zhang Dan and Luo Jie, and various researchers at the Yunnan Academy of TCM, have continued with nationality medicine research of their own, incorporating some anthropological methods as they go. Though few of these research associates were truly insiders in the areas where most of our visits to healers and clinics took place, they were helpful with dialects and local background information. More important, all of them helped us to think about contemporary medical work and showed us how to perceive much more than our training had prepared us to see. We two authors are so grateful to all of them!

As funding from the SATCM and our several US-based grants became sparser over a period of five years, our connections to government in Beijing became more attenuated. We nevertheless continued to rely on the research staff and sponsorship of local government agencies and medical institutions across the south.[63] This positioning confirmed our undeniable identification as PhD researchers from elite academic institutions in Chicago and Beijing, bearing with us, perhaps, our own form of "royal science." Expressed in standard social science terms, because of our starting point within state institutions, our sample of interlocutors was undoubtedly biased. Among the healers we were able to visit at any length, it is certainly the case that the majority were village doctors, medical administrators, herbalists who had collaborated with *materia medica* surveys, and recognized culture experts. Fully aware of the partiality of the connections we could establish from our very specific social locations, we had to constantly reevaluate the social location of the targets of our research: Were our chief interlocutors "wild mountain healers"? "Agents of the development state"? Or perhaps "local elites" with (possibly) self-aggrandizing "minority" agendas? Obviously, how we answered such questions had implications for the everyday work of our research. Choosing whom to interview, deciding what parts of long explanations and historical stories could be credited, noting the social positions of all participants in a complex encounter—all these concerns inform the narratives from which this study is woven.

As we have emphasized throughout this introduction, the putative field of minority nationality medicines did not present us with self-evident sites and experts to study. Leaving behind the policy certainties of the SATCM and its concern with fifty-five national minorities, we quickly began to attend to what *other people* took our project to be. In most cases, we were dependent on officially connected local contacts to put us in touch with interviewees. But as we became interested in the interests of our health department and hospital hosts, the topic of our anthropology began to shift and adopt multiple points of view. As a result, this book is not exactly an anthropology of seven local or nationality forms of knowledge, or of the Chinese developmental state, or of the human and nonhuman networks that play across the fields of medicine and public health in China. Yet the project draws all of these together in an ethnography of a present situation, a nation caught in the act of constructing a set of complex social and epistemological things, minority nationality medicines.

CONCLUSION

When, in 2014, we asked our friend State Follower Wang, with whom we spent a delightful morning in a Lisu self-governing county, whether he had seen any evidence of a "Lisu medicine," he expressed uncertainty about whether Lisu medicine was a thing. He nevertheless cheerfully proposed to Lili and Judith that we all work together to create it. As a village doctor in his seventies, he probably had a deep historical sense of the contemporary need for salvaging and sorting, synthesizing and elevating Lisu medicine, in the manner of Han nationality TCM. And he had spent enough time talking with and learning from other healers in the region to be confident about the potential richness of that not yet actual thing, Lisu nationality medicine.

Enjoying Dr. Wang's optimism, respecting his long life of gathering medicines in the mountains, and appreciating his energetic service to the people under the aegis of the Ministry of Public Health and its local arms, we felt a special kinship with him. Meeting him only near the end of our fieldwork itineraries through the south, we felt we had found someone who, like the Masked Philosopher and our fellow anthropologists, could dream of a new age of curiosity, one that would multiply the paths and the possibilities of comings and goings. He was not the only minority nationality healer who tried to teach us this lesson: The things to be known are infinite. This book gathers some of them.

[CHAPTER 1]

Institution

The People's Republic of China has instituted public health services in unique ways. "Complementary and alternative medicines" are legal and available in many countries, but China was the first nation to make a "traditional" medicine formally available to its people as a part of official public health services.[1] The modern history of medical pluralism in China, and the development of traditional Chinese medicine (TCM) as a state-supported institutional complex, form a backdrop to the minority nationality medicines tracked by this study. Institutionalization, we argue in this chapter, is a key moment in the overarching process of salvaging, sorting, synthesizing, and elevating (*fajue, zhengli, zongjie, tigao* 发掘,整理,总结,提高) Han TCM, first, and more recently minority nationality medicines.[2]

The public health and nationality activists currently at work in China have seen how a nationality form of medicine can be assembled, as most of them participated directly or indirectly in the instituting of TCM. Having benefited from the establishment in the 1950s and 1960s of a corpus (*tixi* 体系) of (Han) Chinese medicine that was (and is) constantly compared and contrasted with "Western (bio)medicine," and in many cases having participated in a renaissance of the TCM field in the early Reform period (which began around 1978), these activists accept that health and medicine are central to the legitimacy of modern government. But they also understand the contingency and precariousness of even the most elite and established medical institutions. They know in their bones that those things recognized as the socially structured components of a medicine, such as clinics, hospitals, specialized literatures, techniques, professional associations, and academic disciplines, are always under construction and often under siege. Especially in the case of "traditional" "non-Western" medicines, which are often put on the defensive about their modernity, effectiveness, safety, and scientificity, nationality medicine experts need to prove, interminably, their social worth. They feel compelled to rescue local expertise from its reputation as trivial "folklore," and they must continually resist a popular image of their expertise as scattered and (at best) "merely empirical." Many of these highly various practitioners, following the example of the large-scale institutionalization of TCM since the 1950s, aim to build a bigger and better system of nationality medicine as they salvage and sort local and ethnic forms of healing.

Gathering a medicine is not a job that can be finished. In this chapter we follow the work of several architects of nationality medicines to show that instituting a nationality traditional medicine in today's China is a difficult and hazardous undertaking, even for those who are passionately committed to the task, and even for those few groups who enjoy generous government support. As local experts have aimed to develop specifically ethnic systems, their strategies have been informed by a modern consensus about the proper structures and functions of laboratories, hospitals, clinics, health stations, pharmacies, health insurance, and doctor-patient relationships. There is a consensus, in other words, about the very nature and form of legitimate medical institutions in a modern state. To turn folk therapeutics, a nomad science, into a state-recognized system of modern medical institutions is a demanding collective labor.

In this chapter we treat *institution* as a process, as a verb rather than a noun signifying an object. Instituting is a style of collective action, and institutions are formations continuously emerging from action more than they are stabilized structures with fixed properties.[3] Translating the kinds of action that interest us into sometimes awkward English, then, we frequently speak of instituting and the process of institution. This research project has tried to catch institution in the act, seeking out nationality medicines while they adventurously, precariously, collaboratively, and lovingly assemble, stabilize, and propagate new social and natural forms as elements of modern Chinese medical and ethnic pluralism. In our field research, then, as we talked with healers and activists, the questions we found most useful were largely practical.

Recall our friend village doctor State Follower Wang—a very practical village doctor in western Yunnan—who spoke to us of instituting "Lisu medicine" in an especially clarifying way. We met him in the summer of 2014, while we were spending time in the mountainous southwest near the Myanmar border. The Lisu are one of China's fifty-four registered minority nationalities. They tend to live as small farmers and hunters scattered over the high mountains of China's southwestern border region, though many Lisu are also town dwellers, storekeepers, migrant workers, itinerant traders, or contract laborers. There is a lot of mobility in this region, both regional and transnational travel for work, and travel for schooling and professional reasons.[4]

Our contacts at the local county health department introduced us to State Follower Wang as a Lisu village doctor practicing in the hills near the county seat of a Lisu self-governing county. A staff member from the township health station accompanied us to the village committee offices where Dr. Wang's clinic was located. Dr. Wang welcomed the three of us warmly to this compound where he and his wife worked and lived. Between patients— there were a lot of them that morning—he told us his life story and described his medical practice. He appeared proud to be identified as Lisu: perhaps having been warned of our research interests in advance by the health department, he was wearing locally made ethnic garments, and he assured us that the village he served was largely inhabited by Lisu nationality people.[5]

Dr. Wang's practice had all the features of an official administrative unit at the lowest level of state organization. He had long held an appointment as the village doctor, and his clinic managed immunizations, medical records, family planning, and public health education for those who lived there. His clinic rooms and much of the village committee courtyard they faced were decorated with health propaganda posters, and a poem of his own composition, entitled "Health Education," was chalked on a blackboard near the village committee's small conference room. His formal training had been minimal. When he was a youth in the 1960s, having had only a few years of primary school education, he had nevertheless been enrolled in barefoot doctor training courses. After that, he was mainly self-taught, consulting about herbals and other natural medicines with other practitioners in the area, and auditing a number of workshops in the county hospital while his first wife was being treated for urinary bladder stones.[6] At some point, he studied hard and passed the county's medical licensing exam; but like many other village doctors we have met, he rather scoffed at the licensing process, saying, "I got my diploma among the common people."

Dr. Wang maintained good clinic records and filed these case-by-case notations with the county on a regular basis, where the basic information was entered into a database. He prescribed and administered the chemical drugs of "Western medicine," and he maintained a large pharmacy of Chinese medical herbal drugs, all—he said—collected in the nearby mountains.[7] He billed all these medical treatments to the "New Rural Cooperative Medical [Insurance] System," and his wife kept the financial records and collected co-pays from patients. He diagnosed illnesses through a combination of traditional Chinese medicine and Western medicine. Yet he knew many local remedies and emphasized flexible matching of local resources to the "ever-changing" challenges of human illness (*rende bing shi qianbian wanhuade* 人的病是千变万化的). He also understood how to manage ghost-induced afflictions and magical attacks, though he preferred to leave this kind of ritual work to the local shaman (who showed up in the clinic the morning we were there, accompanying his wife who had come for a checkup).

We were interested to note that our companion from the township health station, Mr. Zhou, was entirely in sympathy with Dr. Wang's eclectic approach to the practice of primary care medicine. Mr. Zhou even acknowledged the importance of knowing how to cope with ghosts. He apparently found no contradiction, nor did Dr. Wang, in a fully licensed village doctor's hosting the local shaman in his village clinic of a morning. Dr. Wang had, moreover, been recognized for his skills by a "China Famous Folk Doctors Committee," which in the late 1990s had declared him to be an "excellent famous doctor" (we saw the certificate). Indeed, he was such a multifaceted healer, and obviously so useful to local patients, that Mr. Zhou worried aloud: "When this seventy-year-old village doctor retires, who will we get to take his place?"

Over lunch, Lili asked State Follower Wang, "If I were to say that your practice represents Lisu medicine, would you agree?" Amused and surprised, he said "Yes!" Then, thinking a moment, he said, "Well, I'm Lisu, after all, and I do medicine." On the other hand, he said he had never heard of any "Lisu medicine" as such, though he knew about Tibetan, Miao, Uyghur, and other forms of nationality traditional medicine. But "Good idea!" he said, "Let's create Lisu medicine!" Then he paused and added: "Now, how would we go about doing that? I have no idea!"

His modest query and his joking recruitment of visiting researchers into a daunting task of instituting "a medicine" reminded us of just how difficult it is proving to be, even for less "scattered" and better-funded groups than the Lisu, to create a nationality medicine. Which is to say, a system of knowledge and services, workplaces and training sites, that can mount a full-blown alternative therapeutics in a medically plural national Chinese public health apparatus.

Lili and Judith also had very little idea of how to "create" an ethnic medicine, especially if creating implies making something from scratch or *de novo*. But we knew something about the *official* answer to Dr. Wang's question: nationalities should gather together their own traditional medicine in that process known as salvaging and sorting, synthesizing and elevating a nationality heritage, with the result being institutions of "minority nationality medicine and pharmacy." The official program presumed that cultural and healing resources were already present in the local environments where the various nationalities lived and worked, and these could be excavated and drawn together to make up a "minority medicine."[8]

Plenty of methods are available to answer Dr. Wang's "how" question. These include the standard techniques of governance that have long been the hallmarks of the Chinese managerial state: field surveys, collaboration meetings, and focus groups; scholarly and social research; professional education and training, regulation of practitioners and their resources (such as drugs and plantations); and subsidies for needed services.[9] Some of these activities were already an important part of Dr. Wang's own practice: he was proud of the formal medical education he had sought out, he voluntarily engaged in "medical exchanges" (*yiyao jiaoliu* 医药交流) with nearby healers, he participated willingly and conscientiously in state regimes of inscription and record-keeping, and he proudly displayed his medical license, earned through passing a difficult written test. Thus far, much of this activity was institutional, or royal, in the sense that it was legal and organizational, but little of it was specifically Lisu. The question remained: What would the institutions of *Lisu medicine* look like, and how should we build them?

Imagine, for a moment, the process of creating Lisu medicine as our colleagues at the State Administration of Traditional Chinese Medicine (SATCM) envision it. First, local knowledge about local things, and the things themselves (the drugs, the tools), would have to be gathered. Persons and places where skills or expertise could be found would have to be determined at the same time — all these things, previously hidden from national public view, would have to be salvaged and brought into more or less public view. Sorting would follow: those elements experts deemed to be specifically Lisu would be marked as such. The scientific, empirical, and known-to-be-effective elements would be distinguished from "the dross" of superstition and "empty" ritual traditions,[10] and everything of nationality and medical value that remained would be grouped together to form a new assemblage, Lisu medicine (sorted out).[11] But for Lisu medicine to have any future (and therefore, arguably, any proper existence in the past or present), education and professional exchange would be required. The newly marked-off assemblage of "salvaged" empirical things would have to be synthesized or systematized.[12] At the very least, theory would have to be distinguished from practice, methodology would have to be understood as a more fundamental corpus than a mere list of techniques. These kinds of knowledge, once rendered as a coherent system, could structure training manuals, textbooks, historical accounts, government reports. Specific natural drugs, formulae, massage methods, needling techniques, and so forth, could be organized and listed under higher-order rubrics, and the medical practice learned in formal training could be disciplined. Finally, the never-absent question of the efficacy of a traditional medicine should be addressed: scientific research must be deployed to elevate the recognized value of Lisu medicine to the level of scientific truth. Clinical trials, chemical analysis of previously unrecorded medicinals, and even social research on "the Lisu medicine clinical encounter" (for example) could slowly build an evidence base for this nationality medicine.

Sitting at lunch with Dr. Wang and Mr. Zhou in the village committee compound, we all shared a great deal of confidence in Dr. Wang's ethical and effective, if rather ad hoc, methods. But the extent to which his practice expressed or represented Lisu medicine was a problem. We suspected that his Lisu medical knowledge just might not offer enough distinct resources that could be drawn on in a salvaging and sorting, or instituting, process.[13] Possibly this Lisu autonomous county (*zizhixian* 自治县), not to mention the whole Lisu nationality population, doesn't have a great many medical resources that could be collected from insider knowledge and turned to account as a well-sorted, systematic, and highly valued medical system. The nationally familiar "integrated" medicine that weaves Chinese medicine and biomedicine together (*zhongxiyi jiehe* 中西医结合) might be able to incorporate a few miscellaneous local or "Lisu" resources into its own system, but the ethnic and local character of Dr. Wang's practical medical expertise would likely be forgotten in the process. In other words, the *successful* institution of a minority medicine might require a more self-consciously distinct local historical and cultural field than the Yunnan Lisu can realistically gather. Perhaps they live in a nationality terrain full of as yet unknown lore that awaits salvage and sorting, and perhaps they work in a field of uniquely local healing that is not yet gathered into "a medicine." But none of us could be sure what that was.

So Dr. Wang's enthusiasm for creating a "Lisu medicine" might have been misplaced. But there is no doubt that he was actively instituting something like a coherent site of grassroots healing, Lisu or not. State Follower Wang can be seen as a condensed node linking the roles and functions of a great many existing government agencies. As a village doctor working side by side with the lowest level of government administration, the village committee, he reports both to the village and to public health units at higher levels. His preventive medicine work, such as immunizations and family planning, is assisted and regulated by the staff of the township health center, and his clinic records are checked and stored at the county level. County health units (the hospitals, the health bureau, the drug quality agency) report upward to the prefecture (which in Dr. Wang's Lisu case is a Tibetan nationality autonomous prefecture), and some resources and regulations are sent down to villages through these lower levels from the Yunnan Province Department of Health. Health insurance premiums must be collected by the village party secretary with Dr. Wang's help, but the county administers the insurance payouts on the basis of claims filed by Dr. Wang. And don't forget, Dr. Wang became a village doctor thanks to a very aggressive institutionalization of health services in the earlier years of the PRC. The health schools and barefoot doctor trainings mandated by the Beijing government in the 1960s and 1970s were central to the construction and staffing of an effective public health apparatus for the whole country.

Considering that he juggles so many direct and indirect responsibilities, Dr. Wang remains quite light on his feet at age seventy. But he is also linked to other social formations, perhaps not so formal or official as his ties through the county to the state. Recall that he "got his diploma among the common people." This was a reference to his long experience of learning alongside the local people as they coped with problems ranging from famine to ghosts, from propaganda and drug shortages to work points and grain quotas. He also credits the local forests with some of his success as a village doctor: like so many of the practitioners we met, he proudly maintains an herbal pharmacy stocked with natural medicines that he and his family and friends collect in the mountains and process themselves. This village health station is gathered from resources that come from near and far and that have deep roots in a shared past. The medicine that Dr. Wang practices is improvised and co-constructed, drawing things together in an effective but highly contingent healing assemblage that is always a work in progress.[14]

STRUCTURATION, STABILIZATION, GATHERING

"Social practices, biting into space and time," Anthony Giddens remarks, "are . . . at the root of the constitution of both subject and social object."[15] Giddens's poststructuralist approach to institution draws our attention to the many "day-to-day" techniques through which society is constructed. Our ethnographic research on nationality medical instituting practices did the same. Giddens's theory of structuration exhaustively outlines the pragmatics of social dynamics in modern societies; the salvaging and sorting of nationality medicines in China certainly count as ways of constituting (modern, Chinese, regional) society. Institution building of the kind we study here need not derive from a vision of *sui generis* society, a discrete formation with rules, structures, a territorial reach, and definitional essences.[16] Society conceived in this way is, as Ernesto Laclau has argued, impossible. Yet a modernist ideology continues to speak of social institutions as if they were fixed objects that press upon and restrict the freedoms of individuals. Rejecting all efforts to suture the social into stable institutions, or social objects, Laclau pushes a practice sociology farther than Giddens would, perhaps: "The social," he says, "only exists as the vain attempt to institute that impossible object: society."[17]

As ethnographers, we are quite content to dissolve structures into practices and see "the wider society" as a product of ideological work.[18] Looked at from the always-local grassroots perspective of the institution process, China's county government agencies are, admittedly, fairly concrete; after all, human officials frequently leave their nearby offices and come knocking on the door of village clinics, claiming to represent the imperatives of government "up above" (*shangji* 上级). The prefecture, province, and nation-state, however, are more abstract; it requires imagination and everyday discursive labor for most people (including us) to realize them as totalizing or framing institutions. Dr. Wang, seizing with delight on the idea of a "Lisu medicine," was not the only healer we met who could begin to imagine hospitals and academies, textbooks and examinations as a yet to be invented world of a nationality medicine. But they tend to think of institution as a challenging task rather than as a stolid set of social objects.

The collective practices that build minority nationality medicines bite into space and time, marking off units that are never stable; the attempt to "institute society" is always "vain," Laclau says. The protean character of the social field, with its "kaleidoscopic movement of differences," is easy to visualize in contemporary China, where everything gathered is an interested project and where most people try to get by without checking in with any instituted authorities. Aware of this social fluidity, we ask: What are the space and time that are constituted in the new institutions of nationality medicines? Seeking to trace forms of agency, we ask: How do the spatial networks of variously embodied actors, and the experiences and memories of historical groups, give shape to the medicine that is being assembled? Keeping the relational and contingent character of society in mind, we ask: How does spacetime take on a "local" character as it gathers into an instituting process particular to southern China and its nationalities?[19]

STRATEGIES OF GATHERING

In the contemporary situation of salvaging and sorting minority nationality medicines, ethnic and health advocates rely on a number of medical development strategies. Some of these are evident already in Dr. Wang's practice, even though he was not (yet) trying to create a Lisu medicine. Others are clearly discernible in the Zhuang and Qiang cases we discuss below. What concrete activities should anyone hoping to institute a nationality medicine undertake? What work is required to suture a large collection of healing resources into a medical system? Here we present some items from the strategic to-do list that we saw at work in the projects of many who were trying to gather nationality medicine.

First, many activists draw on prior medical institutions, especially (in this part of China) those of TCM and public health education. In chapter 5, "Encounters," we emphasize, for example, the historical importance of health ministry and health department "health schools" (*weixiao* 卫校). Most of the "ethnic" practitioners we met had begun their medical careers with these training courses that covered biomedical primary care, TCM herbal medicine, and acupuncture, in intensive sessions lasting from three months to two years. A few such schools were run by local experts, who taught their teenage students a great deal about how to collect and use the unique natural drugs that could be found in their area. One Lisu healer we met—also a village doctor—showed us his treasured notes, decades old and repeatedly studied, from his short time spent in such a locally oriented school.

Second, as this doctor's notes attested, writing is central to any Chinese instituting process. Indeed, the national experts on minority nationality medicines tend to divide the medicines of the fifty-five minority nationalities into two major categories, those that have written languages and those that don't. Six groups—the Tibetan, Mongolian, Uyghur, Dai, Korean, and Yi nationalities—have had written languages for a relatively long time; as a result, they can search cultural archives, gathering relevant medical materials, sorting, interpreting, and republishing them as a medical system. Because most nationalities don't have historical records in their own language, however, they must draw on random writings scattered in literatures written by Chinese officials or literati (who were mostly Han). For the ethnographer, there are less ambitious texts that certainly relate to the gathering of a medicine: recall Dr. Wang's inscribed certificate of award from the "China Famous Folk Doctors Committee," and the poem of health advice he had chalked on the village committee blackboard in his own careful calligraphy.[20]

A third strategy: instituting in modern highly mediated state societies participates in a politics of recognition.[21] This is why writing and publishing are so important: an ethnic social formation counts for little if it is not acknowledged as legitimate by agencies of the state.[22] In the realm of medicine, in China, a great many healers of various kinds have practiced unrecognized, e.g., without so much as an officially inscribed license; it is not always illegal or undesirable to fly under the radar of the biopolitical state.[23] But if the "infinite play of [ethnic, medical] differences" is to be fixed in an effective institutional form, it helps to make alliances with other institutions—as they also emerge—while representing one's own name, place, population, and culture. The nationality activists who have achieved a recognized public presence have written proposals, newsletters, research reports, and, as we shall see, histories in their quest to achieve official status as a recognized medical association. Indeed, all sorts of writing—not least emails and conference announcements—are involved in the collective work that develops a medical system from a loose network to a hobbyist society (*xiehui* 协会) to a recognized disciplinary association (*xuehui* 学会) that can sponsor and staff agencies made of bricks and mortar.[24]

A fourth item on the instituting to-do list is a term that took an important place in our research from the beginning, partly because government researchers thought it was important: "medical exchange" (*yiyao jiaoliu* 医药交流) is a practice that is widely thought to be essential to the process of building a medicine. When we were beginning this project in Beijing, for example, we heard that some groups (especially, in our sample, the Lisu and the Li of Hainan) were not interested in medical exchange; these scattered healers were considered to be quite jealous of their secrets, unwilling to compare notes, record their emblematic cases, share their drug formulae, or collectively sort and systematize their knowledge. This stereotype of the atomized Lisu was not entirely wrong. In our experience, State Follower Wang stood out in the Lisu context as a lifelong student, seeking to learn from all kinds of experts, including other rural practitioners. However, even some who impressed our collaborators as particularly reluctant to share their "secrets" told us about their careers practicing medicine in public. In a socialist bureaucratic state, almost any medical career would involve "exchange" in the form of conferences, policy workshops, and on-the-job training. All such forms of exchange contribute to the ongoing work of instituting.

There are a few other things on the to-do list: Drs. Huang Hanru and Huang Jinming, for example, whose work to institute Zhuang medicine we explore below, realized that they needed to do considerable conceptual work to define their emergent field. They wrote and lavishly published the results of their careful thinking. They also organized extensive scholarly exchanges and shared study, tracing the roots and resources of local healing formations to delimit and gather an archive that could inform the medical practice they were in the act of defining.

Further, the diverse collection of healers, scholars, and administrators working to institute a nationality medicine insist that they are thinking toward the future of health, that of their ethnic group and region, and that of the Chinese nation. Nationality medicines need to be salvaged and sorted, people say, for the sake of a future community. The practical wisdom of elders both near and far should not be lost. In this aspirational mode, institution demands that experts, even as they are inventing their own expertise in a self-cultivation process, find students and teach. Teaching in schools requires curricula, textbooks, examinations, internships. Mentoring in a more traditional master-disciple relationship requires time spent together, gathering medicines and clinical experience and embodying a healing habitus. The instituting, or gathering, of a medicine is a reproductive process, and it is hard, skilled work.

THE GRASSROOTS OF ZHUANG MEDICINE: WONDERFONT ZHAO

We felt the contingency and dynamism of instituting practices especially acutely when, in the course of our travels in search of nationality medicines, we met Dr. Wonderfont Zhao of Tranquility Town, Guangxi. Lili and I had been advised by Zhuang medicine contacts in the big city of Nanning, the capital of Guangxi Zhuang Nationality Autonomous Region (广西壮族自治区), to seek out Dr. Zhao. He is, we were told, an influential leading activist in the region-wide development—that is, the salvaging and sorting—of Zhuang nationality medicine. Zhuang medicine is currently among the best-organized forms of minority medicine. Since the 1980s, specialists have taken full advantage of an administrative climate that encouraged the development of minority nationality institutions. It has been especially important for Zhuang medicine that legal and financial support has come from the province level: Guangxi is a Zhuang nationality autonomous region, and its department of health encouraged nationality cultural and administrative developments earlier than many other provinces.

In the southern city of Nanning there is a Zhuang medical school and research institute, and across the street is a large Zhuang hospital. Clinics, private practitioners, and freelance researchers are scattered in large and small installations around southern Guangxi. Histories, textbooks, and research journals have been assembled. Zhuang branded herbs and decoctions are sold in stores and street markets; and Zhuang ethnic medical techniques are studied by clinicians. Presently we will examine some of the processes through which Zhuang medicine has come to be so impressively institutional, especially in Nanning. But first, Wonderfont Zhao has something more fundamental to teach us about instituting at the grassroots.

When experts in Nanning expressed their respect for Dr. Zhao's contribution to the development of Zhuang medicine over the past couple of decades, we felt we should pay attention. So we took a five-hour bus ride out to Tranquility County town where Dr. Zhao practices. He met us in his old, small van and was clearly worried when he realized that our party included a foreigner. (He called his wife before leaving the bus station to organize more food shopping, so they could later offer us a more impressive meal.) At first, distracted with these anxieties, he didn't seem like a very formidable expert at all.

Indeed, Dr. Zhao's panic on seeing us arrive at the bus station had a lot to do with contemporary institution-building processes far beyond Tranquility County. He had been warned about Lili, and he knew she was coming from a high-status remote location, Peking University Health Sciences Center. So he would have been nervous about her anyway. But Judith's presence was evidence that news of his authority, responsibility, and status had gone global. On this occasion, then, he probably realized that he would need to perform his Zhuang medicine authority persuasively. In other words, he was even more challenged than usual to demonstrate (or institute) his respectability and authority.

When we got to Dr. Zhao's clinic and home on the edge of town, his daughter and clinic partner hurried out to meet us, shrugging on her white coat. Entering the clinic room under the carved sign "Tranquility Clinic of Zhuang Medicine," we were surprised to encounter mostly dust and neglect. The clinic appeared derelict. No medicines were stored there, and no one had used the tables and chairs for quite some time. There were a number of signboards stored inside the old clinic, so we could see that this disused room had long *claimed* to be the site where some important Zhuang medicine institutions were located. Next door, in a shopfront building facing the street, and housing a walk-in clinic, newer signs announced some of Dr. Zhao's Zhuang medicine institutions. But Wonderfont rents that shop out to former students for their use as a consulting room; he said he never uses it, and his daughter was relieved when he led us back to the living areas of the house, away from all these magnificent signs and dusty cabinets.

Dr. Zhao's name card, thick with information and including his color portrait, turned out to be a better place than his clinic to see his ambitious instituting activities presented together:

Wonderfont Zhao
Principal, Zhuang Medicine Academy, Tranquility County, Guangxi
Director, Institute of Zhuang Medicinal Research, Tranquility County
Committeeman, All-China Consultative Committee, Tranquility County
   Branch
Secretary, Guangxi Nationalities Medicine Commission
Resident Physician, Tranquility County Zhuang Medicine Clinic

This translation of the front of his name card announces that Dr. Zhao is, first, the principal of a Zhuang medicine and pharmacy *academy*; second, he is the director of his town's Zhuang medicine *research institute*; third, he is a committeeman for his town's *national consultative committee* (this is the local branch of the National People's Congress); fourth, he is secretary of the Guangxi *Nationality Medical Association*; and finally, he is resident physician in his own Zhuang Medicine *Clinic*. This list is pretty comprehensive: all bases are covered—teaching, research, government relations, ethnic community organizing, and the all-important clinic. On the reverse side his name card lists at length the "service programs" he provides, which include educational, institutional, and therapeutic activities, all depicted— in keeping with his self-chosen given name Wonderfont—as quite wonderfully effective. Most of the diseases he treats are listed with biomedical labels, and he notes that his clinic combines Western, Chinese, and Zhuang forms of medicine. As you can imagine, once we saw this name card with its great claims, much of our conversation with Dr. Zhao was aimed at learning what activities corresponded to the practical life of the institutions he headed, or embodied.

Though we felt he was performing for us a kind of authority that exceeded the reach of formal institution, Dr. Zhao was not at all distant or pretentious in person, and he was very kind in hosting us for most of a day in his large and comfortable home behind the clinic. His spacious family sitting room is the site where he does most of his work. He was happy to explain to us how his Zhuang medicine academy works. This extraordinarily productive school has, since the early 1990s, trained hundreds of practitioners of Zhuang medicine. To run this intensive training course in Zhuang medicine, Dr. Zhao rents a hotel conference room for a few weeks each year, and he writes and assembles his own textbooks covering areas like internal medicine, gynecology and obstetrics, pediatrics, dentistry, and eye/ear/nose/ throat medicine. These pamphlet-sized texts are reissued every year for the academy's use, with revisions. Sometimes Dr. Zhao invites another experienced practitioner or two to teach along with him.

In its peak year of popularity, the school graduated fifty-two trainees; that was the early 1990s, when any diploma from recognized formal training would allow its holder to practice medicine. But numbers of trainees are down since 1995, the year the county health department began to issue and require medical licenses gained by way of a standardized test administered in the county seat. Nowadays, Dr. Zhao tells us, he is training and awarding diplomas to only four to ten students a year. He says they come to him out of a "love for learning" rather than a need for a medical license; his diploma, after all, has no legal authority, even though it certifies that training took place. Even so, through this seasonal school Dr. Zhao has provided the county and the region with an impressive cohort of practitioners of Zhuang medicine, most of them now legally licensed.

He was also not dissembling when he claimed to be the head of a research institute. Research in local or nationality medicine in China combines field research (knowledge exchange with healers, plant collectors, market dealers) with botanical classification, clinical experimentation, and even legal-archival investigations. Dr. Zhao has a network of co-producing researchers: family members in his home area, about a half-day journey away, help him search out, collect, and process plants; and like State Follower Wang he seeks out other local healers to share techniques and formulas. His many former trainees also serve as research allies to help him assemble more medicines, methods, case files, and insights about Zhuang medicine. This research institute, in other words, doesn't really need a building with labs and offices; it needs only to be drawn together in Wonderfont Zhao's travels and conversations, in his textbook editing and teaching, and in his notes and records, most of which are stored in the second floor of his family home.

His role as clinic director—the last major role listed on his name card— showed Dr. Zhao's instituting process at its humblest but perhaps most consequential level. He sees patients in his sitting room rather than his clinic (several patients came looking for him while we were there, though he asked them to come back later). He has an herbal pharmacy upstairs, where he keeps his notes and files, and he grows a few common herbs along the side of his house. He also embodies, as we shall see, his family's heritage of skilled healing.

During our visit, Dr. Zhao frequently ran upstairs to fetch a document to show us. Many of the items Dr. Zhao wanted to show us were grateful testimonials from patients who had found his treatments effective, some of them using the standard language of "wondrous hands, youth restoring" (*miaoshou huichun* 妙手回春) to describe his healing abilities. An even more important document, though, was a draft of the preface to his next textbook of Zhuang medicine. The draft had been edited and annotated by none other than Huang Hanru, one of the founders of Zhuang medicine and a highly placed scholar in Nanning (his biography is discussed below). Dr. Huang's interest in Dr. Zhao's writing, made concrete in his marginal notes on the paper, turns this scribbled-over essay into a palpable link, an instituting agent. Dr. Zhao is connected upward, as it were, through a collegial project of writing for teaching.

As we learned about Dr. Zhao's organizational and medical activities, and admired the paperwork proofs of his multifaceted efficacy, we began to better understand his self-presentation as leading a full set of Zhuang medicine institutions. We could easily picture him as a man capable of wearing many hats, even though the social roles he occupied might still be seen as having a more precarious existence than the imposing buildings housing Zhuang medicine in Nanning. But we couldn't help wondering about deeper sources of his efficacy (and his reputation) as a healer, teacher, and researcher. Though, as I have said, Dr. Zhao was not pretentious or arrogant, he was nevertheless supremely confident of his abilities, just as our more metropolitan sources in Nanning had been when they sent us rather far out of town to see him. Why was he both recognized and confident? Where did his authority come from?[25]

What he really wanted us to recognize about his practice, in the end, had little to do with official organizing or recognition. It had more to do with heritage, efficacy, and place. In other words, after he had shown us his name card so we could appreciate his institutional hats, he showed us a wilder side, sharing with us some of the unofficial resources that he folds into his instituting life.[26] We asked him, for example, about ritual (*fashu* 法术) aspects of his practice, and he quite cheerfully and openly told us about his involvement in divination, written spells, numerology, and ritual dispositions of bodies in space. Indeed, he opened our conversation by announcing that he was a "thirteenth generation" ordained Daoist priest. This aspect of his expertise remained mostly unwritten; it had not made it into the textbooks for his academy's training sessions. He told us he regarded ritual intervention to be knowledge for family inheritance rather than for public or academic transmission. But Dr. Zhao's interest in announcing his ritual practice suggests that he has deliberately made these skills a part of his wide reputation, and it may be one reason he still attracts a few students each year, for sheer "love of learning."

He attributed much of his healing ability to knowledge he had inherited from his father, a Daoist legacy that went far beyond the medical and the secular. One of the documents he fetched from upstairs was a notebook kept by his father. He wanted us to read and admire a long prose poem his father had written about their home village in the mountains several hours away. He was making it apparent that much of the wondrous efficacy of his own and his family's healing power derived from a special rootedness in a place—a beautiful place rich in medicines, local knowledge, family stories, and unrecorded history, a place to which Dr. Zhao often returned to be with family and gather herbs. Also in his father's notebook, though, were some pages Dr. Zhao had not intended us to see. They were records of mantras (*koujue* 口诀) meant to be chanted in healing and other ritual encounters. Happening upon these pages, of course we asked Dr. Zhao to explain their uses to us; it became clear, though, that he hadn't meant us to see these powerful texts, and he declined to go into any detail about any of his ritual procedures. When we pressed him, he replied, maintaining his ordinary air of good cheer and down-to-earth practicality, that "today is not a propitious day" to engage with these texts. We could only accept this explanation and stop asking awkward questions. And, of course, it takes a special kind of expertise even to know the difference between lucky and unlucky days.

Reflecting on the practical reality, or the institutional weight, of Dr. Zhao's projects, we began to feel that his teaching, learning, and healing assemblages—which stick pretty close to Tranquility County, which center on his own frail person, and which are anchored in a network of plants, texts, students, colleagues, certificates, and communal lore—are not very different from those of the Zhuang Hospital and the Herbal Medicine Research Institute in Nanning. Indeed, the more we learned about the bricks-and-mortar schools, hospitals, and clinics of the most widely recognized forms of nationality medicine, the more these large institutions appeared to be highly contingent, even precarious, conglomerates patched together from heterogeneous resources, claims, and alliances. Even though Wonderfont Zhao's many institutions in some respects seemed to be in decline, he had nevertheless already achieved an organizational longevity that is enviable in the uncertain world of minority nationality medicines. His academy in particular could be credited with having provided a next generation of young Zhuang doctors to the proliferating clinics of Zhuang medicine in Guangxi.[27]

But Zhao's twenty-plus years of running an academy and issuing diplomas were not even the kind of longevity he was most proud of. Rather, he presented his authority and efficacy to us with special reference to his Daoist heritage and lineage discipleship, his and his father's writing, the gratitude of his patients, and his frequent practice of gathering medicines in the mountains. Even the cooling pine-pollen tea he served us when we visited was making a point about healing power. Healing—he seemed to be arguing—happens in particular places and among particular (perhaps "ethnic") bodies. A future can be carved out through teaching and publishing, scholarly exchange and clinical mentoring, but the deep continuities and authoritative foundations of a medicine are not confined within an instituting process.

As we leave Tranquility Town and Dr. Zhao's institutions and projects, turning in the next section to big-city Zhuang medicine, note that naming is a key tool of instituting, specifically, in this case, Wonderfont Zhao's name. His surname, Zhao, is generic, it is the Smith or Jones, the Tom, Dick, or Harry of Chineseness. But his given name is something else. In fact, it is not a given name, it is a taken name. The legal name registered to him is not "Wonderfont" at all, and some of the diplomas and licenses he displays are issued under a different name. Rather, Wonderfont is his "style name," a name he chose for himself. The kind of wondrousness it suggests is an everyday enchantment, an expectation of the extraordinary,[28] a way of keeping an ear out for what is wonderful and amazing about the actual world, a claim to cosmic authority. And the font part? The word we translate as font means source or spring, an origin of an event. Perhaps Wonderfont reminds us of how a certain wildness springs up in the peripheral vision of our institutions, our recognitions, our well-lit public world of impressive name cards. The magic that Wonderfont offers to his friends, students, and teachers is an inarticulate moment of amazement before it is pushed away — institutionally! — into the obscurity of an out-side.[29] This was, after all, "not a propitious day" for representatives of state agencies and international science, like us, to read the esoterica from Dr. Zhao's upstairs archive. It is hard to imagine how any healing, in and beyond any institution of any size and degree of stability, anywhere, can take place without people like Wonderfont on the job.

A FLOURISHING MINORITY MEDICINE:
ZHUANG, NANNING CITY

Even though Wonderfont Zhao's claims to head key Zhuang medical institutions may be weakening, Zhuang medicine flourishes in Guangxi Zhuang Autonomous Region. As a nationality and public health project, it remains an impressive example of salvaging and sorting, synthesizing and elevating — that is to say, instituting. Numerous activists, not all of them ethnically Zhuang, have collected and recorded specialized local knowledge through exchange with folk healers and ambitious field surveys.[30] Committees have produced well-organized textbooks and reference works that sort Zhuang medical knowledge into subfields and clinically useful categories. A few leading intellectuals in Guangxi have done the conceptual work to represent Zhuang medicine *as* a medical system (rather than just a mass of *materia medica* and folklore), one that is founded on theory and that works from a self-conscious "theoretical foundation," or ontology.[31] And specialists in Nanning's nationality medicine research institutes patiently analyze, classify, and test natural drugs and therapeutic techniques, seeking to render these knowledge resources as science. In this section we want to particularly elucidate how these key processes have worked by focusing on the life and work of a few individuals. Most important among these for building the institutions of Zhuang medicine is historian, teacher, and administrator Dr. Huang Hanru.

Professor Huang is proud to be a historian.[32] He is of the opinion that historical scholarship is needed if a medicine is to be gathered, especially when it must be constituted from an archive that is scattered and written in the majority language, Chinese. Much is at stake in this work: He says that his background in medical history has given him a certain vision: "If you understand a thing's past and know its present, you can envision its future. Given Zhuang medicine's past and present situation, it should have a rather bright outlook for development."

Above we noted that the Zhuang nationality is one of those that, traditionally, have not had their own written language and thus have no proper "nationality" archive.[33] This makes the project of salvaging and sorting a traditional medicine especially challenging. Modern Zhuang medicine found its beginnings in the early 1980s, and under these conditions it was clear to Huang and his colleagues early on that some assembly would be required. One could even say that these historically inclined practitioners of a local medicine needed to engage in a sort of bricolage, pasting and folding together a variety of preconstrained objects from diverse sources—which is to say, historically real but scattered—to achieve a social formation that could be called Zhuang medicine. Professor Huang understood in his practice that the instituting social practices involved in gathering a medicine bite into both space and time, Zhuang ethnic areas and their cultural pasttimes.[34]

But Huang's biography shows that he is not just a scholar; his work as a medical doctor is an important component of his influence. He graduated from the Guangxi College of Chinese Medicine in 1965 and worked as a TCM doctor for thirteen years in a county hospital in Guangxi. His rich clinical experience and seniority as a practitioner partly account for the respect accorded to him, both nationally and in Guangxi. In 1979—a time when advanced education in medicine had just been reopened to academically qualified experts—he was able to go to Beijing to pursue postgraduate study at the Chinese Academy of Chinese Medicine and Pharmacy. (This institute later became the Chinese Academy of Chinese Medical Sciences.) While he was studying the history of medicine there, he took at least one class with professor Cai Jingfeng, a noted authority on the history of minority nationalities medicines. Professor Cai mainly specialized in the salvaging and sorting of Tibetan medicine, a process that had already been underway in Beijing and in Tibetan areas for a few years by the late 1970s. So the very concept of a "minority nationality medicine" was available to

Huang before he returned to Guangxi in 1982, even though there were few if any clinical sites devoted to nationality medicine yet established, so early in the Reform and Opening Up period.

After graduating in 1982, Dr. Huang went back to work in the Guangxi Hospital of Chinese Medicine, where he successfully proposed to establish a research office (*yanjiu shi* 研究室) devoted to Zhuang medicine. Beginning in 1983, working from this small research base, he started to carry out a field study of Zhuang medicine on behalf of the Guangxi (provincial-level) Health Department. For a historian like Huang, this kind of field survey included locating and "salvaging" personal collections of manuscript sources on medicine and culture. This preliminary survey was mostly based in Tranquility County, where Wonderfont Zhao works.[35] Articles he published from this research drew the attention of the public health establishment to his argument that a "Zhuang medicine" really did exist, even though it needed to be sorted, "preserving the essence and discarding the dross," as everyone used to say about the TCM development process.

The year 1984 witnessed the First All-China Congress on Nationality Medical Work, in Inner Mongolia. Often referred to as "the Hohhot meeting," this congress was initiated jointly by the Ministry of Public Health and the State Committee on Nationality Affairs. The event is widely considered to have been the launch point for nationwide nationality medicine development, including all the instituting that has ensued. The Guangxi Nationality Medicines Research Institute was one of the agencies that quickly sprang up in response to the enthusiasms and alliances that developed in Hohhot. By 1985 the State Committee on Science and Technology had approved Guangxi's application to establish a provincial-level research institute; Huang Hanru became its first director.

Enjoying considerable support from Guangxi leaders, the newly established institute received a big piece of land, was awarded a quota of thirty staff members, and was allocated 3.8 million RMB in financial support. Among the thirty staff members, fifteen in the first group were Zhuang medicine doctors from all over Guangxi, some of whom had only an elementary education. These "less literate" practitioners were nevertheless considered to be important authorities in local medicine. When these "folk" practitioners came to work in the institute, they were all granted licenses to practice medicine (the autonomous region's law allowed province-level regulations and priorities to override all national licensing procedures, of which there are still very few). The other fifteen staff members were conventionally trained college graduates. The institute set up a clinic right away. Now this Guangxi Zhuang research institute runs its own famous hospital, and the number of staff altogether has reached over 156.[36]

One of the first projects of the institute was a large-scale field survey, the "Nationalities Medicines Sorting Survey" (民族医药普查整理), begun in 1986. The project was sponsored by the Guangxi Planning Group on the Editing and Publication of Nationality Literatures, and directed by the Guangxi Department of Health's Leading Group for the Editing of Minority Nationality Classic Literatures.[37] (The word used for editing in these titles is *zhengli*, the same term we have been translating more often as "sorting.") The names of these organizational sponsors remind us that the gathering of a nationality medicine has been significantly conceived as a work of building an archive and sorting out the history of practices. A writing function, in other words. But this project was not really, or only, a survey of "literatures." Fieldwork throughout the autonomous region was collaboratively conducted by the Guangxi Nationality Medicines Research Institute (already led by Huang Hanru) and the Research Office for Zhuang Medicine of the Guangxi College of Chinese Medicine. (This last organization was headed at the time by Dr. Huang Jinming, another important founder of Zhuang medicine and a longtime collaborator of Huang Hanru's.)[38]

Surveys of this kind have been very important in the instituting of minority medicines, and, as we will discuss again in chapter 5, they have a deep history. They involve identification, inscription, collection, and preservation of medicinals; collection of historical "literatures"; and—as Huang Hanru and Huang Jinming would insist—conceptual work all through the process.

To conduct this project, which lasted six years, an office was established at each prefecture and county level; Guangxi government offices at all levels supported the survey as part of their official duties. About three hundred people participated. Many local doctors turned over their secret and effective formulas to fieldworkers, probably because they felt it was important to cooperate with this government program, though Huang also pointed out that some of those doctors hoped to build useful connections with large government agencies in Nanning, as a kind of *quid pro quo*. The survey recorded 4,000–5,000 minority nationality medical practitioners, archived more than thirty thousand "folk formulas," and collected and classified tens of thousands of individual herbal specimens. The outcome of this project was the *Catalog of Effective Formulas of Guangxi Nationality Medicine* (广西民族医药验方汇编), published in Nanning in 1993.

Huang Hanru's historical work at the institute he led was, like this huge survey, also collective and rather large scale. He organized a team to conduct an extensive literature review of all local historical records (in this part of China this would be a vast collection of administrative records and literati writings), excerpting every mention of local medicine. A sorting practice par excellence! This group compiled a book, *Collected Zhuang Nationality*

Historical Medical Materials (历代壮族医药史料荟萃). This volume, edited by Wang Bocan and an editorial committee of twenty-five other researchers, took a long time to finish;[39] it was finally published in 2006 by the Guangxi Nationalities Press. Published research of this kind is widely taken to be proof that a uniquely Zhuang medicine has existed in the past.

Huang Hanru repeatedly emphasized to us that it was never enough to simply compile the scattered historical records of Zhuang medicine, nor were the many objects collected in the 1980s field survey enough to add up to "Zhuang medicine." All these resources would have to "be elevated to theory." He told us: "These copied out records are of no use unless you also press forward with rational analysis. Otherwise no Zhuang medicine can ever be abstracted ["refined out," *tilan buchulai* 提炼不出来]. A bunch of records are not theory."

Huang Jinming was, as we have noted, an important partner for Huang Hanru in their shared project of subjecting Zhuang medicine to "rational analysis," thereby elevating it to the status of a true medicine. Huang Jinming also graduated from Guangxi College of Chinese Medicine in 1965, and he stayed on there as clinical faculty. In 1974 he received "reformation and thought education through labor" in a May 7 cadre school,[40] where he got to know a cadre who practiced what he now calls Zhuang medicine in his spare time. This was Long Yuqian, a folk medicine doctor who was so well-known that many patients came from long distances to consult him. Huang Jinming started to follow his work, in particular mastering the technique of cautery using a medicinal thread burned at acupoints (*yaoxian dianjiu* 药线点灸). (The end of the thread forms a glowing, smoking ember that is held just above an acupoint, heating the skin while vaporizing the herbal medicine in which the thread has been soaked. This is like the moxibustion practiced throughout China in TCM clinics, but there are many technical differences.)

After Huang Hanru established the Research Office of Zhuang Medicine in 1983, both Doctors Huang served as associate directors of that office. They conducted preliminary surveys of Zhuang medicine together in the countryside outside Nanning from November 1983 to June 1984.[41] After this survey was complete, Huang Jinming chose to focus his research on the very characteristic local therapy of medicinal thread cautery, once again collaborating with Huang Hanru. Together they went to Dr. Long Yuqian's hometown in Liuzhou Prefecture to conduct a social survey (*shehui diaocha* 社会调查), including some genealogical research, and discovered that the Long family had been practicing healers for over one hundred years, at least three generations. In this trip they also gathered many case records.

Even before Huang Hanru's establishment of the Guangxi Nationality

Medicines Research Institute in 1985, the two Huangs were able to open a Zhuang medicine clinic at the Guangxi College of Chinese Medicine and Pharmacy. The clinic was established at a time when not many people in Nanning were familiar with anything called Zhuang medicine. Huang Jinming became the director and chief practitioner in that clinic, and he invited Long Yuqian to work with him as a doctor there. This unusual arrangement, inviting a "folk doctor" into the formal institutions of health care delivery, received administrative support from the leaders of both the college and the provincial government. In 1986 Long moved over to the Zhuang Medicine Hospital. At the same time, Huang Jinming was researching and promoting Long's signature technique of medicinal thread cautery.

It might seem odd to found a full-blown nationality medicine on the efficacy and uniqueness of one technique, medicinal thread cautery. Indeed, this is not the only resource the two Huangs were able to gather as they salvaged and sorted Zhuang medicine, even as early as the 1980s. (See chapter 2, "Knowledge.") But they saw depths in this efficacious technique, and one of their strategies was to seek wide recognition for Zhuang medicine by way of research on medicinal thread cautery. The two Huangs say that they collaborated on the medicinal thread burning technique from the beginning of their first field survey in 1983. In 1986 they published a textbook, *The Medicinal Thread Cautery Therapy of Zhuang Medicine* (壮医药线点灸疗法). This is considered to be the first "theoretical systematization" in the field of Zhuang medicine, as well as the first formal textbook that could be used for training and promoting Zhuang medicine.

After this first book on medicinal thread cautery was published, Huang Jinming continued to study the technique, not only by collecting case records but also through clinical trials. Reflecting on his work of that time, he said what he did was basically collect data on extant clinical practices, writing analytical and synthesizing articles as he did so, then experiment with the technique he was articulating while treating patients, in order to assess efficacies for himself. Huang Hanru indicated to us that formal clinical trials were also being conducted during the 1990s.[42]

In 1996 Huang Hanru published an article based on these various surveys and research results, entitled "Summary of the Zhuang Medical Theoretical System," in the *China Journal of Chinese Medical Foundations* (中国中医基础医学杂志). This article tends to be seen as marking the successful synthesis of the theory of Zhuang medicine.[43] And Huang Hanru himself sees the theory he summarized as a key element of his group's effort to achieve official national recognition for their minority nationality medical system.

In 2002 Zhuang medicine was formally reviewed by a panel of experts convened by the State Administration of Traditional Chinese Medicine. Those serving on the panel included scholars and practitioners of Tibetan, Mongolian, and Dai nationality medicines as well as experts in both (Han) Chinese medicine and Western medicine. This formal evaluation process was called "The Salvaging and Sorting of Zhuang Medical Theory and Clinical Experimental Research." In one of our meetings, Huang Hanru recalled the work that led to this triumph. He said they knew that they needed to make Zhuang medicine such that "even the moderns could accept it" (要给现代的人也能够接受). For the formal review, the Guangxi Institute submitted about one hundred research papers reporting both clinical and laboratory research. He said, laughing, "even the Western medicine doctors found Zhuang medicine miraculous [*hen shenqi* 很神奇]."

Only after this official approval was gained was it possible for the Guangxi College of Chinese Medicine to establish a school of Zhuang medicine and begin to recruit undergraduate students to study in it. (Medical degrees in China are awarded with five years of undergraduate education.)[44] Also soon after the approval, twelve textbooks of Zhuang medicine were published. The Guangxi government instituted the "Regulations for the Development of TCM and Zhuang Medicine in the Guangxi Zhuang Autonomous Region" in 2008, and the Food and Drug Administration of Guangxi issued a quality standards document for Zhuang medicinal drugs at about the same time. Last but not least, in 2008 the National Medical Licensing Examination Committee approved a Zhuang medicine licensing exam, to be held annually starting in 2010.[45]

This series of instituting acts in the early 2000s sets Zhuang medicine apart from the great majority of nationality medicine movements. One of the projects through which all these new "social objects" bit into space and time was the founding of schools, that is, the effort of activists to guarantee a future for the field. Huang Hanru's master's degree program (begun in 1985) aimed to produce teachers who could train qualified practitioners who could, in turn, train yet another generation of Zhuang doctors, teachers, and researchers.

Huang Hanru thinks about the historical sequence of these instituting practices as somehow necessary or foreordained. He laid out a kind of order of emergence for us. "After theoretical sorting has been done, a clinical system must be established," he began. His own history, and that of his close colleagues like Huang Jinming, suggest that salvaging and sorting must go in this order: history, then medical history, then theory, leading to a clinical system, and (perhaps more or less simultaneously) the proliferation of clinics, trainings, and research institutes. After all of these, he says, comes the legislation. "Without theory there can be no discipline formation; without a discipline, research and teaching cannot routinely develop and [the field] cannot be propagated for larger-scale usefulness."

There is much more that could be reported from the Zhuang medicine instituting process led by the two Huangs and many other Zhuang and Han visionaries. A few other accomplishments of which Huang Hanru is proud include the formation of a Zhuang medicine society (the Guangxi Nationalities Medical Society, 广西民族医药学会), which morphed through official recognition into the China Nationality Medical Association (中国民族医药学会) (1994). He also emphasizes the 1989 founding of a national journal, *Nationality Medicine Reports*, one of the first periodicals in what is now an ambitious publication program housed in the Zhuang Hospital in Nanning. Professor Huang told us that the journal functions both as a platform to support minority nationalities medicines and as a front to defend the field against attacks from medical skeptics.[46]

Perhaps one reason we have dwelt so long on Huang Hanru's career in developing Zhuang medicine is that he so often steps back and reflects on the significance of this personal and collective history. He told us, for example, that "Marx's *Capital* and Engels's *Anti-Dühring* and *The Dialectics of Nature* are extraordinarily important, especially the last." These books taught him how to look at things analytically and gave him confidence that he could succeed in "(re)producing" the Zhuang medical system. "There are twenty million Zhuang people living in this country, and it would have been impossible for them to reproduce and multiply [*fanyan shengzhi* 繁衍生殖] without the protection of [their own] medicine." He also expressed his strong attachment to being Zhuang himself:

> [We Zhuang have] a population of twenty million, but with much less population the Mongolian, Tibetan, Uyghur, and Dai all have their own medical systems. I have confidence in [the heritage of] my nationality, even though the past traces of Zhuang medicine we have salvaged and sorted have been relatively few. But, think about it, in the past there were hardly any Chinese medical services in the whole countryside of Guangxi. Our survey in Tranquility County showed that when it was first liberated in 1950 there were only one or two Chinese medicine drug stores in the county town. You tell me, how did the masses deal with illness? It had to be the herbal medicines that we now identify as Zhuang medicine.[47] Truly, the people make their own history.

And he went further, in a nationalist vein: "People, to tell the truth, need to have a certain nationality feeling; if a person lacks all nationality feeling, how can they be patriotic? The territories of the minority nationalities occupy more than 60 percent of the nation, the majority of the land is occupied by minorities, so what about their culture? If it is not passed down and promoted, this is a great loss for the nation."[48]

The buildings and libraries, medical experts and legal documents, textbooks and classrooms that so effectively institute Zhuang medicine in Guangxi and beyond are impressive. They seem to stabilize and naturalize this form of healing practice in ways that are no longer subject to debate. Even so, on one of the occasions when our research group was to have a meal with Huang Hanru, he arrived late to our meeting, full of apologies. He had been trying to meet a midday deadline with a report on the Guangxi Institute's research activities; this last-minute report was to be an important part of funding applications for additional clinical trials. We were surprised. "But aren't you retired?" we asked. "Why do you still need to do this kind of work?" His amused answer was that, like any institution, Zhuang medicine must always do the work of instituting; nothing can be taken for granted.

EARTHQUAKES AND LANDSLIDES:
FOLDING AND FRAYING QIANG MEDICINE

Most Qiang nationality people are located in northwestern Sichuan province, in the same area (Maoxian and Wenchuan) where a devastating earthquake struck in 2008. In our several visits to this relatively rural area between 2011 and 2013, we were especially impressed with a continuing sense of instability in the area. Heavy summer rains often produce landslides that block the one highway leading from Chengdu to Maoxian; government road crews can't keep up with the demand for clearing roads and restoring downed utility cables. As we talked with Qiang medical and public health experts in the area, memories of the earthquake, which collapsed whole towns and filled the river valleys with mud and boulders, were fresh, even after massive national and international relief and reconstruction efforts. Even as outsiders who were elsewhere in China in 2008, we recall one important form of bitterness visible in media coverage of the earthquake: Parents who lost their children in collapsed school building publicly protested the government corruption that had permitted poor-quality construction for educational facilities. The controversy reminds us that even institutions like schools, stabilized in buildings, employing professional staff, and propagating rulebooks and disciplines, might fall apart in a moment and be difficult to reproduce.

Looked at historically, Qiang medicine would seem to have developed and stabilized well. This nationality's institution process enjoyed many of the same strengths and resources as Zhuang medicine did: talented and committed leaders, generous government funding, a rich local *materia medica*, and a positive public health and ethnicity policy environment. Yet as we have followed the recent fortunes of Qiang medicine, we have been more impressed with the precariousness of this promising field than with its institutional progress.

The modern history of Qiang medicine instituting begins later than that of Zhuang medicine. In 1992, TCM doctor Bao Xifu (who is not Qiang but of Han nationality) acted on his long-standing interest in the local healing practices in Maoxian to found a Qiang medicine research institute.[49] Dr. Bao (now widely addressed as Hospital Director Bao) had been working in Maoxian since 1979, having been assigned there from Chengdu after earning his TCM medical degree. He thought of himself as working at the "base" level, a perspective from which he could appreciate the many local medicines and techniques that were in use. Though his institute was not formed until the early 1990s, he told us in interviews that he had been "collecting data" on Qiang medicine since his move to the county before 1980.

Hospital Director Bao is only one of the medical experts providing significant leadership in the development of Qiang medicine. His strengths as an organizer of a Qiang medical system were supplemented in the 1990s and 2000s by the research and writing of several collaborators: Yang Fushou, a clinician in Chengdu, is known for his theoretical investigations; TCM academician Zhang Yi has been establishing the discipline of nationality medicines for Sichuan province (he has devoted much recent work at the Chengdu University of Chinese Medical Sciences to Tibetan medicine); and a specialist in pharmacodynamics, Wang Zhanguo, has contributed to the scientific systematizing of Qiang medicine. In reflecting on the research careers of these men, we note the extent to which they have relied at key moments in the instituting of Qiang medicine on the preexisting organizations devoted to Han Chinese medicine. In particular, the SATCM in Beijing has been a key supporting agency throughout the development of Qiang medicine.[50]

Director Bao's Qiang Medicine Research Institute began with a staff of four, and their first project was ambitious, given their resources. They spent four years, with some funding from the SATCM, in surveying—that is to say, salvaging and sorting—medical practice in a large number of Qiang villages in Sichuan. This program of medical exchange, in which they systematically interviewed and learned from rural healers, paid off in recognition from above: the research project received an award from both the State and Provincial Administrations of Chinese Medicine in 1997. In 1999, Director Bao followed up with a proposal to the State Ethnic Affairs Commission and to the SATCM, applying to expand their archive of materials. He argued that they could "sort [the medicine] to achieve a theory" that would then be published in an authoritative book on Qiang medicine.

This plan fit well with some national priorities that were developing at that time. The SATCM was planning to publish a series of books on minority nationalities medicines, sixty in total. Qiang medicine was thus to be included in a national publication series for the first time.[51] In 2002, the SATCM awarded a research grant of 40,000 RMB to the institute; at the same time, they appointed Professor Zhang Yi of the Chengdu University of Chinese Medicine to form a team (including Yang Fushou and Wang Zhanguo) at the university that would collaborate with Bao's project based in Maoxian.

With Zhang Yi's team on board, there were now experts in pharmacognosy (*shengyaoxue* 生药学), medical history and literature (*yishi wenxianxue* 医史文献学), medicinal plant resources (*yaoyong zhiwu ziyuanxue* 药用植物资源学), and ethnobotany (*minzu zhiwuxue* 民族植物学) at work. It took the group two to three more years to collect the data for the book. Though they especially emphasized ethnobotanical methods, they also interviewed and surveyed a diverse collection of Qiang doctors and healers about their "styles of practice" in using drugs. In their efforts to sort the medicine to achieve a specifically Qiang theory, they selected ten to twenty healers for more intensive study, including clinic practitioners, herb farmers/collectors, and shamans (*shibi* 释比).

Though one of the researchers, Yang Fushou, had a lot of theories of his own, which have been made central to the work of synthesizing and elevating Qiang medicine, Bao's research group in the early 2000s insisted on continuing to work at the "base level." Recognizing the limitations of drawing Qiang theory mainly from one clinician, however brilliant and erudite he might be, the project paid close attention to the "locally specific therapies" (*tese liaofa* 特色疗法) that could be found in the work of practitioners like the renowned Bright-Right Cai of Wenchuan County. Wang Zhanguo made this clear in an interview: the SATCM specified that the gathering of local therapies was an important preliminary step in the promotion of nationalities medicines. By this time in the national salvaging and sorting process (the early 2000s) national authorities no longer required ethnic medical activists to demonstrate that they had "their own" medicine awaiting salvage. Intellectual leaders in Beijing tended to assume that every nationality—perhaps especially those in a naturally drug-rich area like Sichuan—already had its own folk tradition of healing. Everyone still acknowledged, however, that it would never be easy to tease out so-called "theory" from the complexities and variations of local practices.

The Maoxian-Chengdu research group published their research results in a major book, *Qiang Medicine and Pharmacy* (羌族医药) in 2005.[52] This was also the year when the national and provincial governments all began promoting nationalities medicines more intensively. For example, the Sichuan Bureau of Chinese Medicine issued a series of policy statements to support the development of nationality medicine. Carving out a local area as a target for institutional policy and some new funding, they recognized Maoxian as the site where Qiang medicine should be based. Also in 2005, Yang Fushou represented Qiang medicine in a speech at the Second International Science and Technology Congress on Chinese Medical Modernization, his first scholarly conference, which was held in Chengdu.

This was not only an important moment for nationality medicines, it was a turning point for Yang Fushou personally and professionally. Or at least his friend Wang Zhanguo believed that to be the case. Yang Fushou's attendance at this "science and technology" conference shaped his whole style of being a Qiang organic intellectual. It also seems to have enhanced his identification with Qiang medicine and his willingness to be recognized as a Qiang leader. Yang often told Wang Zhanguo that Qiang people should be the major force (*zhuti* 主体) in the development of Qiang medicine, partly because it would be more natural for a Qiang researcher to collect cultural materials among his own people and in his own homeland than for a Han researcher. Yang came to feel that he had a "deeper base among the masses" than any Han researcher could. Han nationality scientist Wang Zhanguo responds by claiming an auxiliary role as research facilitator, while explaining Yang's ethnic identification to us: "Really, regarding their own innately rooted things, you absolutely can't interfere, you feel deep down that there is no way to enter into their roots."

Qiang ethnicity may have been deeply felt by activists like Yang Fushou for quite a long time. But we had the distinct impression when we started to visit this area in 2011 that Qiangness became more important to many more people after the 2008 earthquake. Maoxian is the Sichuan county with the largest majority of Qiang residents, and it follows that the largest proportion of the dead in Maoxian, Wenchuan, and Beichuan (reports number more than 69,000 deaths) belonged to this ethnic group. Our colleague Zhang Dan, who brought her background in religious studies to our collaborative project, explained to us that Qiang religion involves a vitalism of the earth itself. The Qiang "white stone culture" she tried to explain to us was in evidence everywhere we went and helped us imagine, beyond the countless casualties and terrible losses, the crisis of meaning—given the importance of earth-beings and the land itself—brought on by this catastrophic earthquake.[53]

The national and international funding for reconstruction that flooded into the earthquake area after 2008 provided new opportunities for the expression of Qiang ethnic pride. A much expanded tourist industry stimulated the expansion of ethnic craft industries. A major museum and cultural plaza were built in Mao County town. And the large new "villages" that were built to replace destroyed housing were self-consciously architect-designed in "Qiang style."[54]

Qiang medicine, though its institution process was already well under way, also benefited markedly from the infusion of cash that came after the earthquake.[55] A new county hospital of TCM was quickly built with Director Bao at its head. Under pressure from the vast medical crisis presented by the earthquake and its aftermath, he persuaded some respected Qiang healers, experts in "local therapies," to open clinics in the hospital, even though they were not licensed. Dr. Virtuefont Li and his disciple son moved down to the county town from their earthquake-destroyed family home in the mountains, "hoping to relieve the suffering of so many injured people" (as Dr. Li told us). And Dr. Bright-Right Cai's township hospital expanded, adding clinics staffed by some of his traditionally trained but unlicensed family members in the Weizhou Township Qiang Osteopathy Hospital.[56]

Despite the vast funding that has landed in Qiang country, and though the funds appear to have been wisely spent by a committed leader, Hospital Director Bao, working with the scientific talent in Chengdu and the provincial TCM administration, all was not well in the world of Qiang medicine when we visited. For example: the "Renowned Senior Chinese Doctor Studio" staffed by Dr. Virtuefont Li in the Mao County TCM Hospital was not formally recognized as a clinic beyond Maoxian. Virtuefont Li despaired of ever passing the health bureau's licensing examinations. Both he and his son were frustrated that Dr. Li's widely respected clinical skills, and his deep understanding of local natural drugs, could not be officially approved.[57] At one point in our time with Dr. Li and his family, the old doctor joked, "If I'm a practitioner of illegal medicine, fine, I'll just treat illegal diseases."

Our fieldwork collaborator Zhang Dan mentioned in an ethnographic article that she found Qiang medicine people constantly at odds. In the course of her research, she often heard people accusing each other of plagiarism, fake research projects, misappropriation of research funds, and more.[58] She thinks these conflicts have to do with increased funding after the earthquake. Perhaps the expansion of resources only increases competition for economic goods.

After we were no longer visiting so frequently, we learned that Director Bao had retired from the Qiang Medicine Research Institute and the county TCM hospital; Virtuefont Li and his son have left their hospital "studio" and practice privately as herbalists in the county town's new housing estates; and a popular "bone-setting" clinic led by Dr. Patriot Sun has also closed. Certain embodied and spatial aspects of the instituting of Qiang medicine seem to have frayed and scattered completely after an impressive post-earthquake gathering.

Yet in other respects, perhaps more conceptual and disciplinary, Qiang medical instituting may be gaining ground. Scientific and survey research on Qiang medicine continues, some of it developing far from the designated ethnic "base" in Maoxian. Director Bao and his team are in touch with quite a few other institutes involved in Qiang medicine research, including units at Southwestern Nationalities University (Chengdu), Sichuan Academy of Chinese Medical Sciences, and units in the nearby provinces of Shaanxi, Qinghai, and Ningxia. These institutional sites suggest that the most committed experts for Qiang medicine now are academics and bureaucrats. Though there is not yet a medical school specializing in Qiang medicine, there may be hope for the formal cultivation of future expertise in the fact that so many of the still-active research units are in academic settings. Eventually, Qiang medicine instituting still might be able to follow the example of the longer established field of Zhuang medicine, even though Qiang medical history does not include any early academies.

Director Bao still prides himself on his work at the authentic "base level" of Qiang medicine, and even though this disciplinary ground may be sliding out from under his feet, his activities with these elite allies still give him hope. Partly to celebrate the achievements of his nationality medicine network, and partly to express his optimism about the field, Bao devoted considerable effort to convening both the first and second National Research Conferences on Qiang Medicine and Pharmacy (held in October 2012 and August 2015, in Maoxian; Lili attended in 2012). At the 2012 meeting, Professor Zhu Guoben of the China Nationalities Medical Association in Beijing delivered an uplifting keynote address. Professor Zhu spoke of the despair he had felt at the time of the earthquake, sure that all the efforts to build Qiang medicine that had been made in Maoxian and Chengdu would be fruitless under the weight of the crisis. Speaking only four years after the earthquake, however, he was deeply impressed at the institution building that had flourished since then.

There were other ritual expressions of support by various dignitaries at these meetings, and even a few research reports.[59] Though the programs were intended to make everyone feel hopeful, Lili found that rural healers like Virtuefont Li and his son were left wondering whether anything would change for the better for them. Still, Dr. Li like his friend Director Bao was convinced that untold medical riches await the serious Qiang medicine researcher. So he (a little grudgingly) welcomed the enthusiastic participation of so many seeking to salvage and sort the kind of medicine he practices.

After the first conference, we spoke in August 2013 with Wang Zhanguo, the Chengdu scientist, about the state of play in Qiang medical politics. He told us that their core task now was to establish the Qiang Medical Association as a section of the China Nationalities Medical Association. To realize this goal, though, the core group needed to produce more publications. The next day we visited again with Qiang clinician Yang Fushou and asked him about publications. He told us that three books were to be published that year, his own on Qiang medicine, Wang Zhanguo's on Qiang pharmacy, and Bao Xifu's on classic drug formulas.

Though on our reading these new publications look like a minor expansion of previous research reports authored by these three key leaders, they have nevertheless been important for instituting Qiang medicine. The Qiang Medical Association was formally inaugurated at the second national conference held in Maoxian in August 2015. It was also announced at the conference that, owing to all the achievements of Maoxian leaders in developing Qiang medicine, the association would be based not in Chengdu but in the Maoxian County TCM Hospital. This must have felt like a victory for those whose work expresses Qiang medicine's local character.

Above we mentioned our collaborator Zhang Dan, who has continued to do ethnographic research on Qiang medicine's social networks. In a conference paper she presented in January 2016, she discussed oral histories she had collected from five Qiang medicine doctors who hold formal licenses.[60] She notes that most of them were formally trained in Chinese medicine, and at least one of these men belongs to the Han nationality. Though she is not herself Qiang, she is skeptical, asking how "genuine" those licensed Qiang medicine doctors could be. Based on her reading and observations, she thinks most of the "legal" practitioners are practicing integrated Chinese and Western medicine. As far as she is concerned, the most authentic Qiang medicine doctor she knows is Virtuefont Li, a doctor who will never be licensed and who has left the formal institutions of Qiang medicine and public health behind.

CONCLUSION

This chapter bristles with the names of research institutes, reference books, government agencies, and professional associations. In a chapter on processes of institution, in a bureaucratic state like the People's Republic of China, this is only to be expected. Even though Wonderfont Zhao's academy, clinic, and research institute are all run from his family sitting room, with

their official-sounding names they nevertheless have been real and important elements in the complex institutional mix that is Zhuang medicine in
Guangxi. Or perhaps we should say, the mixed ethnic and medical project
that is always *becoming* Zhuang medicine in Guangxi. Dr. Zhao's practice
effectively bites into space and time to build and configure institutions, at
least some of the time.

In the partial histories of Lisu, Zhuang, and Qiang institution offered in
this chapter, there is ample evidence that the work of salvaging and sorting, systematizing and elevating a nationality medicine requires some of the
same practices wherever it appears. Thus, activists must draw some of their
authority from involvement with already more or less established institutions; they must write, and publish the writings they gather in formal texts;
they must play politics, seeking recognition from above; they must engage
in medical exchanges "at the base," or at least claim to do so; they must do
important conceptual work, defining the essential features of a discipline
and delimiting its archive; and they must teach, thereby assuring a future
for their always nascent field.[61]

With this to-do list we have been able to answer State Follower Wang's
question, "How would we go about creating a Lisu medicine?" But who are
the "we" he is imagining? We were of course flattered that he seemed to include us, two outsiders belonging to other ethnicities, in his playfully proposed project. But we were also not certain that a few human beings could
actually "create" a nationality medicine. We prefer the idea of *gathering* a
medicine because of the complex and multiple agencies, or actor-networks,
implied by the process of gathering. Things are gathered in deliberate collective (human) projects. And things also gather spontaneously (or naturally) to manifest as relatively discrete formations and functions. At the
same time, as the early sage Zhuangzi knew and accepted, living things like
human institutions are always under threat of scattering: "Human life is a
gathering of qi: when it gathers, this is life; when it scatters, this is death."

The gathering of a southern Chinese nationality medicine would be
impossible without alliances and resonances (*ganying* 感应) between human herbalists (*caoyi* 草医) and the forests, between healers, patients, and
natural drugs. Wonderfont Zhao showed us this: Quietly recognizing that
his academy and publishing, his province-wide reputation and his village
clinic—these were his more official "institutions"—were gradually falling
on harder times, he preferred to draw on an even more diverse network
of powers: the medicines he gathered in the mountains, the forests of his
hometown, the knowledge-exchanging friends and colleagues he kept in
touch with, the possibly ancient texts that informed his family's Daoist practices, and (we're pretty sure) the family's ancestors and local gods. He de-

rived not only his public authority but his all-important healing power from participation in a broad and not entirely human, not entirely social network.

And he is not alone in this. We also see a cosmic dimension to salvaging and sorting, or instituting, in the willingness of Qiang activists to include shamans in their pool of experts, and in Zhuang reliance on field research with deeply rooted rural healers. We have discussed amulets and the healing-cum-poison powers of drugs with nationality healers in the Yao Mountains, which are known to be so full of magic; in our travels in Tujia nationality country we have learned that ghosts attack researchers and their jeeps; and we have seen how, even in more thinly networked and less instituted groups like the Lisu, Li, and Achang, healing power is taken for granted as a mixture of nature and culture—all these encounters persuade us that instituting is a form of life: when it gathers, this is life.

CHAPTER 2

Knowledge

Knowledge is everywhere a practice, a collective effort unfolding in time and yielding facts and interpretations that, in an interested way, center some matters and obscure others.[1] The knowing practice of Chinese traditional medicines presents problems that are epistemological (how do experts know reliably?), ontological (what is "disease" in a tradition that has roots in a nonanatomical body?), and pragmatic (how is medical action made effective?). When we reflect on the vast archive of writings on medicine in Chinese, and the debates, with their truth claims, that fill that literature and have occupied experts for hundreds of years, we inevitably begin to see written texts less as representations of physiological and pathological concepts, accurate or not, and more as effective tools and resources that assist the work of healers. They might be thought of as collections of rules of thumb, heuristics, and useful mnemonics, none of which seek to be comprehensive. What interests us first in this chapter, then, are the practices through which the embodied knowledge, or skill, of the practitioner is rendered as formal and textual information that can be conveyed in a modern pedagogy.[2] And then we turn to some of the informal uses to which the resulting written knowledge is put in modern healing settings, both institutional and verging on the "wild."

The traditional Chinese medicine (*zhongyi* 中医, TCM) that has been thoroughly instituted in modern China claims particular kinds of clinical and popular authority in its self-representations. Experts in the TCM field still fight for the legitimacy of their field in public life and in the everyday life of hospitals, clinics, and pharmacies, despite official recognition and significant support from government. The field's popularity with patients, however, tends to center on respected practitioners and their healing experience, rather than on the scientific evidence invoked in professional journals and policy documents.[3] A tendency to privilege the wisdom of embodied experience is not confined to the cultural or popular sphere of TCM, however. Among the nationality medicine experts we have visited, a reputation for efficacy, good judgment, kindness, creativity, and intimate familiarity with drugs and techniques count for more than mastery of modern science or years of formal schooling. These less textual forms of knowledge are understood as the personal fruits of healing experience. For scholars as for practitioners, embodied skill and accumulated experience seem to contrast with the systematic, standardized bodies of textual knowledge required in, for example, formal medical education.

In chapter 1 we traced a similar contrast, between the official institutions of nationality medicine and the wild healing, even magical powers, that underpin the authority of healers perceived as partly nomadic, both in and outside of institutions. We also suggested that institution and the wild, royal science and nomad science, are modes of existence that both define and constitute each other in contemporary Chinese social life. Turning now to questions about knowledge, we maintain and problematize a similar distinction and generative relationship: we trace a complex traffic between formal knowledge constructed as medical textbooks, curricula, and information, and slowly accumulated experiential lore, skills, and tacit knowledge that can be conveyed only through discipleship, which is to say, time spent working and studying together.

Embodied understanding and skill, the form of knowledge derived from experience of healing work, is often felt, in the worlds of China's traditional medicines, to be under threat and in danger of disappearing.[4] This despite the fact that "traditional" Chinese medicine has grown especially rapidly since the beginning of the Reform Era (i.e., since the late 1970s), and notwithstanding TCM's effective organization as an integral part of China's national public health system.[5] TCM is, after all, a form of official medicine in the PRC, functioning legitimately alongside and often within the institutions of "Western" biomedicine. When we compare TCM with both biomedicine and the minority nationality medicines that are now being sorted into systematic existence, China's unique situation as home to the first fully state-supported and state-fostered non-Western modern medical system — i.e., TCM — comes into sharp focus.

A comparison with medical diversities in contemporary India is instructive: David Hardiman and Projit Mukharji contrast "statist medicines" like the officially recognized Ayurveda and Unani in India and TCM in China with the scattered, eclectic, and nomad practices that flourish in Asian markets, villages, kitchens, and gardens.[6] These latter modalities the historians and ethnographers of medical marginality in South Asia call "subaltern therapeutics," invoking a postcolonial historiography that can attend to forms of healing that have been occluded, or violently excluded, in previous histories. Studies of marginalized medical traditions concern themselves not only with class hegemony and state domination in the multicultural field of medical pluralism; they also closely examine the kinds of knowledge that coexist, sometimes with considerable friction, in places where healing tactics and embodied skills always exceed those disciplines encouraged and recognized by the state.

Acknowledging with subaltern studies, and with Foucault's comments on modern biopolitical governmentality,[7] that modern states and postcolonial orders are fully engaged in the production of legitimate knowledge, in this book we ask, in addition: How do novel forms of state or royal medicine come into existence in a medically plural place like China? Where "folk healing" has been rich and various, often part of a literary heritage, and practiced by many different classes of people, how can those who would salvage and sort minority medicines locate, study, or understand "subaltern" therapeutics? Can subaltern healers "speak" to those whose imagination extends only as far as established statist forms of medical knowledge?[8] And most important for this chapter, how do the many forms of knowledge change as new systems of medicine are self-consciously carved out of diverse landscapes full of nomad, subaltern, or wild healing practices?[9]

EDITING THE FUTURE: PEDAGOGY AND TEXTBOOKS

Medical education, and the systematic, standardized body of knowledge its pedagogy requires, is a major—if sometimes only implicit—target for those seeking to establish an official minority nationality medicine by gathering together the folk therapeutics characteristic of a locality.[10] Many in China's nationality areas feel that locally embodied healing knowledge has no future. Aging doctors complained to us that their children are not interested in learning Zhuang, or Tujia, or Yao medicine by spending time at the sides of their elders as they cope with illnesses. Every healer we interviewed acknowledged the importance of having a disciple to whom they could transmit their special local expertise; but only about half of our interviewees actually said they had a disciple working with them. Recall for example Wonderfont Zhao: he had a teenage son and an older daughter. The daughter was assisting in the clinic and appeared quite keen to carry on her father's various projects, including his clinical work. But Wonderfont told us that he currently has no disciple, and as for his son's potential for taking on the family's Zhuang medicine and Daoist ritual heritage, he was awaiting some evidence that the boy was fated (*yuanfende* 缘分的) to be a healer. Dr. Zhao saw this as a dilemma in spite of the hosts of students he could claim, scattered around Guangxi, all practicing versions of the Zhuang medicine he had taught them.

In this chapter, then, we will attend first to the processes of salvaging and sorting, systematizing and elevating that have yielded textbook nationality medicine knowledge.[11] These editing projects render existing knowledge formal, carving it into discrete bits of transmissible information and structuring facts into a more or less coherent system.[12] The medical pedagogy that relies on this new library of published resources is thus the privileged practical arena in which formal knowledge takes on its power to make a future.

After brief attention to a fundamental question we encountered while doing research on a relatively marginal group, the Achang nationality of Yunnan province (the question was, "what is 'medicine' anyway?"), we will focus most of the chapter on the formal knowledge that is taught as Zhuang medicine in Guangxi. We read and analyze introductory summaries, classifications of types of information, and comparisons with TCM and other nationality medicines, all of which orderings of knowledge are found in textbooks, to attempt an answer to the most general question, "What is Zhuang medicine?" Then, in an effort to get past the settled bodies of knowledge handed to students and the general reader as finished packages, at the end of the chapter we accompany Zhuang doctor Laborjoy Wei in his clinic and his field investigations, asking not only how he practices his sophisticated Zhuang medical knowledge but also what world of things he practices in, and how he gathers an eclectic and idiosyncratic medical corpus of his own.

Of the seven nationality groups focused upon in this book, it is the Zhuang who have advanced furthest along the path of salvaging and sorting, systematizing and elevating their nationality medical system. As we showed in chapter 1, Zhuang medicine is a well-documented field of knowing practice that has enjoyed the leadership of brilliant scholar-doctors since the early 1980s. It has benefited from generous province-level support since the early 2000s, and ZM experts have developed a significant library of authoritative published works we can consult. The contemporary history of the nationality medicine movement is more legible in the Zhuang medicine literature and in its institutions than it is in that of any of the other southern groups we studied.[13]

As anthropologists of knowledge, we are prone to ask both epistemological and pragmatic questions as we trace the development of Zhuang medicine: What sort of medical knowledge has been salvaged and sorted in Guangxi Zhuang Autonomous Region? What are its logics or basic assumptions? How has this knowledge been rendered authoritative and useful as practice? How does the knowing practice of Zhuang medicine, emerging formally over the past few decades, differ from the knowledge practices of other minority nationalities? How does it differ from traditional Chinese medicine? What sorts of objects and processes are known to Zhuang medicine experts? How do practitioners develop confidence in the ways they know what to do about any given illness? What is taught to aspiring doctors in a systematic way, and what is more often left to their own clinical explorations with patients?

Some of these questions have been addressed by Zhuang scholars and practitioners writing in Chinese, and we will rely on their findings and their ways of representing Zhuang medicine. We cannot provide a comprehensive short course in Zhuang medical knowledge, which is marvelously complex and extremely various in its applications. (Tables 2.1 and 2.2, and the translation attached as an appendix, summarize some of the technical details taught in Zhuang medicine medical school courses, however.) Instead, entertaining the epistemological and practical questions above, we here follow the lead and paraphrase the thinking of some committed scholars and doctors practicing in Guangxi Zhuang Autonomous Region (a province-level government unit). These experts have emphasized and refined a local form of healing knowledge and practice into a literature of great technical detail. Rather than attempt to present an essential Zhuang medicine philosophy of knowledge and reason, or seek to delineate a Zhuang ontology of the body and the causes of its suffering (but see chapter 3), we here seek to appreciate the ways local experts have themselves represented and analyzed Zhuang medicine in writing. We attend both to the process of sorting out knowledge and to the stabilized products of that intellectual and practical labor: To this end, much of this chapter is an analytical reading of parts of several important textbooks.

Before taking up the textbooks, however, some readers may wish to turn to the appendix. There we translate in full a 2015 summary that rather comprehensively describes the key features of Zhuang medicine (ZM). This essay, "The Emphasis on 'Three Ways and Two Roads' in Zhuang Medicine and Pharmacy," recently published in a Chinese medicine journal by Zhuang historian Huang Hanru (with Rong Xiaoxiang), is an excellent summary of formal Zhuang medical knowledge. It includes a brief history of the modern development of Zhuang medicine, which began in the early 1980s; and it helps the reader to visualize a Zhuang body that is spatialized as the "three ways and two roads," and that is provided thereby with a set of functional organs knowable through Zhuang medicine. The essay is technical but accessible to relatively novice Chinese readers. It is an authoritative expression of a well-sorted nationality medicine. Rather than paraphrase Huang Hanru's summary of the mature and modern field, however, for this discussion we turn to textbooks, which we read as evidence that the field is still being sorted.[14]

Table 2.1 *Du* ("Poison") Diseases and Their Therapeutic Methods

Type of *Du*	Typical Symptoms	Therapeutic Methods
Sha Du (Subacute fevers)	Whole-body distension and pain, cloudy head, vexing oppression of chest and abdomen, nausea, fatigue, *sha* papules on chest and back	Dissolve *sha du*, clear heat, eliminate dampness, regulate qi function
Zhang Du (Miasma)	Intermittent shivering, feeling cold, high fever, sweating	Dissolve poison and eliminate miasma, expel *xie* (pathogenic evil) and interrupt malaria, regulate qi function
Gu Du (Poisonous worms)	Enlarged abdomen with prominent veins, distension pain in the ribs/side, eating and drinking less, heat vexation and bitter taste in the mouth, belching, loose diarrhea, brief urination, swelling of the face and lower limbs, lassitude and fatigue, fear of cold	Expel *xie* (pathogenic evil) and kill the worms, free up the Water Way and the Grain Way, bolster qi and blood
Duwu (Toxins)	Acute onset, vomiting, diarrhea, convulsions, coma, bleeding from orifices, dyspnea	Various specific antidotes
Feng Du (Wind)	Fever, headache, sweating, avoidance of wind, numbness of the limbs, itchy skin, body spasms, convulsions of the limbs, opisthotonus	Dispel wind-*du*, clear heat, free up the two Ways
Han Du (Cold)	Fear of cold, fever without sweating, nasal congestion with clear phlegm, cold pain in the abdomen, vomiting, diarrhea, cough, shortness of breath, menstrual pain, amenorrhea, infertility	Dispel cold-*du*, warm bowels and viscera, warm limbs and body, combining with other therapeutic methods at the part where cold-*du* has invaded
Re Du (Heat)	Fever, bleeding, ulcerative carbuncles, sweating, thirst, yellow urine, constipation, red tongue, yellow tongue fur, forceful rapid pulse	Clear heat-*du*, abate heat, while giving attention to other untoward effects caused by heat-du
Shi Du (Damp)	Jaundice, arthralgia syndromes, clouded heavy head, fullness and oppression in chest and stomach, slimy mouth and lack of thirst, no pleasure in eating, diarrhea, nausea and desire to retch, heavy, cumbersome, or aching limbs, fatigue and sleepiness, heavy vaginal discharge.	Eliminate damp-*du*, free up the Three Ways, abate jaundice, soothe the joints

Table 2.1 Continued

Type of *Du*	Typical Symptoms	Therapeutic Methods
Tan Du (Phlegm)	Cough with expectoration, thick sticky phlegm, fullness and oppression in chest and stomach, nausea and loss of appetite, vomiting of phlegm, dizziness, weight gain, unclear mind with phlegm rales in the throat, dementia with withdrawal, or mania, imbecility, epilepsy, scrofula, goiters and tumors of the neck, mammary lumps, node lumps, etc.	[Treated like phlegm disorders in TCM]
Yu Du (Stagnation)	Stabbing pain, swelling, cyanosis, bleeding, chapped skin, rough pulse	[Treated like stagnation disorders in TCM]

MEDICINE IS REASONING (*YIZHE YI YE* 医者意也)

While Zhuang medicine serves as the most extended case study in this chapter, it is not alone in its efforts to carve formal medical knowledge from the unruly terrain of local healing practices. A much smaller group, the Achang nationality, is also involved in a process of salvaging and sorting. Their story, thus far a much less elaborate history than that of ZM, very clearly presents a fundamental problem in the carving out of knowledge. This is the problem presented to knowing practice by the *category of medicine* itself, as we encountered it with a research team led by our friend Academy Director Resolution Ma.[15]

As head of research at the Yunnan Academy of TCM, Director Ma was frustrated. When we first joined his field investigations of minority nationality medicine in 2010, he had been focusing for more than a year on the Achang nationality, specifically one village—which has since then erected an ornate gateway announcing itself as "the Achang homeland"—near the town of Caojian. Director Ma and his team of survey researchers had located a group of healers linked by ties of discipleship and locality and showing some medical practices in common. Most of these healers and their families had registered, relatively recently, as members of the Achang nationality, one of China's least populous minorities. Ma had established good relations with senior medical practitioners and local health department officials, and he had funding from the SATCM in Beijing to salvage and sort Achang medicine. But after making several visits to Caojian for field research, he was not satisfied. Although practitioners of Achang medicine had been generous in sharing their herbals and techniques with him, he still complained that no one in this local group had been willing to teach him their "medicine." Director Ma felt that Achang healers were withholding a deeper level of local knowledge.[16]

He was not alone in making a distinction between (deep) medicine and (merely instrumental) pharmacy and body manipulations. Minority medicine researchers at the national level, with whom Director Ma often meets, work with this distinction as they lead efforts to develop minority medicines. The medicine-pharmacy difference partly reflects a politics of knowledge long evident in the recognition struggles of traditional Han Chinese medicine (TCM), in its process of becoming and holding its ground as a state or royal medicine. Beginning in at least the 1920s, scientifically inclined modernizers argued that biomedical science could make sense of TCM pharmacy using modern methods like chemistry and clinical trials. These critics insisted that the classical conceptual framework—the "medicine"—according to which traditional practitioners diagnosed disorders and used drugs was outmoded, irrational, and could safely be discarded by the whole profession. As numerous historians have shown, however, this strain of argument and field of research was strongly resisted by more conservative and nationalist—but still, perforce, scientizing and statist—interest groups allied with traditional Chinese medicine.[17] The TCM that was salvaged and sorted, epistemologically crafted and widely institutionalized, in the course of the twentieth century, and that continues to be contested and challenged by scientifically inclined critics, is a deeply theorized system of medicine, not "just" acupuncture and pharmacy. Every introductory textbook in the field begins with a "basic theory" chapter, with—at a minimum—subsections discussing the natural yin and yang dynamic, the classificatory and interactive rubrics of the five phases (*wuxing* 五行), and the basic substances of the human body: germinal essence, qi, and blood (*jing qi xue* 精气血). The TCM body is known to rely on circulation tracks (or meridians, *jingluo* 经络) that cover the surface accessible to acupuncture and connect to interior viscera, and it is visualized with yin and yang organs that serve as core nodes for disseminated and particular forms of activity. All this is thought of as theory; all this is what modernizers and scientizers have long argued should be discarded with all the other imaginary dross associated with traditional healing in East Asia.

But when the grassroots knowledge of minority nationalities is a matter of concern, when activist systematizers try to "salvage" nomad expertise for state recognition, TCM theory can be both a resource and a model against which to work. Zhuang medicine, for example, strongly emphasizes yinyang theory but devotes little attention to the five phases or the TCM-standard

circulation tracks. Instead it posits a different system of internal-external relationships, with, for example, notions like the "three ways and two roads."[18]

If the history of TCM is any guide, nationality medicine researchers
would be expected to presume that some form of clinical reasoning and
critical evaluations of strategy are always involved in any proper medicine.
"Medicine," an ancient source asserts, "*is* reasoning" (*yizhe yi ye* 医者意也).[19]
This formula is often quoted in the conversations of specialists in China's
traditional medicines; it seemed to us that Director Ma—who was trained
in TCM—had it in mind as he sought to deepen the findings of his survey
research, questing after "medicine."

Thinkers and clinicians in TCM explain and control pathology with reference to a number of unique entities (qi, channels and collaterals, functional
viscera) and forces (pathogenic qi, yinyang oscillations) not recognized in
the biosciences. Many "traditional" doctors, even as they enthusiastically incorporate elements of biomedical knowledge and technique in their teaching and practice, carefully preserve a Chinese imaginary of the human body
and its logic of pathological change.[20] These ideas inform the reasoning process that guides their flexible and effective use of both natural and chemical
drugs. The "medicine" in "TCM" is much more than a list of effective drugs
matched to a list of disease symptoms by way of a modern controlled experimental system. Along with other philosophically inclined medical practitioners, traditional medicine doctors in China insist on thinking beyond
the protocol: They know that they know the art and craft of medicine, so
medicine is reasoning *above all*.

Before we turn to the conceptual depths edited into the textbooks of
Zhuang medicine, let us return for a moment to Resolution Ma's continuing
research on Achang medicine. We traveled with Director Ma and his rather
large research team to Caojian to interview Achang nationality healers and
cultural activists. After our daylong drive from Kunming, Ma convened a
planning meeting in the hotel. He emphasized to all of us that we needed to
push informants a little harder than we had in the past, to encourage them
to disclose the theories, principles, and systematic relationships expressed
in their practices. He said, repeatedly, in several ways, "We want to find the
medicine among all this *pharmacy*."

Assigning one researcher to interview local seniors on the history of the
Achang, Ma pointed out that he didn't mind if memories were flawed or
even if informants recounted pure legend, it was still important to have a
better sense of the Achang past. Another researcher was directed to focus
on modes of heritage transmission: Director Ma's hope was that Achang
healers, in teaching disciples, had found ways to articulate some theoretical
aspects of local knowledge. A third researcher was asked to use interviews

to tease out the principles informing diagnosis and treatment; these might serve as a kind of theory. And Director Ma assigned "pure pharmacy" to a fourth researcher, who was expected to collect samples, take good photographs, and record the vernacular names of all specifically Achang medicinals in local use.

The last of these four tasks turned out to be the easy part, as it had been in earlier visits.[21] Although field researchers of nationality medicine projects expect ethnic healers to "keep secrets" and to withhold the details of their local herbs and "secret formulas," in our collaboration with these projects we found nationality medical experts to be quite forthcoming about the medicinals they used. In the case of the senior Achang healers we visited with Director Ma, these elders were a bit nervous to be hosting so many scientific urbanites, but they offered warm hospitality nevertheless, and they willingly answered all our questions. If they were "keeping secrets," they were doing it in a very mannerly way.

At one point we asked Director Ma to compare an earlier phase of herbal medicine surveys (1968–72) with the habits of the present. He recalled those earlier years, before the end of Maoist collectivism, as a time when folk healers came forward voluntarily to serve the people by revealing and recording their effective herbal treatments.[22] Not so nowadays. Though many people appear to be grateful that enforced collectivism is a thing of the past, Director Ma nevertheless regrets that knowledge has been so thoroughly reprivatized, made proprietary and even secret in support of individual careers and medical businesses.

So he kept pressing us to "go deeper." And Judith and Lili tried, but we were skeptical. We didn't see any particular reason why the "medicine" Director Ma was seeking would be explicit in the practice or the conversation of Achang doctors. We tried to persuade him that a philosophy or a system of Achang medicine could result only from the analytical work of researchers like him and his team.[23] Few clinicians anywhere, we argued, bother to theorize diagnosis or therapeutics, even when they have students to teach and colleagues to argue with (which many folk healers do not). But Director Ma was old enough to have witnessed the salvaging and sorting, synthesizing and elevating of more than one Chinese traditional medicine. He knew the TCM textbooks in which the fundamental theories, the principles of diagnosis, physiology, and pathology, and the rules of drug formulary were neatly laid out for students. And he knew that some other medical systems (Tibetan, Zhuang, Dai, Mongolian, Uyghur come to mind) had produced well-sorted and well-analyzed publications along the same lines in recent decades. In engaging with Achang healers, he believed that he had found a genuine "current" (*liupai* 流派) or living tradition of practicing, effective, and intelligent nationality doctors.[24] So he kept wondering, why wouldn't they share the principled foundations of their medical practices with him?

Sometime after we witnessed Director Ma's epistemological frustration with the Achang, his desire for depth in medical reasoning was echoed in interviews with two other leaders in the field of nationality medicines. They agreed with their friend Resolution Ma that "theory" is a central concern of state-supported projects for salvaging and sorting medicines. Both theoretician/clinician Huang Jinming and historian Huang Hanru, in separate conversations in Nanning about the development of Zhuang nationality medicine, assured us, "If your minority medicine doesn't have theory (*lilun* 理论), there's no way you can get the state to take you seriously." Understandably, since they were seeking recognition from a Han-dominated national government, their remarks echoed the TCM mantra, "medicine is reasoning."

This interest in theory is not only an expression of anxiety about recognition of ethnic cultural heritage, or availability of state resources for clinics and schools, or the proper management of licensing examinations, though it is certainly all that. It is also a Chinese way of accepting a modernist epistemological imperative.[25] Perhaps it is an aspect of the modern constitution that we tend to assume a certain tacit structure inherent in any formal knowledge:[26] at least there must be a difference and an interdependency between "theory" and "practice"—in this case, between "medical" reasoning and the instrumentalism of "pharmacy." Director Ma's Achang dilemma arose from this dualistic modern imaginary, as he discerned group-specific practices but could find no group-specific theoretical foundation.[27] What was Director Ma looking for as the "medical" knowledge that continued to elude his grasp?[28] What kind of "theoretical" propositions or first principles would have been powerful enough to organize, to his satisfaction, the details of pharmaceutical practice? What sorts of folk philosophy or lay medical reasoning do official nationality medicine researchers look for as they articulate new (and old) therapeutic systems? And how do those who sort healing practices carve local lore into recognizable and transmissible clinical reasoning and official knowledge? Ultimately, how do they answer the question, what is a nationality medicine? The recent history of Zhuang medicine holds some possible answers to such questions.

ZHUANG MEDICAL HISTORY: EXCAVATING THE ABSENT ARCHIVE

The textbooks of Zhuang medicine usually include this historical observation: "The origins of Zhuang medicine and pharmacy were early, but the formation of the theoretical corpus [*lilun tixi* 理论体系] was late. For a long time, Zhuang medicine could not achieve the synthesizing inductive logic [*zongjie guina* 总结归纳] enabled by written language [*wenzi* 文字]."[29] This is a complex observation. At least two "medicines" are invoked: the Zhuang medicine and pharmacy that has ancient origins is a scatter of idiosyncratic usages belonging to the "precursor population" of the Zhuang (*zhuangzu xianmin* 壮族先民) in the region now known as Guangxi. This medicine is knowable from archaeological finds of ancient fine acupuncture needles and gazetteer biographies of renowned local doctors, for example. We could call these practices that left traces prior to modern salvaging and sorting a subaltern therapeutics or a nomad science. The other Zhuang medicine invoked in this framing observation is a more coherent entity, a "corpus," or *tixi* (体系, lit. interwoven body); it is represented here as a medical system with theoretical foundations (*lilun jichu* 理论基础). And it is on its way, through a "synthesizing" process, to being recognized as a set of state-certified medical institutions.

We will usually refer to this latter formation as ZM. Prior to the modern systematizing efforts that yielded ZM, presumably a profound popular understanding of medical healing languished, unrecognized as such, for several thousand years among the people of the mountains and rivers of Guangxi, being transmitted orally in local speech between mentors and disciples but longing for a written language in which it could be summed up and rendered logical. Only in the 1980s, thanks to a few educated activists, did an ancient Zhuang medicine and pharmacy undergo transformation to find coherence and completeness as the corpus (*tixi*) of ZM.

As we noted in chapter 1, those who seek to develop a systematic nationality medicine often lament the absence of records written in their own language.[30] Some large and successful minority medicines (Tibetan, Mongolian, Uyghur, Dai, and Korean, mainly) have old writing systems and thus substantial cultural archives. Most other minority nationalities need to rely on historical records written in Chinese. There is a Zhuang written language, but it was recently invented and is little used. ZM activists must assemble their medicine from ancient fragments translated through a language of empire. Everyone believes that Guangxi has a rich oral heritage of expert healing. But without an archive written in Zhuang language, it is difficult to find, in the scatter of subaltern therapeutics, a specific style of reasoning that could be translated into a modern nationality medicine.

The "Zhuang medicine" that had "early origins" in the hands of the "precursor population" of the Zhuang nationality, then, could be seen as episodic in historical time and as distributed over the space belonging to a pre-ethnic "precursor population." Sorting (or editing, *zhengli* 整理) is required if this medicine is to be gathered up (or salvaged) and stand as a "synthesized" and "logical" system. Zhuang medicine activists learned this lesson from the modern history of (Han) TCM. Historians have traced the many ways a modernizing field of "national medicine" (*guoyi* 国医), during the period that the Chinese nation-state was forming in the nineteenth and twentieth centuries, changed and reorganized into "traditional Chinese medicine" (TCM) alongside expanding biomedical services.[31] As we have noted elsewhere, the contemporary official historiography of medicine in China recalls this complex history as a process of salvaging and sorting, synthesizing and elevating native knowledge and techniques—"preserving the essence and discarding the dross"—under the legitimizing rubrics of science and public health. But the modern state-sanctioned sorting process that gathered, regulated, standardized, and institutionalized a medical system—"TCM"—from the vast Chinese-language archive, from the thousands of texts that could be classified as in some sense "medical," has been very complex; it also has been an occasion for considerable polemic, debate, and creative experimentation among practitioners.[32]

We were frequently made aware as we conducted the field research for the present study that nationality medicines are self-consciously following a TCM model of historical development. Those who are seeking to establish a new system of medicine in the present historical context—clinicians and intellectuals like Huang Hanru and Huang Jinming, and health researchers like Resolution Ma—face a somewhat contradictory strategic situation: *first, Zhuang medicine must resemble TCM, and second, Zhuang medicine must be different from TCM.*[33] The new field must present itself as a body of knowledge that is structured in a clinically and pedagogically useful form, just like Han medicine.[34] But it must also be unique to a nationality group, in depth.

Lacking an archive comparable to that of TCM, however, Zhuang medicine developers have had to be historically creative.[35] Ancient and popular fragments, scattered across a rather vast and populous homeland, have been placed into relation with each other with reference to a more unitary matrix. Ancient acupuncture needles, local wild herbs, secret formulas, ritual texts, spoken language, and stories of cures have been treated as indexes of larger and deeper epistemological formations that must have existed but have not been recorded. What is the worldview that can be imagined to make sense of these scattered traces? How should one sort and synthesize practice in a way that will reveal larger and deeper formations, and ultimately give voice to the thus far relatively silent "medicine" among all this "pharmacy"?

ZM THERAPEUTICS: MEDICINE, YES, TCM, NO

Above we quoted both Huang Hanru and Huang Jinming, architects of modern Zhuang medicine, saying that without "theory," no "medicine" will be taken seriously. What is the essence of the theory they and numerous colleagues have salvaged and sorted for developing ZM? There is a breathtakingly rapid summary of "the essentials" in the modern history section of a 2006 textbook, *History of Zhuang Nationality Medicine*.[36] The modern history section is entitled "The Establishment of the Scholarly Field of Zhuang Medicine," and it gives substantial credit to Huang Hanru for "undertaking the complete explanation and systematic construction [*xitong goujian* 系统构建] of Zhuang medicine's theoretical corpus, [thus] laying the foundation of the theoretical system [*tixi*]."[37] Here is one of this history book's summaries of Zhuang medicine theory:

> The essentials of Zhuang medical theory are as follows: it centers on the worldview of a heaven-human relationship that takes "yinyang as the root and synchronizes the three forms of qi" (heavenly, earthly, and human). It takes teachings on "yin and yang organs, qi and blood, bones and flesh," and on the "Three Ways" and the "Two Roads," to form the theory of physiology and pathology. With respect to disease causes and disease mechanisms, Zhuang medicine holds that "poison" and "depletion" bring on the manifold ailments [*baibing* 百病]. With regard to diagnosis, it emphasizes combining multiple diagnostics, but especially ocular orbit examination [*mu zhen* 目诊]. As for therapeutic principles, it privileges "adjusting qi relations, breaking down poisons, and supplementing depletions." With respect to knowledge of disease names, these are summarized as the six great types of *sha*, *zhang*-miasma, *gu*-parasites, *du*-poison, *feng*-wind, and *shi*-damp [see also table 2.2]. Clinically, it is strong in combining disease diagnosis with [TCM-style] pattern differentiation, but it leans toward the former. Therapies are divided into the two broad types of "internal methods" and "external methods," with external methods being especially rich and complex. In the use of drugs, it [follows] the principle that "supplementing with food is better than supplementing with drugs" (with a bias toward meats), and the principle of "similar processes seek each other out."[38]

There are several agendas at work in a dense summary paragraph like this one. One aim is to assert the completeness and coherence of Zhuang medicine *as* a medical system. Like biomedicine and like Han TCM, ZM includes a philosophical worldview, a vision of the physical body, a short list of functional entities belonging to the body (the Three Ways and Two Roads), an account of disease causes and mechanisms, a diagnostic technology, and a nosology, or a list of diseases with their proper names. The summarizer does not even forget to mention drugs and therapeutic body manipulations, the most concrete expressions of a clinical medicine.

Even though the Zhuang medicine summarized in this way is not said to be a structured system as such, there is an implicit hierarchy in the order in which the elements of ZM are presented: beginning with the foundation in a "worldview" (*tianrenguan* 天人观), the list works its way along a chain of theoretical relationships: the Zhuang medical body (grounded in a "holistic" worldview) is the foundation on which the Three Ways and Two Roads find their function; and all the practical categories (causes and mechanisms, diagnostics and therapies, diseases and drugs) can be seen as guided and channeled by the logically prior functional processes of the Ways and Roads.[39]

This summary passage makes it clear that Huang Hanru and his colleagues in Guangxi have done a job that Director Resolution Ma may never be able to complete for the Achang: the Zhuang group has gathered a systematic medicine from fragments. Zhuang medicine's theoretical completeness is still limited, however. We could propose plenty of "foundational" metaphysical orientations that are not mentioned here: the relationship between hidden natural sources and perceptible bodily manifestations, the correlational logic that classifies things in order to put them into interaction with each other, a "geographic" awareness of the therapeutic value of local (and thus "nationality") things, the "scattering" tendency of natural entropy in parallel with the human action of "gathering" beings into correlated sets,[40] and much more that is buried in locally specific cultures and practices. But these unstated metaphysical assumptions are not needed to recognize that a form of *medicine* has been assembled. Sources and manifestations, correlational resonance, the gathering of forms of being, and the rest are issues for classical epistemology and ontology in East Asia, themes for ancient metaphysical speculations. They are in some sense kept alive in modernity in the discursive life of traditional medicines, which are the premier surviving expression of premodern Chinese knowledge. With its technical complexity and profound philosophical reflection, medical theorizing still makes cosmology and ontology explicit—up to a point—in its citations of literatures that were gathered into text form several thousand years ago.[41]

The medicine that Zhuang experts have gathered, then, has a worldview, an account of the body, ways of reading the body's signs, and lists of causes and diseases, drugs and therapies. These things make it medical, or perhaps we should say, these things are the essential elements of any modern medical system. Some of them, such as taking yinyang as the root, make ZM look very similar to Han TCM. But an ontological question remains: what *things* make this new system specifically "Zhuang"? This question too is being answered in the summary translated above, but it speaks of different emphases rather than radically different worlds. In the passage cited we can see, for example, that ZM uses a lot of diagnostics but especially emphasizes ocular orbit examination. This is a technique not usually taught in the TCM curriculum. Further, in table 2.1 we have listed the disease factors that double as disease types and disease names for Zhuang medicine. In its emphasis on poisons and just a few of the classical TCM illness factors, the list is notably different from any such tabular summary that could be made for either TCM or biomedicine.

ZHUANG MEDICAL THINGS: A TABLE OF CONTENTS

Textbooks are a particularly good place to see the sorting process at work, or, more properly, to see how a self-consciously constructed framework orders information so that it can be transmitted to students as formal knowledge. Conceiving of their task as producing a next generation of well-trained practitioners, editors of ZM textbooks have felt obliged to distinguish basic theory from all manner of other details: historical events, accepted techniques, local drugs, folklore, and so forth. On the whole, theory and practice are kept distinct in the textbooks.

The detailed and hierarchized tables of contents of such comprehensive textbooks reflect a great deal of careful thought and lively debate. These books are authoritative for students, and they play a central role in the professional life of recently trained doctors. But the information they present, bland as it first appears, is contested among experts and even within the large editing committees that convene to produce the standard textbooks. Frequently revised, textbooks continue currents of scholarship that have divergent orientations and express ongoing research with often inconclusive results. Authors sometimes do not concur on the definitions of terms, on recommended clinical priorities, or even on the existence of medically salient things.[42] But textbooks also provide the stable matrix within which newly trained practitioners can craft their own creative clinical tactics, making new medical knowledge as they work and accumulate their own experience.

If we examine a table of contents we find evidence of the different levels and categories into which Zhuang medicine folklore and experience have been sorted, by committee compromise and consensus, over the past thirty years. The table of contents is the tidiest part of a recent authoritative text-book, *Zhuang Medicine (vol. 1)*; it is translated in table 2.2.[43] A clinician or student intern interested in finding, for example, the three most classic treatments for "Grain Way" indigestion can locate the exact passage she needs without extensive browsing. Facts are neatly sorted into categories, and the categories are listed with brief, clear headings. This tidiness mirrors the order of TCM textbooks. Indeed, the four main sections of this Zhuang medicine textbook—"Basic Theory," "Diagnostics," "Pharmaceutics," and "Formulary"—look identical to those of many TCM textbooks. When we actually read the text, however, and especially when we read it along with other Zhuang medical works (needling guides, histories, theoretical works, pharmacology texts, and so forth), we can discern some of the continuing tensions, contradictions, and practical struggles that textbook writers have been unable to keep at bay.

The meaning of the word *du* 毒, "poison," is a good example. *Du* is highly ambiguous throughout the ZM library, and it is made more complex by a popular reading that fears magic and witchcraft, which is to say, poisoning by hostile others. Yet *du* remains a very important object and concept for a resolutely modernist, secular, and technical ZM (this is reflected in table 2.1). The various forms of poisoning may not quite resemble the ontological diseases for which biomedicine is well-known, but they are legitimate medical entities nevertheless.[44]

We suspect that neither medical students nor clinicians find the contradictions and ambiguities turning up in the study of nationality medicines to be a weakness of ZM; rather, even the most systematically organized books can be read as listing diverse resources for an eclectic medicine able to adopt tactics that respond to an illness situation. The usefulness of tools, concepts, and correlations is in their variety; perhaps orderliness is required only to help practical people find the elements they need to put to work, each in his or her own way.

There is a great deal of overlap between the apparently discrete categories of the table of contents we translate here. The classification achieved by this table of contents is of the usual mixed sort. In keeping with points made by Geoffrey Bowker and Susan Leigh Star, who list the requirements of classification as (1) having consistent principles, (2) using discrete categories, and (3) being complete, we can agree that "no real-world working classification system meets these 'simple' requirements, and we doubt that any ever could."[45] A real-world working classification that includes some of the same things under different headings is maximally useful in practice. If you're looking for a guideline or a correlation, chances are you'll find it in the first place you look, providing the table of contents is messy and redun-

Table 2.2 TABLE OF CONTENTS.
Leading Group Bureau, eds., *Zhuang Medicine,* Volume 1,[1] 2013

Table 2.2 Continued
Leading Group Bureau, eds., *Zhuang Medicine*, Volume 1,[1] 2013

Part One Continued		
		(1) Drugs for the Dragon Road
		(2) Drugs for the Fire Road
	Unit 8	Drugs for treating the *qiaowu* (brain functions)
	Unit 9	Drugs to stop bleeding
	Unit 10	Drugs to relieve pain
	Unit 11	Drugs to attack parasites
	Unit 12	Drugs to relieve astringent effects
	Unit 13	Drugs used in subspecialties
		(1) Drugs for external use
		(2) Drugs for gynecology
		(3) Drugs for pediatrics
		(4) Drugs for treating sense organs
		(5) Drugs for treating wounds
Part Four	*Formulary in Zhuang Medicine*	
	Unit 1	General
		(1) Formulas and therapies
		(2) The composition of Zhuang medicine formulas
		(3) Model formulas
	Unit 2	Formulas
		(1) For Qi Way disorders, (2) for Grain Way disorders (3), for Water Way disorders, (4) for Dragon Road and Fire Road disorders, (5) for *sha* disorders, (6) for *zhang* disorders, (7) for *gu* disorders, (8) for heat poison disorders, (9) for cold poison disorders, (10) for wind poison disorders, (11) for damp poison disorders, (12) for depletion disorders, (13) for *qiaowu* disorders, (14) for blood disorders, (15) for pain disorders, (16) for parasitic disorders, (17) for broken bones and injuries from falls, (18) for external and skin disorders, (19) for children's diseases, (20) for gynecological and obstetric disorders, (21) for treating sense organs, and (22) Zhuang medicine formula design

1. Volume Two of *Zhuang Medicine* is a lengthy catalog of diagnostic and therapeutic procedures organized under the names of diseases. It has five sections: Internal Medicine, External Medicine (Injuries and Skin Treatments), Gynecology, Pediatrics, and Acumoxa.

dant enough. If, moreover, there are disagreements between members of the textbook editing committee, many problems can be solved by scattering different references to the same thing, which will lead to different practical consequences, into different sections of the text.

The highly redundant explanations found in the body of the *Zhuang Medi-*

cine teaching text remind us of some basic principles shared with TCM, but they also teach us some locally known entities—*sha* feverish disease, *gu* poisonous worms, the Three Ways and Two Roads, and so forth. These medical things, some foundational and some just frequently seen in the Guangxi clinic, both distinguish ZM from Han TCM and initiate us into a world that has its own way of configuring bodies, causes, and matters of concern.

Our first pass over the table of contents translated in table 2.2 showed a clear distinction between "basic theory" and other aspects of medicine and pharmacy. The book has four major sections, and, quite conventionally, only part 1 is announced as theoretical. But a closer look reveals that many things listed in this first part, "Basic Theory of Zhuang Medicine," are not especially theoretical: units 1.1 and 1.2 are both historical accounts, for example, and unit 1.5 is a description of "characteristic therapeutic methods" (*tese liaofa* 特色疗法). Moreover, part 3, which should be more or less devoted to the empirical details of pharmacy, includes a "Basic Theory of Zhuang Pharmacy" unit (unit 2). Even where the word theory (*lilun* 理论) isn't used for a heading, we can see that certain fundamental principles are (re)articulated in the later sections of the book. For example, part 4 (Formulary) unit 1 (Introductory) has a subsection (4.1.2.1) near the beginning entitled "therapeutic principles" (*zhize* 治则). The rather lengthy discussion provided there attempts to relate various techniques to three specifically Zhuang kinds of action on the body, all of which we consider to be specific to the terminological system of Zhuang medicine, and all of which are plausibly theoretical: dissolving poisons, supplementing depletions, and regulating qi.

Ontologically specific principles like these three make sense only in relation to the Zhuang *things* that are named and defined in Zhuang medical theory. We argue below, for example, that poisons (*du* 毒) exist clinically in particular Zhuang (or at least southern) ways; they are disease factors, disease mechanisms, and disease names all at once, and they differ from either the pathogenic qi (*xie* 邪) of Chinese medicine or the infective agents and chemical toxins of biomedicine. *Du* poisons are differently understood even among different Zhuang medicine practitioners and textbook authors. Further, the "depletions" that need bolstering in Zhuang therapeutics are (elsewhere in the same textbook) conventionally read as depletions of normal (*zheng* 正) qi. "Normal qi" is a very particular organization of the body's energies that is more theorized in TCM than in ZM, but in its local use it is, like *du* poison, a concept embedded in a Zhuang semantic system. And finally, the qi that can be regulated using Zhuang medicine techniques is a famously theoretical problem for TCM and the history of science in China. Qi is both force and form, matter and energy, structure and function;[46] wherever qi appears in even the most concrete or descriptive Zhuang medicine writing, it drags a whole metaphysics along with it. In other words, when you read either the chapter headings (table 2.2) or the text, looking for Zhuang-medicine-specific entities and forces, there is almost no part that is not in some sense theoretical. (This assertion could be tested with a reading of Huang Hanru's summary account of Zhuang medicine in the appendix.)

Disease causes, for example. Zhuang medicine has a strong tendency to analyze and classify disease according to its cause, or *bingyin* (病因). And it is standard for textbooks to declare that *bingyin* are of two main types, poison (*du* 毒) and depletion (*xu* 虚). Some textbooks classify all diseases that are thought to result from attack by another agent as forms of poisoning. Thus in *Zhuang Medicine* 3.9.1 (Diagnosis, Main Points of Diagnosing Common Diseases, Main Points of Diagnosing Poison Diseases), the list of poison-caused diseases is as follows: *sha* (痧) poison, *zhang* (瘴) poison, *gu* (蛊) poison, poisonous things (*duwu* 毒物), wind poison, cold poison, hot poison, damp poison, phlegm poison, and *yu* (瘀, stagnation) poison. The disease category is ruled by and named according to the *bingyin*, the kind of poison that has attacked. Even if we could know immediately what all these diseases "are"—we can't, but see table 2.1 for a rough guide—the list is problematic. If all these disease factors are poisons, why is number 4 a separate item on the list (*duwu* 毒物 translates as "poisonous things")? If poisons tend to be those *bingyin*-others that attack a "self"—whether from outside or as an internal alien agency—are the last two items, "phlegm poison" and "stagnation poison," forms of attack from within? Are they poison-bearing others that originate on the inside of the body, and if so, how "other" could they really be? It would seem plausible, in other words, that stagnation and phlegm have their roots in weakened normal qi, rather than in a poison-style exogenous attack. But this ZM textbook is nothing if not consistent in labeling almost all diseases as forms of poisoning.

Du-poison, in other words, is a series of entities carved from the flow of climatic influences, bodily manifestations, and dangerous forces and drawn to the attention of ZM specialists as they target pathology. *Du* is not the same thing as *xie* qi, or pathogenic qi, in TCM, though the comparison is tempting. Han TCM theory is explicit about the *bingyin*: there are external disease causes (especially including the six climatic factors, the six *yin* [六淫] of wind, cold, humid heat, dampness, aridity, and fire) that, in excess, attack. And there are also internal and "neither internal nor external" causes. The most important internal causes are "the seven emotions" (joy, anger, anxiety, pensiveness, fear, and startle are always on this list), and "neither internal nor external" causes include pathogens entering the body from food and breathing. This is a tidy and rather complete list that, in fact, little interests working TCM clinicians; they pay more attention to the pathological process they can discern at work in the presenting symptoms than to the original or antecedent "cause" of the disorder.[47] Zhuang medicine, on the other hand, by combining cause and pathogenic mechanism under the headings of the various *du*-poisons, works with diseases that are known, named, and classified with reference to a disease cause and a disease mechanism: *sha* feverish poisoning, miasmic poisoning, wind poisoning, and so forth (table 2.1).

Histories and medical texts have unfailingly reminded us that poison looms large in the climate and cultures of China's warm and humid south;[48] it is a vague and broad cultural anxiety. Even though medical *du*-poison is a much more capacious category than a mere "toxin" (such as snake venom or foxglove), it has nevertheless proven useful as a way of understanding diseases in the modern sorting and systematizing of ZM. Though there is overlap in the contents of the pigeonholes in table 2.1, and *duwu*, poisonous things (item 4), leaps out as rather incommensurate with the series, the list itself shows evidence of thoughtful carving. Perhaps once in China's southern climes, "poison" was an undifferentiated global fear that was inseparable from a whole imaginary of threat and vulnerability. Now, with the rise of Zhuang medical theory, this threat to health can be captured, diagnosed, classified, and correlated with a series of treatments ranged in parallel.

ZHUANG MEDICINE, RELATIVELY SPEAKING

The textbooks discussed here, and Huang Hanru's summary essay (see the appendix), seek to define their field in a variety of ways: inevitably, they respond to the question, what is Zhuang nationality medicine? Thus far in this chapter we have addressed this question through an epistemological lens, asking how ZM authorities represent the knowledge belonging to Zhuang medicine in writing, while we have also referred to the knowing practice of scholars and teachers. Given that ZM is on its way to becoming a full-fledged state-recognized medical system, its very nature is subject to contestation and compromise, as reflected, for example, in the murky but useful classification scheme of a textbook's table of contents. The historical, institutional, and practical question facing nationality medicine developers seeking state recognition immediately calls for more specific expressions of the problem, however: What is Zhuang medicine *now* (in a multicultural, medically plural China with a changing health-funding landscape)? What is Zhuang medicine *as opposed to* TCM, biomedicine, or other nationality medicines? All definitional fiats aside—"medicine is reasoning" makes few discriminations, after all—an institutional and epistemological system becomes something positive and specific mainly through relationships with what it is not.

ZM scholars understand, then, that *comparison* is a necessary part of their institutionalizing and knowledge production task. The frequently invoked special features of Zhuang medicine (perhaps especially because perforce expressed in standard Chinese language) do not stand on their own. Certainly, historical accounts like that of Dai Ming cited above emphasize the ethnic and local coloration (*tese* 特色) of ZM and seek to articulate an essence (*hexin* 核心) for the field. Official recognition of a nationality expertise is at stake,[49] and Dai Ming represents ZM both as a medicine (structured like other recognized medicines) and as a nationality specificity (found in Guangxi, among the Zhuang people and their local pathogenic qi and natural medicines). But Dai and his collaborators also define ZM in relation to its epistemological, institutional, and practical others: the book *contrasts* Zhuang medicine with TCM and several other nationality medicines. (See table 2.3.)

With such comparisons, Huang Hanru, Huang Jinming, Dai Ming, and other textbook-writing systematizers may be, underneath it all, resisting their relegation to the status of "minority nationality" subalterns in the domain of world medical systems and medical knowledge. Perhaps, as knowing experts on a local therapeutic tradition, they are rejecting the hegemonic royal authority of the knowledge systems of both TCM and biomedicine. But precisely because there have long been *two* fully recognized state medicines in China, "Chinese medicine" and "Western medicine," certain claims to universally true knowledge, coming from any quarter, have been made more difficult to sustain. The Triple Burner and the Life Gate, for example, are real organs for much of TCM, but they go unrecognized in biomedicine (and they are not mentioned in any minority nationality medicine we have studied). And the treatment of anxiety and agitation with neurotropic drugs in biomedicine makes no sense for TCM doctors. Instead they tend to treat affective disorders with reference to a system of yin and yang organs that manage "essence, energy, and spirit" (*jing* 精, *qi* 气, *shen* 神) as whole body physiological processes.[50] Nationality activists crafting new traditions of medicine are invited by the unique medical pluralism of modern China to propose new anatomies, new disease causes, new forms of therapeutic efficacy—new, at least, to the authoritative world of modern biomedicine.

And speaking of biomedicine, and its tendency to universalize its version of biophysical human nature, few in contemporary China reject the idea that biomedicine is more effective against many diseases than tradi-

Table 2.3 Zhuang Medicine, Relatively Speaking

Knowledge Domain	Han TCM	Zhuang Medicine (ZM)	Mongolian Medicine
Basic Theory	Yinyang & Five Phases cosmology	"Yinyang is the basis"	Yinyang & Five Phases cosmology
	Body composed of channels & collaterals and interlinked yin and yang visceral systems	Bodily microcosm of "Three Qi in synchrony" (heaven, earth, the human)	Three Roots, or material capacities, in balance:
		Functional organs: Three Ways & Two Roads	*he-nong, sha-la, ba-da-gan*
	jing-essence, *qi*-energy, and *shen*-spirits are basic substances	Body of organs, qi, blood, bone, & flesh (and *qiaowu*, ≈ nerves)	Seven Essentials & Three Excreta sustain the Three Roots
		Du-poison theory	Six Basic Illness types
			Body has 12 trunk channels plus auxiliary channels
Disease causes & mechanisms	6 External Evils, 7 Inner Feelings, plus food & drink, overwork, injuries	*du*-poisons & depletions	6 reasons for disease: *he-nong, sha-la, ba-da-gan*, blood, urine, sticky parasites
Diagnostic methods	4 Examinations (looking, asking, listening/smelling, pulse palpation)	Ocular orbit exam, nails exam, Master Nong's abdominal exam	Looking, asking, pulse palpation
	8 Rubrics, 6 Channels, 4 Sector correlations, etc.	Diagnosis of Southern Diseases, especially *du*-poisons	

Table 2.3 Continued

Knowledge Domain	Han TCM	Zhuang Medicine (ZM)	Mongolian Medicine
Treatment Methods Therapeutics	Pattern Discrimination and Therapy Determination "Seek the root" "Support normal qi, expel pathogenic qi" (etc.) Systematic formulary using classic *materia medica*	"Regulate qi, dissolve poisons, bolster the depleted" Achieve through-flow in the Ways and Roads Simple heritage formulas, fresh wild herbs	Preventive medicine; roots-seeking, pathogen expelling-depletion bolstering measures Regulate the Three Roots Herbal treatments plus bone-setting techniques, blood-letting, moxibustion, herbal baths, etc.
Typical Diseases	All, but Cold Damage disorders especially central	Warm Factor illnesses of the south, and especially *Sha, Zhang, Gu*, Toxins, Wind, Damp	
Areas not emphasized	Inattentive to Southern Diseases	Little emphasis on emotional causes, mental illnesses; organs not dynamically interlinked, no reliance on Five Phases theory; spleen organ unimportant; no emphasis on pattern discrimination	

Comparisons taken from Dai Ming (2006, 102–13). These lists of keywords are incomplete and only roughly translated, but minor differences that might be evident in this simplified representation are important to nationality medicine authors.

tional and nationality medicines are, but we have nevertheless seen some clever resistances to "Western medicine's" acknowledged dominance in Chinese public health and science. In 2011, for example, we were amused to note the labeling we found in a Nanning (Guangxi) bookstore above a few shelves of biomedical textbooks. These works on technical topics formed only a small section in a bookstore substantially devoted to minority nationality studies, including, of course, traditional medicines. Our friends at the

Zhuang Medicine Hospital had recommended we visit the store in search of nationality medicine publications. The label on the two shelves holding books like *Handbook of Neonatal Clinical Care* and *English for Hospital Use* was "Foreign Nationality Medicine" (*waiguo minzu yixue* 外国民族医学). This is a charming relativizing joke, one that insists on the local and ethnonational character of *all* medicines. Classifying biomedicine as a "nationality" medicine invites a symmetrical historical approach, even if the label is only a joke: both modern science and traditional local knowledge should be contextualized in their dependency on particular historical conditions. In a symmetrical historiography of knowledge, nothing acknowledged by any collective—nothing that is "in the true" somewhere—needs to be denounced as untrue, though it might still be worth denouncing as dangerous or wrongheaded. Many incommensurate forms of knowledge can be seen as contingently meeting the intellectual and practical needs of particular people, times, and places.[51]

"Foreign nationality medicine" expresses a relativizing view that makes sense in the context of medical pluralism. Even before science and technology studies, with its commitment to explanatory symmetry in the history and sociology of science, became an important inspiration for ethnographies like the present study, anthropology's commitment to the comparative method advanced an unsettling relativism and a willingness to see deep differences cohabit in "multicultural" situations.[52] A historical view also seems to *require* the work of comparison. So let us return to Dai Ming's *History of Zhuang Nationality Medicine* to consider his more extended and explicit comparative sorting of minority medicines.

The major comparison that must always be done by minorities is between the nationality medicine being taught and advocated by a local interest group and the nationally institutionalized system of TCM. Dai's section headed "Comparing Zhuang Medicine with the Medicines of Various Nationalities" (pp. 102–13) begins with a justification of historical comparison in the domain of medicine. Writing as both historians and medical experts, Dai and his co-authors argue that the various strengths and weaknesses of culturally diverse traditional medicines can be assessed through comparison, ultimately to the greater benefit of sufferers, who are, after all, dependent on a public health system that can be enriched by minority medicines. The text then turns to brief accounts of the "history of development" of nine emblematic forms of nationality medicine, first repeating at some length the long and thoroughly studied history of Han TCM, with an emphasis on developments in the southern parts of historic China. Repeating historical material included in earlier sections of the book, the discussion distinguishes the more limited history of ZM development within a broad (but

Han-dominated) East Asian historical framework. The text especially notes that the "theoretical system" of TCM dates from Warring States, Qin, and Han Dynasty times (from around the fifth century BCE to the third century CE), while Zhuang medicine's theory, by contrast, was articulated and synthesized only in the 1980s and 1990s. Despite the embarrassing difference between these chronologies, however, "in the process of its historical development, Zhuang medicine also made a vigorous contribution to the formation and development of [Han] Chinese medicine."[53] This turning of the tables is typical for Zhuang ethnic activists, who like to claim civilizational priority in East Asia: we were often told in Guangxi that the actual origins of Han civilization could be found among the "precursor populations" of the Zhuang people, so "China" is really, at root, Zhuang.

The minority nationalities whose medical systems are compared in this section of *History of Zhuang Nationality Medicine* are (always in this order, and always after a consideration of TCM) Tibetan, Mongolian, Uyghur, Dai, Korean, Yao, and Miao. After brief sketches of the "historical development" of each of these nationality fields, the text turns to "Basic Theory," i.e., disease causes and mechanisms, diagnostic methods, and theoretical system. These sections are followed by comparative discussions of "clinical therapies." We can best discern Dai et al.'s comparative strategy from the "theoretical corpus" section (3.5.2.3, 107–8). Here is how the section opens:

> The basic theory of Zhuang medicine takes as its core essence [*hexin* 核心] the teachings of "yin and yang are the root, synchronizing the Three Qi, the yin and yang organs/qi and blood/bones and flesh [body], the Three Ways, and the Two Roads," and it emphasizes the doctrine of "*du*-poison qi." Zhuang medicine's teachings of "yin and yang are the root" and "synchronizing the Three Qi" are a worldview that chiefly explains the relation between humans and nature, man and heaven, and the internal interconnections of the human body. Zhuang medicine basically ignores TCM's five phases theory, however, and doesn't use the generation and constraint relations of five phases theory to explain the physiological and pathological phenomena of the human body.

In this initial list of theoretical elements, there are several terms obviously shared with TCM—yinyang, and the "yin and yang organs/qi and blood/ bones and flesh [body]"—and there are several that are unique to ZM. The Three Ways and Two Roads, for example. *Du*-poison is known in Chinese medicine, but this text notes that ZM includes a much greater emphasis on this notion than TCM does. It is interesting, however, that one key feature of TCM, five phases theory, is said to be "ignored" by ZM. Not only is this feature of TCM theory an especially ancient and very abstract method for explaining the actions and interactions of the myriad things, it is operationalized in the TCM body (but not the Zhuang body) as the physiology of the interacting yin and yang organs, or visceral systems.[54]

If five phases logic is ignored in ZM, then, perhaps the "yin and yang organs/qi and blood/bones and flesh body" its theorists claim as a "core essence" is not quite the same body as that theorized in TCM. Our comparing authors are ahead of us in addressing this problem:

> Yin and yang organs/qi and blood/bones and flesh are Zhuang medicine's outlook on physiology and pathology, and Zhuang medicine considers that these form the major material basis of the human body. Zhuang medicine does have a notion of organs [*zangfu*], but it doesn't make a very definite distinction between the *zang* [yin organs] and the *fu* [yang organs]; there are no [theorized] linkages between the *zang* and *fu* by way of the collateral channels, nor do they link up in interior-exterior relations.

Nor, as has been pointed out, are the interactions of the five *zang*, or the five great organ systems of TCM, understandable for Zhuang medicine in terms taken from the five phases. There are a lot of negatives in this comparative discussion! Apparently many of TCM's "core essences" cannot be found in Zhuang medicine.

Is Zhuang medicine little more than a gap-ridden analog of TCM, then? Obviously, the Zhuang authorities writing texts like this would not like to convey this impression. After noting the features of TCM that are emphatically not shared by Zhuang medicine, the authors turn to a positive characterization of unique elements of Zhuang medicine theory:

> What Zhuang medicine calls the Three Ways refers to the Grain Way, the Qi Way, and the Water Way; the Two Roads designate the Dragon Road and the Fire Road. Zhuang medicine considers that the "Three Ways" and the "Two Roads" are the basis of preserving the synchrony of the Three Qi of heaven, earth, and the human.

Though it is elsewhere pointed out that the Three Qi are drawn from the same ancient cosmological writings that give shape to TCM, the closely allied functional organs—the Ways and Roads—theorized in Zhuang medicine are not found in TCM. They are not only a spatial organization of body functions but also a local or ethnic way of "preserving the synchrony" of humans in the cosmos. Let us attempt our own positive definition: the Three Ways and Two Roads are names for the patterns of flow and transformation of qi and other substances, such as food, water, blood, and even emotions and thoughts, through bodily space and time. These things are like functional organs that configure the life of bodies in a way that clinicians can understand and use. As Huang Hanru explains in his 2015 summary of ZM (see appendix), "at the heart of the Three Ways and Two Roads is [the concept of] *tong* (通), or through-flow." And, as he also explains, pathology most often takes the form of a poisoning that must be therapeutically "dissolved" or "freed up" so that *sha* or *zhang* or *gu*-worm pathogens will not clog pathways or hamper the movement of the Three Qi in the human body. (Look again at table 2.2, keeping *tong* through-flow in mind.)[55]

But comparison of medical systems, even when it discovers a positive knowledge in a "minority" system that is not shared by the more hegemonic royal medicines, cannot so easily banish nationality medicine's minority status. This text persists, resistantly, with some further observations about how Han TCM and Zhuang medicine differ:

> Actually, ZM doesn't much emphasize the function of the spleen yin organ (*zang*). In Zhuang language the spleen is called the *milong* 咪隆 (which means "the easily forgotten organ") or the *mimenglong* 咪蒙隆 (which means "the organ we don't know the function of"). TCM, on the other hand, strongly emphasizes the function of the spleen *zang*, holding that the spleen is the root of the Latter Heaven [postnatal factors], it is the *zang* or yin-organ of the Earth Phase, the Earth that gives rise to the ten thousand things.

This remark is one of the few observations we have found in print that suggests that nationality medical theory might have roots in the oral language of the nationalities that "lack a writing system." And this oral language, rather than denying the reality of the spleen *zang*, merely displaces the Earth organ's centrality for Zhuang people, who slyly present themselves as forgetful or a little confused, compared with those Han TCM authorities who make great pompous ontological claims.

The *History of Zhuang Nationality Medicine* textbook, after these comparative opening paragraphs, then turns to a paragraph-by-paragraph juxtaposition of Zhuang medicine with TCM and seven other nationality medicines. These are positive characterizations that allow the "theoretical systems" to be compared and contrasted. The passage devoted to TCM remains the most interesting to us:

The core of the TCM theoretical system is yinyang-five phases theory, yin and yang organs and channels-collaterals theory, and a holistic sensibility; pattern differentiation and therapy determination are its two great unique features. Its yinyang and five phases theories are mainly used to explain the relationship of dynamic equilibrium between humans and nature, and balance in the internal interconnections of the human body; as soon as this kind of equilibrium relationship is damaged, there is a disease state.

The attentive reader will note that Zhuang medicine has its own way of worrying about "the dynamic equilibrium between humans and nature," one that involves the tripartite "Three Qi" (heaven, earth, human), which need to be synchronous (*tongbu* 同步). The similarity is noted explicitly in the next sentences.

Yin and yang organs and channels-collaterals theories are a core part of the theoretical system of TCM; they are the basis that guides pattern differentiation and therapy determination. Strictly speaking, though, it is not only TCM that has a holistic sensibility; in reality, the medicines of many [of East Asia's] nationalities emphasize knowing the heaven-human relationship and the internal connections of the human body from a holistic point of view. Relatively speaking, then, it is TCM's yin and yang organs theory and channels-collaterals theory that stand out as rather unusual (*tuchu* 突出).

This is an interesting move. Rather than placing TCM on the traditional medicine high ground, positing it as the most ancient, developed, complete, and systematic center against which all other medicines are to be tested, this textbook presents Han medicine as a theoretical and historical anomaly. Its core methodology of pattern differentiation and therapy determination (actually quite a modern approach),[56] along with its highly differentiated human body of interacting organ systems and linked channels and collaterals, *belong only to it*, while a much more general "holism" characterizes the medicines of most of China's nationalities. Maybe "pattern differentiation and therapy determination" are, for Zhuang medicine practitioners, the "theoretical system" that is "easy to forget"!

With our reading of textbook comparisons of theoretical systems we have argued that the "What is Zhuang medicine?" question is perhaps most effectively answered through the work of comparison. Table 2.3 summarizes the characteristics of Zhuang, Han TCM, and Mongolian medicine as they are revealed in the brief comparisons of two textbooks.[57] As with table 2.1, we consider these summaries to be quite rough; they are at best codes,

mnemonics, or indexes of something known in other ways, not full representations of knowledge itself, not even reliable sets of stripped-down and
neatly packaged information. Yet substantive differences between systems
of medicine *are* reflected in this simplifying table. The authors of Zhuang
medicine textbooks have a stake in differentiating their specialty from the
medicines of other nationalities in East Asia (and "the West"); table 2.3
shows at least how synthesizers have attempted to take up a specific institutional and epistemological role in this multicultural and local—but also
thoroughly medical—work.

WORDS OR THINGS?

The work of comparison among the nationality medicines may be an essential task for the politics of knowledge and of health services in a multicultural and medically plural state. For better or for worse, however, from
either a patient's point of view or an anthropological point of view, a multiculturalism of words is not a satisfactory settlement of the interests at play in
medical knowledge production, either for healing or for harmonious life in
a plural society.[58] Rather, the things that are present at hand for healing and
knowing practice—organ systems, viruses, channels, environmental forces,
poisons, tumors, worms—cannot all be equally possible or impossible. This
is precisely because they are things: paraphrasing twentieth-century soci-
ologist W. I. Thomas, we presume that medically salient objects are elements of a situation that have been defined as real, and as such they are
"real in their consequences."[59] Considering that medicine is a field of activity in which consequences (of pathogenic invasion, of therapeutic intervention) are of fundamental concern, it would seem that the objective status
of medical things matters a great deal. Medical situations raise ontological
questions, in other words. Where state-recognized medicines compete for
scarce Ministry of Public Health resources and official status, as well as for
the patronage of the ill, it matters to practitioners what things actually exist
in the world because they need to act on and with them as they intervene in
illness. As Shigehisa Kuriyama has helped us to see, when we acknowledge
that medical interventions and strategies have varied profoundly in history,
we are led to inquire historically into the bodies and disease agents on which
medicine acts. These entities have been differently known in ancient Greek
and classical Chinese, Ayurvedic and Himalayan medicine; they are different things.[60]

But the historians of ZM do not quite agree, or so it would seem. Huang
Hanru closes the comparative section of his 2001 masterwork on ZM with
four pages devoted to all the things that Han medicine and the minority

medical systems have in common,[61] refusing to highlight differences even as he accords ethnic ownership of new systems to Zhuang, Miao, Korean, Dai, and a number of other nationality medicines. Dai Ming, writing a few years later, refuses ontological differences in a more pointed way. Here is a long and diplomatic summary that appears near the end of Dai's comparative section:

> The theory of each of the nationality medicines has its own ethnic and local distinguishing features, it's just that some are more complete, some are only a rather rough framework, and some have systematized only some aspects of theory. Looked at in general, the theory of every nationality medicine has features in common. The most obvious of these is that every nationality medicine without exception describes human physiological and pathological phenomena from a macroscopic holistic point of view; this forms a distinct contrast with the microscopic point of view taken as the starting point of *modern medical theory*. Another outstanding distinguishing feature is that all the nationality medical theories strongly emphasize relations of equilibrium between humans and nature, as well as the internal balancing of relations of interconnection within the human body. At the same time, it is damage to this kind of equilibrium that is the basic mechanism of the appearance of disease. *Only the ways of wording [these assumptions] differ.* [Consider, for example] TCM's yinyang balance, Zhuang medicine's synchrony of the Three Qi, Tibetan medicine's Three Elements theory, Uyghur medicine's Four Material Types, Mongolian medicine's yinyang and Five Sources theory, Dai medicine's Four Great Elements [*si ta* 四塔], Yao medicine's balance between waxing and waning, etc. These essentially all emphasize relationships of balance between humans and nature and between every part of the human body.[62]

This would seem to express a turn to a very general and widely accepted underlying culture of cosmic harmony, but note that (unlike Huang Hanru in his comparative discussions) Dai Ming does attempt a contrast with "modern medical theory." Even this deepest conceptual chasm, however, is presented as only a contrasting "point of view." Meanwhile, the holistic harmony-centered assumptions shared by all the nationality medicines (but not biomedicine) are hardly differing at all: "Only the ways of wording differ."[63]

We see the power of this formulation, but we think the problem of difference runs deeper than wording. Practical knowledge is more than words on textbook pages, as practitioners of East Asian traditional medicines are always willing to demonstrate. Here, for example, is an account of how ZM knowledge arose from clinical work with the medicated thread cautery technique, or how, in other words, certain ZM entities and processes came to be carved into existence in medical practice. In a biography of "renowned senior" clinician Huang Jinming, the author describes how Huang articulated some basic theory for the field of Zhuang medicine as it was being synthesized:

> After many years of research and analysis, Huang Jinming proposed the Zhuang medicine theory [*xueshuo*] of qi-blood balance. He holds that [since] *du*-poison and depletion cause diseases, *du* and depletion are the two great factors in the occurrence of disease, even to the extent that it is their interaction that becomes disease [*qie xiangyin wei bing* 且相因为病]. The occurrence, development, and changes of disease are all brought on by qi-blood imbalance—if qi and blood are not balanced, then the Three Qi of heaven, earth, and man cannot move in synchrony, and disease is the result. In therapies, then, it is important to balance qi and blood, regulate and improve qi [flow], break down *du*-poisons, bolster depletion, and dispel *yu*-stasis: [these are] Huang Jinming's "keywords" [*ba zi* 八字] for treatment principles.[64]

All these actions—balancing, regulating, breaking down, bolstering, and dispelling—act on something: if not anatomical objects, at least very material processes; if not a concrete bounded thing, at least a composite body situation. If the disease these treatments address is real (and it would hardly be medically advisable to suggest otherwise), then so are the physical conditions that have gathered to make this a state of illness. In this passage, those pathological conditions and processes have been carved, together and apart, and named as qi and *xue*-blood, *du*-poison and *yu*-stasis.

It would seem at first that only the Chinese words in this list, qi and *du*, would be problematically (un)real; surely "blood" and "stasis" can be imagined in the commonsense physiological imaginary of biomedicine? Qi and du can be directly translated, moreover: "energy" and "poison" are nouns, or names for things, that seem to work in an English sentence—they do not raise metaphysical red flags. But it has long been argued in studies of Chinese medicine that the "blood" (*xue* 血) of Chinese medicine cannot simply mean the red liquid that flows from a wound, precisely because it is part of a yinyang dyad that governs physiology far beyond the vascular system. (The other term, the yang to blood's yin, is qi.) And especially in the passage translated here, the term for stasis (*yu* 瘀) covers much more than, e.g., a blood clot or kidney stone. Rather, "stasis" is the generalizable enemy of *tong*, the desired healthy through-flow so emphasized by Huang Hanru (appendix, table 2.1).

Huang Jinming's biographer, then, identifies in this historical-biographical note an act of not only theorizing but also clinical crafting of a certain body. "Qi-blood balancing" is not only a "theory" (*xueshuo* 学说, or a scholarly teaching), not only a "principle" of treatment that can conceptually inform strategies of using drugs, needles, and medicated threads to treat concrete illnesses. Rather, Huang's "keywords" drag real things into play in real practical clinics.[65] For ZM (and TCM too, for that matter) "disease" (*jibing* 疾病) is not ontological, but there are plenty of ontological things in play nevertheless. The fact that qi and blood, stasis and *du*-poison are carved out of the material life of the body in a different way than the vascular system or the immune system, the appendix or the brain, does not make them unreal. They are not only "ways of wording that are different"; these practical things are all too real in their consequences.

We were impressed with the stubborn actuality of some rather unfamiliar things when we witnessed ZM practitioners at work. Dr. Laborjoy Wei, for example, said that he was needling and pinching a "leaf" when he was using a needling technique on a patient's back. He was presuming that we could visualize the spread and the veins of an actual leaf structure or shaped current of flow.[66] Let us turn, then, to Dr. Wei, in the hope of reexpanding knowledge beyond the debates, the comparisons, and the careful textual hairsplitting of historians and medical school curriculum writers.

DIAGNOSING *SHA*

Laborjoy Wei is a full-time resident physician in the Zhuang Medicine Hospital in the big city of Nanning, Guangxi. Dr. Wei is licensed to practice traditional Chinese medicine (TCM) and Zhuang medicine, having taken examinations in these specialties in 2003 and 2008, respectively. He was one of the first younger doctors to benefit professionally from early efforts, discussed in the previous chapter, to salvage and sort, and institutionalize, a specifically Zhuang nationality medicine.[67] He is certainly a product of the medical education system supported by the textbooks we have discussed above. Now, having practiced and studied for several decades, he considers himself to be "an innovative force" in Zhuang medicine.

Wei's interests range far beyond any particular style of practice; he is not *just* a nationality medicine doctor. He stays current with biomedical research in his specialty areas, often enrolling in medical continuing education courses and attending conferences where he engages in exchange with others, both in infertility medicine (his major specialty) and in nationality medicines. He told us he has been in correspondence with a biomedical doctor from Hebei who also uses herbal medicine, and they are sharing techniques. He studies various medical and scholarly literatures on his own, and meeting us, he became quite intrigued by anthropology as well. He tells us he is interested in constructing protocols for Zhuang medicine therapies, and he has worked on standardizing treatments for a locally common illness called *sha* (痧).

During one of our visits to Nanning, Dr. Wei invited us along on one of his "social survey" road trips to visit healers who have informal medical practices in storefront clinics and in their own houses. He told us he was always seeking to "learn from the old doctors." We also learned from him, of course, both while observing him at work in his hospital clinic and while on the road, as he shared his network of informal experts. What most impressed us was Wei's insatiable curiosity and his eclectic experimentalism. He wanted to understand the logic and the technical details of therapeutic practices—adding them to his accumulated knowledge, as it were—and he wanted to incorporate new procedures into his clinical toolkit, if he could determine that they were safe and effective, to better help his patients. He was also planning publications in the professional literature—such as his proposed standardization of *sha* diseases—that would add to the formal knowledge available to students and more junior specialists in Zhuang medicine.

At the beginning of this chapter we introduced Laborjoy Wei as a very knowledgeable practitioner of Zhuang medicine. A clinician in a large urban ZM hospital, he not only sees patients but reads, writes, and teaches. He is in frequent touch with the activists who are carving, editing, and synthesizing Zhuang medical knowledge. And as the son of two rural Zhuang nationality doctors, he speaks with some authority about ZM's "special features," the kinds of things summarized and compared in the textbooks we have discussed above. One of these special features is "sha" disease (痧); it is listed in our table 2.1 as *sha-du* (a "poison"), and roughly glossed there as "subacute fevers."[68] When we first met Dr. Wei, we had read in textbooks about *sha*; but it was only when we traveled with him to meet other Zhuang healers that *sha* became a significant reality for us.

Almost everyone we met on our road trip with Laborjoy Wei spoke about *sha* disease and *sha* qi. Generosity Luo, a storefront doctor in a market town (about the same age as Dr. Wei and also formally trained), was particularly clear: he said that *sha* qi is the kind of thing that modern medicine can't explain, but he's known about it since he was very young. *Sha* disease expression involves all sorts of little aches and pains, dizziness, and minor discomforts. Hearing this, we recalled that hospital practitioners in Nanning had also told us that they often see *sha* in the clinic. As a frequently occurring and sometimes hard-to-manage disorder, this local disease generates a lot of patient visits to clinics at all levels.[69] And presumably Zhuang medicine, both the royal textbook and wild nomad versions, is the specialty best set up to manage the disorder.

In 2012 Laborjoy Wei told us that one of his research and writing projects is an effort to standardize the characterization and treatment of *sha* 痧 for ZM. A couple of years later, with a co-author, he published a note in the *China Journal of Nationality Medicines*. This is an excerpt from it:

> Three methods to examine for *sha* disease on the upper back:
> 1. "Cross" examination: expose the upper back, using both hands, the thumb and index finger facing each other, pressing to make a cross mark on the skin. Lifting hands after about 10 seconds, observe the subtle color changes where the marks are: if the fine hair is yellowish, it's "yellow-hair *sha*"; if the fine hair is reddish, it's "red-hair *sha*"; if the fine hair is blackish, it's "black-hair *sha*"; if the fine hair is whitish, it's "white-hair *sha*"; if there's no obvious color change of the fine hair, then it's common *sha*.
> 2. One-finger pressure examination: expose the upper back, search for the suspected eruptive point of *sha* by following along the skin surface; when you have found it, then press on the point with one fingertip for about 10 seconds. Suddenly lift the finger and observe the mark on the skin: if the suspected *sha* eruption point disappears for a moment but soon reappears, this is then the eruptive point of *sha* disease.
> 3. Fingernail pressing examination: expose the upper back, press along both sides of the spine with the right thumbnail from top to bottom, and from the middle outward toward the two sides, at points one inch apart. If the muscles are tight, if the patient complains of unusual pain, or the back's surface is bumpy and rough, accompanied by unevenness in the thumbnail marks at different places on the skin, these signs might result from a blockage of the Dragon Road and the Fire Road. Once the Dragon and Fire Roads are returned to freer flow, *sha qi* usually recedes.[70]

Technical writing like this, a detailed description of hands-on diagnostic procedures, makes the ontological point better than any literary analysis could: the things engaged by medicine are "real in their consequences." The way in which these actions assemble *sha* as a clearly perceived disease involves an indirect elicitation of multiple indexes, which is to say, a gathering of signs arising from the thing itself.[71] *Sha* expresses itself in ways that can be read by the diagnostician: *sha* changes the color of fine surface hairs, *sha* erupts and withdraws and erupts again at points, *sha* makes pain under fingernail pressure, *sha* disrupts the smoothness and resilience of healthy skin. The concreteness of these signs of an excess of "*sha* qi" testifies in turn to the simple existence of the Dragon and Fire Roads. It is these functional pathways, classic in Zhuang medicine (see appendix), that can be blocked by feverish *sha* poison, they are patterns of qi flow that need to be freed up. They are not, in other words, just concepts or terms in a "theoretical corpus," not just different "ways of wording" that might be translatable into the channels and collaterals of TCM or the vascular and central nervous systems of biomedicine. The Two Roads are things that flow or become blocked, and Laborjoy Wei can show us how to know, with our hands and eyes, what state they are in.

On the other hand, detailed as Dr. Wei's diagnostic instructions are, as we translated them, we found them somewhat lacking as guides to hands-on work with concrete things, such as patients' bodies and doctors' hands. The color change of the fine hairs in method 1, for example. Presumably these are subtle differences requiring good light and a keen eye; would we compare the "blackish" hairs along the pressure "cross" with their previous color, or with the color of hairs in other parts of the patient's back? When using method 2, how is the "eruptive point of *sha*" discerned, visually or with the fingers? By color, or by surface texture, or perhaps by temperature? And though method 3 seems ideal for the work of two hands, the instructions specify only the right hand.

Puzzled by these gaps in a piece of technical writing, we contacted Dr. Wei to ask him to clarify. He was amused by the gravity of our queries. Rather than add more words to his already detailed description, which might fill out our knowledge of *sha* disease and its diagnosis, he laughingly asked us why we were so surprised by these ambiguities. "I learned these techniques at the side of Zhuang medicine practitioners," he said. "They showed me the color changes, and the unevenness in pressure marks; they showed me where to put my fingers and what responses I could expect when the patient had some type of *sha*. How could this kind of experience be conveyed in words?" He was not being facile, or lazy; nor was he simply reminding us of the truism that textbook knowledge is not as reliable as learning by doing in the clinic.

Rather, he was speaking from a particular moment in the development of Zhuang medicine and from a particularly fecund orientation to medical knowledge and practice. Like other leaders in the ZM field, he seems to feel that it is imperative to sort the knowledge of Zhuang nationality medicine into things and methods that can be taught to the next generation of professional (and licensed) ZM doctors. Hence his publication of an inspection protocol with a colleague in a medical journal. But he also lived contentedly with a mostly inarticulate corpus of ZM knowing practice, and he slipped away from the hospital in Nanning as often as he could to engage in "medical exchange" with various nomad experts. Dr. Wei told us, for example, that he had learned at least the first of these techniques from a healer named National Treasure Fan, an eighty-two-year-old practitioner whose body-surface manipulation techniques and herbal medicines had been passed down through his family, "in the old way" (*gudao jiachuan* 古道家传). When he took us to meet Dr. Fan, the two Zhuang doctors spoke mainly about diagnostic techniques useful for *sha*. Dr. Wei wanted to learn a technique and took off his shirt so the old specialist could demonstrate on his back. The pinching and pressing that we saw (and that Dr. Wei felt) looked a lot like method 1 above; even with light from the doorway falling on Wei's back, it required a special talent for visualization (*shi* 视, Wei called it) to see the changes taking place under Dr. Fan's fingers.

We were a little surprised on this occasion, perhaps mostly because we had been thinking of Laborjoy Wei as an authoritative leader of the field in a very modern and systematic hospital-based Zhuang medicine. We were not prepared to see him as a humble student submitting himself to a series of hard pinches in the dark and smoky sitting room of an old "folk healer." But his interest in Dr. Fan's methods was growing increasingly clear. By the time Dr. Wei had put his shirt back on and the two of them were grubbing around in the old healer's herb garden, discussing the qualities and efficacies of some medicinal plants, we felt we were participating in folk medical exchange at its most respectful. Perhaps this was a good example of the "salvaging" moment of Zhuang nationality medicine's development process.

Dr. Wei also told us, after we left the Fan household, that he was sure that National Treasure Fan has not taught him everything, or even most of what he knows. No wonder Wei keeps going back and worries about his old teacher's failing health. In his visits, he sees and learns from a different world of knowing practice. National Treasure Fan himself explained this to us: in trying to help us understand what *sha is*, he said that it coexists without being commensurate with biomedical diseases: "Patients may come to me with a Western medicine diagnosis, and that diagnosis may be right; but it has nothing to do with whether or not they *also* suffer from *sha*."[72]

Laborjoy Wei not only "salvages," though, he also sorts and synthesizes. He has incorporated Dr. Fan's methods into his own practice, and as noted, several years after our shared visit he published a paper reporting on some of the things National Treasure Fan had demonstrated to him in 2012. He continues to work in the ZM hospital, though he has considered opening a

private storefront clinic where there would be less paperwork, less regulatory attention, and more personal profit. He is clearly ambivalent about his
clinical and "knowing-practical" life inside the institutions of an increasingly statist medical system. He is far from the nomadism that has brought
authority to his parent's rural clinic, and he is certainly not a voiceless subaltern in Guangxi's medically plural environment; he's too well trained and
institutionally influential for that. But he is an eclectic and curious practitioner of ZM (and more), interested in anything that might help the very diverse patients and illnesses he encounters in various places in Guangxi—at
his parents' village clinic, in the Nanning hospital, drinking with old classmates, and even (during a tourist moment on our 2012 road trip) in a restored
temple with an ailing caretaker. His practice embodies the two sides—the
relatively institutional and the relatively wild—of nationality medicine development: He excels in the royal knowledge he has learned from medical
textbooks, curricula, and other information sources, to which he contributes through publication. And he gathers the experience, skills, and nomad
knowledge that can be gained only through time spent working with those
who know, looking at illness together in its home places.

"MIRACULOUS ZHUANG MEDICINE IS GOOD"

In our 2012 Guangxi field trip with Laborjoy Wei, we stopped to visit his
parents in Gu Peng village. When we arrived they were seeing patients in
the large village clinic where they have both practiced for several decades.
This is also the setting where Laborjoy honed his clinical skills under his
parents' guidance, but his name is the only one on the clinic's shingle at the
front door. Inside the main room, which was open to the quiet street, there
were desks and chairs for consultations and many red silk testimonial banners, some of them handmade by amateur calligraphers, hanging around the
walls. The praise formulas one finds on such banners are predictable, but
they were not quite standard in this family clinic. "Medical Efficacy Spreads
Its Fragrance, Miraculous Hands Bring Back Youth," might have been found
in many clinics, but others referred indirectly to the Wei family's shared specialty of infertility medicine. One banner read "Elevated and Noble Medical Talents, A Healer's Gourd That Serves the Generations." With its image
of the healer's gourd, this testimonial invoked the herbalists of southern
medical lore,[73] while also referring to the many people who had sought out
the medical services of this family to help them have children. "Medicines
That Assist Reproduction," and "The Talents of a Child-Sending Goddess
of Mercy, Medicines That Banish Low Spirits" were even more direct, the
latter of these formulas also praising Dr. Everlucky Wei (Laborjoy's father)

for his treatments for emotional disorders. One simple handmade banner simply writes, "Miraculous Zhuang Medicine Is Good."

Indeed, "Zhuang medicine" was a specialty the Wei family was happy to claim. Also hanging around the walls of the main clinic room were framed (but somewhat decrepit) handwritten introductions of the doctors practicing there. These included panels for the late patriarch Calm Succession Lao, born in 1896, and his wife Clan Member Lan (born 1903), as well as for Everlucky Wei and his wife, Noble Phoenix Lao, and for Laborjoy Wei himself. In different ways, we are told by these accounts, each of these healers has practiced Zhuang medicine, both the nomad and royal varieties. The three family members still living all announce a specialty in treating infertility with Zhuang methods. Wei father and son have both taught and lectured on the subject of medical theory and techniques, and the whole family has been formally trained in various schools and workshops, some of them part of the ZM development and institutionalization movement. The shingle standing outside their village clinic door announces simply that this clinic, the "Springtime Herbals Hall," offers Zhuang medicine and pharmacy.

Everlucky treats mental disorders (*jingshenbing* 精神病) as well as infertility. When we arrived, in fact, he was seeing a patient complaining of headaches, diagnosing the pathological process by holding his two hands at a slight distance from, and moving them around, the man's head.[74] These "miraculous hands"—praised in several banners—were obviously important in even the mundane activities of this village clinic. Later, when Dr. Wei Sr. took us to the edge of the village to see the "Zhuang Medicine and Pharmacy Research Base" (an herb farm and processing plant he and the family had established), he directed our attention to a photograph pinned to a wall there. The fuzzy image showed a female patient reclining on a box bed, with Everlucky Wei standing at a slight distance and holding his left hand out toward her. There was a caption: "Dr. Everlucky Wei exclusively performing his hand technique for treating mental illness in 2008. Immediate effectiveness in this case." We asked him how this hand technique worked; he said that his hand conveys "information," and that in fact there was an "information exchange" between him and the patient via his hands. This approach to sending and receiving some form of qi calmed this patient down very quickly, and Dr. Wei was then able to write a prescription for some medicine, which she took with further good results. He reiterated, standing there looking at the snapshot, that his form of medicine was very good for mental cases, and this was important because "there's one in every village." But he hastened to add, without the herbal medicine, it would just be "superstition."

There was one other kind of display in the Wei family clinic. Dozens of snapshots of happy healthy babies and parents holding new infants were pinned up in several large frames. One picture was labeled "the 1,740th infertility patient treated." Of course this label does not indicate how many of those thousands of treatments resulted in a pregnancy and a healthy baby.

These pictures did not go unnoticed by some other patients who came in while we were visiting. These out-of-towners were a married couple from a village an hour away. They were taking a break from contract labor much further away, in Guangdong, and they had been having no luck getting pregnant. Anxious to have children, they paid close attention to Dr. Lao's quiet advice and waited a long time for her to prepare thirty packets of powdered compounded medicine for them, a three-month's supply they could take back to Guangdong with them. During this wait, we all admired the baby pictures on the wall.

The satisfied parents who kept in touch with Drs. Wei and Lao by sending their children's pictures were surely believers in Zhuang medical magic. Conception is, after all, little different from magic, and a healthy baby is nothing short of a miracle. Many medical systems offer medicines that "assist reproduction," as one of the Weis' testimonials said, but desperate families learn quickly that such drugs often don't help. Patients understandably have little confidence in expert knowledge in this area, but they also feel that they have no choice but to consult the experts. The statist Zhuang medicine practiced in Laborjoy Wei's Nanning hospital, and taught at the provincial medical school across the street, may look clumsy, contradictory, and full of lacunae from the point of view of a family heritage clinic in a Guangxi village. We might even appreciate the charm of this bucolic clinic by classifying it as an instance of nomad therapeutics, successfully resisting the salvaging and sorting projects of the state. But we have seen how, in the working lives of Laborjoy Wei and his family, specifically Zhuang medical things (*sha* poison, the Two Roads, locally grown, gathered, and processed herbs, and all manner of textbook objects) impose their authoritative existence in practice. For Drs. Wei and Lao, and for their patients, there is no necessary divide between textbook knowledge and effective practice. It is in the practice of knowing (medically, eclectically) that new worlds—such as adored new babies—can be made and then, in family snapshots, represented.

CHAPTER 3

Bodies

In July of 2016 we found ourselves in Donglan, Guangxi. Luo Jie, a collaborating researcher from the Guangxi University of Chinese Medicine, was with us. She had arranged introductions to several local officials, leaders of the Donglan Health Department. We hoped they would tell us about the state of development of Zhuang medicine (ZM) in this pleasant river town, which we had been told by many is "the homeland of Zhuang medicine." As it happened, these administrators were more interested in biomedicine and official Chinese medicine (*zhongyi*, Han nationality TCM) than in any local nationality practices, saying that Zhuang medicine in the area had fallen on hard times as the true folk experts have aged and passed away. And they worried about unregulated itinerant charlatans.

Their views, so suspicious of wildness, contrasted with some we had heard in Nanning. A few days earlier our research group had been impressed with the extraordinary "nomad science" resources invoked by a highly placed ZM leader in Nanning. He had called these matters "earth medicine" (*tu yi* 土医) and said he had learned much of value in his earlier career, which had been spent in Donglan.[1]

Strolling along the riverside streets before sitting down to dinner with Health Department Vice Director Wei, we had immediate proof that ZM, or at least "earth medicine," was active here. We encountered a woman patient sitting on a stool, her back bared, receiving a cupping treatment (*baguanr* 拔罐儿) from a female practitioner who (the two of them told us) often worked at this spot. (Also routinely installed on the riverside close by was a diviner who used his calendrical tables and cosmic correlations tables to calculate the fate of clients.) This treatment was a bit different from the cupping methods we had witnessed both in the herb market in Nanning and in the ZM hospital there. Instead of using bamboo tubes steeped in a warm herbal bath, this practitioner had a basket full of metal soft drink cans. These long tubes were open at one end, like the more usual bamboo tubes, but they were not stored in any sterilizing liquid. In the usual *baguanr* manner, this folk doctor used an alcohol-fueled torch to consume the air in the tube before slipping its open end quickly onto the skin of the patient. The tube opening immediately formed a seal and drew skin and underlying tissue into a bulging circle. By the time ten tubes were in place, presumably positioned at acupoints, the patient's back was bristling with long metal cans.[2] After leaving the tubes in place for five to twenty minutes, the cupper later used her index finger to break the attachments with the skin, and the tubes were then easily and painlessly removed. The patient's back showed several rows of round, inflamed circles. Unlike some cupping treatments, this procedure left her with little broken skin or leaking blood.[3] In a few days, all these marks would fade, and the whole procedure did not seem to be painful. (This despite the fact that the metal mouths of these cans must have been rather sharp and hard.)

This discovery of a "folk medicine" treatment in a provincial town proved especially memorable for Judith, who, though she had been aware of cupping as a medical treatment for some time, never really understood its rationale or desirability. Indeed, it was learning about the haptic techniques—touching and surface-manipulating modes of perception and intervention—of East Asian medicines that began to persuade her that there is a difference between a conceptual representation of a medical technique and an embodied understanding of its value. All medicine, perhaps, seeks to "grasp" pathology beyond the visible, but we began to feel that Asian and southern mountain therapeutics showed a special reliance on touch and surface manipulations. Abandoning for a while the relativism required of an anthropologist, Judith tended to experience cupping and some forms of needling as a kind of personal attack. Her anxiety about the haptic techniques typical of various East Asian medicines highlighted for her some embodied assumptions about her own habitual, lived body.

In Donglan, the substitution of metal cans for sterile glass globes or herbally prepared bamboo tubes only heightened Judith's discomfort with the procedure. Lili had less difficulty, however: she occasionally gets a *baguanr* treatment herself with a massage, on the advice of medically trained masseuses. Moreover, the worth of cupping is readily stated by experts. According to Huang and Rong, for example (see appendix), "working through the strength of the medicine, the heat, and the pressure of the suction, [cupping] facilitates the functions of expelling poisons and moving qi, dispelling cold and stopping pain, driving out winds and dampness, and enlivening blood and relaxing muscles." These authors see one local version of the technique, using medicated bamboo tubes, as particularly Zhuang—though a Nanning hospital cupping technician told us that the same method is also used by Yao medicine experts, possibly cooking the tubes with different herbs.[4] But Huang and Rong's characterization of the functions of the technique is applicable across many medical traditions, including Chinese medicine and European folk medicine.

But for Judith, and even to some extent for Lili, the expert explanation only deepens the mystery: what kind of body is this from which poisons can be expelled, and wind and dampness driven out, with the application of heat suction at the surface? More specifically, what is the nature of the body surface on which nationality medicine practitioners — across the mountain south, we found — are so focused in their practice? Watching the work of a riverside "village granny" in a Zhuang medicine homeland, as she toiled with hot tubes over the surface of a sufferer's body, Judith was forced to examine her own assumptions about the "natural" human body.[5] Perhaps skin is not just a sensitive envelope for muscle, blood, organs, tendons, and nerves, not just a thin membrane that unequivocally marks the line between a person's insides and the outside world. Perhaps qi and wind, or static clumps of dampness and cold, are actual pathogenic forces that should be grappled with, drawn outside of the body, nudged into motion with sucking, scraping, or needling. And perhaps more parts of the body know how to sense, breathe, and excrete than those few orifices (eyes, ears, anus, etc.) we can list on one hand. In this chapter, then, we ask: How do "southern bodies" happen? What can the practices of nationality medicine in China's mountainous south teach us about lived bodies? Are the bodies treated by ethnic medicines local and different from those we have observed in TCM clinics or biomedical examinations? How are suffering and enjoying bodies made in practice? Can the bodies of others be understood with reference to some common ground of human physicality? Or must the discomforts and pleasures of others remain a mystery? Our answers to these questions are empirical rather than theoretical. And there is never only one answer.

SOUTHERN BODIES

Throughout the course of our field research in the southern provinces, with various ethnic groups, we asked practitioners of the healing arts if they thought that local bodies — local to their places of work — had any special characteristics. Sometimes we even asked if they thought there was such a thing as a "local body" (*bendide shenti* 本地的身体). Almost universally these health care practitioners answered no, arguing that their herbal medicines, manipulations, and explanations would be just as effective with Beijingers or foreigners as they were with the villagers and townspeople living nearby.

Their position was logical: if the same physical interventions work the same way with all patients, then the patients must in some sense have the "same" body.[6]

This view of a universally similar human body was consistent with medical modernization in China, a complex development over many decades that has quietly imported from world biomedicine a universalist understanding of the human body seen as a structured and autonomous closed system.[7] Even the most "remote" healer, working from his farmhouse sitting room, has been influenced (and trained, see chapter 5) to think about bodies and medicines with a modernist ontology.[8]

But we persisted with our questions about local bodies. After all, both of us had been reading and writing about historical and practical bodies, situated bodies, for quite some time. In a 2017 conference paper, for example, Lili summarized her explanation of the use of the term "embodiment" (*tixian* 体现) as follows:

> If we take the body [*shenti* 身体] to be a contingently formed temporal, spatial, and material field [*changyu* 场域], then every kind of practice, discourse, institution, visual image, specific site, and matter of concern can become united in an emergent 'embodiment' [体现 *tixian*]. To use the term embodiment to speak of bodies makes for a difference with the steady state human body that is of significance in medical anatomy. Rather, *tixian* emphasizes understanding the temporality of the body. Bodies are continuously located in specific times and places. Not only is body emergent in each specific moment of a life course, at the same time each body's changing life is also located in specific social and historical processes.[9]

Judith also continues her efforts to propose an approach to embodiment that is dynamic, historical, and practical (and thus local by definition). In a published interview with Guangzhou anthropologist Zhang Wenyi, she said:

> Eventually I developed a way of thinking about bodies as concentrations of practices which extend beyond the skin-boundary and put the whole body—inward turning and outward-reaching—into motion, treating it as a condensation of life rather than as a structure. So I began to talk about embodiment or bodiliness, not "the body," trying to emphasize the active contingency and specificity of all manner of bodies.[10]

With ideas like this on our minds as we did fieldwork, we could only be hyperaware of all the contingencies that might have been making some very particular bodies: Zhuang or Qiang bodies, bodies under magical attack, porous bodies in tune with the mountain forests, damp and hot southern bodies, and so forth.

Others have found reasons to think locality, medicine, and embodiment together. The basic logic of our own research for this chapter, for example, can be found in Shigehisa Kuriyama's influential book *The Expressiveness of the Body and the Divergence of Greek and Chinese Medicine.* There he notes, the very fact that medicine has a history challenges our casual assumption that "the workings of the human body are . . . everywhere the same."[11] Medical knowledge and practice have varied historically and geographically, "accounts of the body in diverse medical traditions frequently appear to describe mutually alien, almost unrelated worlds."[12] Kuriyama proposes that the world's "different ways of touching and seeing the body were bound up with different ways of *being* bodies."[13] His method, his historical curiosity and eye for difference, his way of reading for lived ways of being that are more often assumed than described in texts—these offer to us a kind of charter for seeking a sense of "divergent" embodiment in the nationality medicines being gathered today in China. By attending closely to medical knowledge and practice, we can better imagine the lived worlds with which healing expertise engages.

In the discourses of traditional Chinese medicine today, there are many ways of considering how human bodies differ, and in what ways they are local. There is a medical specialty called "constitution studies" (*tizhixue* 体质学), for example, the textbooks of which list nine qualitatively distinguishable types. Along with body types notable for their tendency toward certain kinds of imbalance (tending toward phlegmy dampness, tending toward blood stasis, tending toward qi depletion, etc.), there is a "mild" or normal and harmonious constitution, and also a congenitally unbalanced constitution type. (This last type shows exceptions to usual patterns of pathology, but it is interesting that the other eight types, by contrast, are not indicated as congenital.) The field of constitution studies concerns itself with the causes that generate bodies of particular kinds, and it focuses even more on methods of diagnosing the constitutional qualities of any given patient, in order that therapy can correct for inherent tendencies. For this field of medicine, environment and habits of life are more important forces than any idea of genetics for knowing and treating diverse bodies.

Judith recalls a clinical encounter in a Guangzhou gynecology clinic in the 1980s involving a patient who was from central China. She suffered from persistent vaginal infections. The doctors in this southern city questioned the patient about her work and travel history. When they learned that she had long worked in the kitchen of a Thai restaurant, they said they understood better why she had chronic "yin depletion" problems. (Yin depletion is one of the body types in constitution medicine.) "No wonder this is hard to cure," they said. "She's breathing all those hot peppers in a sweltering kitchen sixteen hours a day!" They added that she did not have the right body type to manage well in a southeast Asian microenvironment like the restaurant kitchen.

Constitution studies scholars and clinicians find their charter for classifying bodies and physiologies, and for adjusting therapeutics to correct for local qualities, in classical explanations in the Han Dynasty canonical work *Plain Questions*. They summarize these *sanyinzhiyi* (三因制宜) doctrines for modern use as "healing proceeds according to the person, the place, and the time" (*yinshi yindi yinren* 因时因地因人).[14] This is not just a textbook rule of thumb; we have found that conscientious doctors often invoke this principle to explain how they customize and individualize treatments in practice, whether or not they think in terms of "constitutions." And then there are the many southern herbalists who ground their practice and expertise on the knowledge they have gathered concerning the specificity of the plants they have personally encountered. The powers of plants and other natural medicines also arise from "time, place, and person."

These commonsense discriminations—of body types, local influences, and wild herbal medicines—known to every well-trained practitioner of China's traditional medicines do two important things: first, they spatialize differences, leading to an implicit medical geography encompassing both disorders and natural drugs. And second, they echo a profound and persistent interest, in China, in the local character, or qualities, of persons. The "time, place, and person" guidelines of the *Plain Questions* presume, for example, that the particular bodies that walk into our clinics should be known and understood in ways that are subtler than can be found in a universally applicable human biology. This second element of common sense could lead, then, to the study of local biologies.[15] Perhaps the nationality medicines movement is precisely that, a development of medicines for the local biologies that, in practice, everybody takes for granted. The local or regional character intrinsic to every body and every self is very deeply embedded in modern Chinese common sense, after all. "Home place" becomes an issue in every conversation with new acquaintances, and localized speaking styles, food preferences, and physical appearances are often returned to as topics of polite conversation.

As we noted, many trained medical practitioners in the south deny that the bodies presenting in their clinics are in any sense "not the same" as those for whom mainstream Chinese medicine is intended. At the same time, they are proud of understanding the special needs of the villagers and townspeople they usually treat, and they expertly address southern diseases, like the many kinds of *sha* (痧) reported on by Dr. Laborjoy Wei in the previous chapter, compounding formulas from drugs that are relatively unknown in the national pharmacopeia.

Historian Marta Hanson has brought a rich historical texture to these forms of therapeutic localism in modern China.[16] She traces a deep genealogy of "the geographic imagination" over several centuries in early modern and modern China, focusing particularly on the development of the Warm Illnesses scholarly current of medical thought. The Qing period theorists of Warm Illnesses, discussed by Hanson, did not, as far as we know, find it important to represent or "anatomize" southern bodies as such. But the variations and debates traced by Hanson allow us to read through a history of medicine and a geography of disease to discern the particular forms of embodied life allied to southern knowledge.

Still, modern medicine seems to require some explicitness about "the body." Contemporary writers charged with salvaging and sorting nationality medicines have often tried to systematically characterize the variable bodies addressed by the particular therapeutic system they present. As we shall see, in their efforts to present a characterization of local practices that can be recognized as legitimate medical knowledge, they detail the structures, substances, functions, and specific vulnerabilities of Zhuang, Yao, Qiang, etc. bodies. These writers (sorters and synthesizers all) do not reduce local characteristics to an "ethnic" or nationality nature—this is not, in other words, a racial logic—but they are acutely aware of differences brought on by the winds and waters, the foods and drugs, and the social and physical environments where people live.

TEXTBOOK BODIES

Medical textbooks, under modern conditions of state-led knowledge production and management, are required to be explicit about "the body." Almost all of the general and basic nationality medicine textbooks we have found begin with a "theoretical foundations" section that characterizes the particular body addressed by the therapeutics in question. These early chapters do not present a simple or neatly sorted body. Indeed, we will show that there are quite different and even contradictory body systems entangled and entailed in the textbooks. But these theorists begin their pedagogy by establishing an ontological foundation for the practices covered by the rest of the book. Because each nationality claims a unique medical system, each nationality medical body is—arguably, with careful reading—different from that presumed by either biomedicine or traditional Chinese medicine.

Take the scarce but authoritative writing on Tujia medicine, for example. Every source seems at first to present a very modernist, concrete, and even narrowly biomedical account of "the structure of the human body." The most influential textbook on Tujia medicine, that of Zhao Jinghua, introduces the field's knowledge of the body with a decidedly materialist and modernist disclaimer:

> The human body is an extremely complex organism, made up of many structuring organs, and all of these structuring organs have their own material foundations and physiological functions. Tujia medicine has gone through thousands of years of life observation and clinical practice, assembling a rather simple anatomical analysis, and slowly developing systematic knowledge of the structure and function of the human body.[17]

Reading this introductory sentence, schooled as we are in traditional Chinese medicine, we immediately notice a rather strong emphasis on structure and function (anatomy and physiology, for classic biomedicine). And we are led to wonder what, exactly, are the implied shortcomings of the promised "rather simple anatomical analysis." The body described in this way is a skin-bounded organism, thoroughly biological, full of discrete and material "organs" (*qiguan* 器官). Fairly familiar to a reader of English, in other words.

What follows this preamble is indeed quite structural: "Tujia medicine holds that the human body is mainly made up of three parts [*sanyuan* 三元], ten orifices, limbs and joints, vessels, and [the fluids] qi, blood, and germinal essence."[18] Zhao sorts the organs (those recognized in Tujia medicine), orifices, and channels of the body into Tujia medicine's "Three Parts": the upper, middle, and lower "yuan." The upper yuan incorporates the brain, the heart, and the lungs; the middle yuan is the site of the stomach (*du* 肚), intestines, and liver; and the lower yuan holds the kidneys (*yaozi* 腰子), the uterus (*yang er chang* 养儿肠), and the germinal essence sacs and urinary bladder (*jingpao, niaopao* 精脬, 尿脬).

The words that name these bodily organs are very concrete. Most of them are as likely to be used by a butcher of pigs as by a medical doctor. And as a nationality medical terminology, these names for organs seem to set Tujia medicine apart from Chinese medicine. We look in vain for that famous processual logic of East Asian medicines, the flow that unifies heaven and the human and emphasizes a continuity of forces and substances between people and their environments.[19] Moreover, even the list of organs differs from the list of visceral systems important to Chinese medicine. Tujia anatomists apparently pay more attention to the brain and its functions than

TCM doctors do, yet one of the most powerful TCM viscera, the spleen, is missing from Tujia experience.

It would seem, at least in the textbooks, that for Tujia medicine every normal function takes place inside the frame of the body. Here's how Zhao, after supplying many details about the work of each of the organs, summarizes his "simple anatomy" of the Three Parts (*sanyuan* 三元):

> The Three Parts are the most important constitutive units making up the organic structure of the human body. The life-material of humans' activity, qi, blood, and germinal essence, are all produced within the inner organs of the Three Parts. All the life phenomena of the human body are managed by the inner organs [*neizang* 内脏] of the Three Parts; and the qi, blood, and germinal essence of the human body circulate back and forth, irrigating [*guan* 灌] throughout the body, so as to sustain the normal life activity of the body.[20]

This summary of the character of Tujia medicine's most distinctive feature, the Three Parts, stops short of expecting any of the three parts to *act* as a visceral system of function. Unlike the Triple Burner of Chinese medicine, which is both a functional and a spatial "organ without material form" (as the TCM textbooks often say), these Three Parts apparently serve only to be the local site of concrete organs; visceral functions properly belong to the organs, not to the Tujia-specific "Parts." Even the circulating fluids that "irrigate" the body are "produced within" and "managed" by the common-sense organs, not by any of the Three Parts directly. Moreover, the "ten orifices" of the body are treated here as localized anatomical structures with very concrete functions (seeing things, breathing air, excreting waste). And the "numberless tiny sweat pores," which count as the tenth orifice, do not so much link the person to the world as provide an outlet for, well, sweat![21]

We have not been reading this "Tujia Medicine Foundations" body very sympathetically, we confess. This is partly because this "Body" section of a key textbook reads as a kind of obligatory interlude, deemed necessary for any modern medicine, and because an account of Tujia anatomy serves as a convenient place to provide long lists of local-language terminologies used by healers in Hunan and Hubei. Moreover, Zhao Jinghua does not seem to be offering a body that is different from that "body with organs" that we presume is to be found in modern biomedicalized societies.

We gain a similar impression from a textbook of Qiang medicine that appeared in 2005 as a result of concerted organizational work by several clinical and public health activists in southern Sichuan.[22] In the early chap-

ter devoted to "basic theory of Qiang nationality medicine," the section entitled "Qiang Medical Knowledge of the Structures of the Human Body"
uses most of the space of a few pages to provide the names (in a romanized
Qiang vocabulary) of body parts. This list, like much field linguistics in an
earlier era, presumes an ease of translation between Chinese and Qiang,
given that those obvious things like the head, eyebrows, palms, toes, shoulder blades, elbows, and so forth should be the same for everyone.[23] But this
fairly obvious catalog is prefaced with quite a different list, having quite a
different ontological character. This is the first sentence of the section on
the body:

> Qiang medicine considers that the human body is made up of stone,
> water, fire, qi, blood, and subtle matter [*jingwei wuzhi* 精微物质], com-
> prising an outer frame and inner organs that are interconnected by means
> of variously sized vessels.[24]

This anatomy is not at all commonsense, even for Han visitors from Beijing to Qiang country, and there is very little context in the book to help us
understand. One might pose many questions: what is the difference between
qi and "subtle matter"? What are the functional relationships between the
elements listed? For example, does Qiang medicine rely on a qi-blood relationship exactly like that of TCM? How does the element "stone" manifest in bodily life?

A reading of the subsection devoted to the location, structure, and functions of the six organs and eight bowels (*liuzang* 六脏, *bafu* 八腑) finds considerable mixing between the concepts of biomedical anatomy, TCM, and
this version of Qiang medicine.[25] But it doesn't get us closer to understanding "stone, water, fire, qi, blood, and subtle matter" as bodily agents or entities. In the end, we must agree with the editors' prefatory remarks, in which
they confess that they really don't understand much about the naturally
occurring theoretical foundations (or, we would add, ontology) of Qiang
medicine:

> In recent years, in accord with the government's emphasis on nation-
> ality medicine research, Qiang medicine has received unprecedented de-
> velopment. With salvaging and sorting, our scholarly framework for re-
> search on Qiang medicine has reached a preliminary understanding. The
> therapeutic activities of Qiang medicine do not simply rely on experi-
> ence; rather, its way of treating disease and using medicines has theoreti-
> cal guidance; it's just that that theory is not well understood by us. We

have performed interviews on aspects of Qiang medicine and have summarized some content ranging from basic theory to clinical techniques.
Although the Qiang medicine content [to follow] is still not comprehensive, we can reflectively sketch an outline of Qiang medicine.[26]

This confession of relative ignorance is rather rare in the textbooks we've
surveyed. It reminds us of the similar humility and philosophical curiosity
displayed by Academy Director Resolution Ma (chapter 2 and 5) as he was
instructing his fieldworkers for research among the Achang in Yunnan Province: "They *have* a theory, they just haven't been able to articulate it to us.
Until we have the theory, we cannot say this is a 'medicine' (as opposed to a
pharmaceutical miscellany)." Looked at another way, the chapter's section
on the Qiang body is rather arbitrarily filling in gaps in the editors' knowledge with a miscellany of words about anatomical bodies. And meanwhile
all Qiang-specific "subtle matter" escapes the medical gaze.[27]

MATURE REFLECTIONS ON EMBODIMENT:
ZHUANG MEDICINE

We have been reading recent Tujia and Qiang textbooks in the hope of discerning a local body, only to find a rather familiar modern body, one with
discrete anatomical organs in the usual places and with the usual jobs to do,
serving as the "theoretical foundation" that seems to be required for any
modern medicine. This "rather simple anatomical analysis," as Zhao Jinghua called it for Tujia medicine, resembles a Vesalian or modernist gross
anatomy (even though there are gaps and redundancies) in that it seems to
be a comprehensive and objective description: one body, made up of structures with functions, enframed with bones and skin, standing apart from its
environment.

We do not think that Tujia and Qiang medicine, as these practices were
passed down over the years prior to all textbooks, are really committed to
this rather mechanical body. A practicing doctor with powerful therapeutic
techniques and with his hands on a suffering patient cannot afford to over-
simplify. Thus, to understand the forms of embodiment that live in these
nationality medicines will require a turn to observations of clinical practices, reflection on the practical healing interventions that respond to the
behavior of bodies in practice. But before we turn to the bodily encounters
that can be found in the clinics of southern nationality medicines, we want
to consider one more piece of systematic writing. Lest readers presume that
the salvaging and sorting writers of nationality medicine textbooks are naïve

about how embodiment can be specific, local, and dynamic, we want to return briefly to Zhuang nationality knowledge of the human, or southern human, body.

Zhuang experts have been working on salvaging, sorting, systematizing, and elevating local knowledge rather longer than Tujia or Qiang medicine practitioners, and the tapestry they have woven is complex indeed. The article cited above and translated in the appendix, authored by historian Huang Hanru, one of the founders of modern Zhuang medicine, and his colleague Rong Xiaoxiang, is meant to introduce Chinese medical readers to Zhuang medicine. It tends to briefly summarize the body, physiology, pathology, and therapeutics, rather than elaborating on any of these topics. After all, by the time this article was published, in 2015, there was already a library of authoritative and highly technical textbooks and research reports available for use in Zhuang medical education. But even the summaries do not deliver a body that is entirely familiar to either biomedicine or Chinese medicine. Here's a catalog of ZM characteristics that appears early in the essay, for example:

> The ZM theoretical system, incorporating the tenets of yinyang as the root, synchrony of the Three Qi, the body composed of visceral systems [*zangfu* 脏腑]/qi and blood/muscles, bones, and flesh, emphasizing the disease causes of poison and depletion and the therapeutic principles of resolving poison and supplementing depletion . . .

As we noted in chapter 2, this list of "tenets" of Zhuang medicine is self-consciously hybrid. "Yinyang as the root" is no different from the same theoretical foundation claimed by traditional Chinese (Han) medicine, though Zhuang nationalists like to point out that the ancient origins of TCM are to be found among proto-Zhuang people and territories, so the similarities should be no surprise. The "synchrony of the Three Qi" (the qi of heaven, earth, and the human), however, is a cosmo-ecological principle centered by Zhuang theorists and neglected by modern TCM. The Zhuang body, further, seems to be made up of "visceral systems" of the same functional type as are found in TCM bodies, but it also incorporates some anatomical parts important in biomedicine: muscles, bones, and flesh. A later paragraph adds the brain (locally called *qiaowu* 巧坞) and gives it a very central role in regulating all manner of bodily activities. This emphasis in ZM is both not very TCM and, when you attend to the details, not identical to a biomedical central nervous system.

A catalog of this preliminary kind is not likely to help a working clinician. How qi, flesh, brain, and the rest actually work in the physiological and pathological processes that might require medical intervention is not at all clear, and yinyang, "the root," is here too vague to be of much use in practice. Instead of providing clinical guidance, Huang and Rong in this essay expand "basic theory" beyond discrete bodies and immediate causes to invoke "a particular medical reasoning": they give us ZM versions of the cosmic forces and processes that flow *through* bodies. The authors rather quickly abandon scientific or anatomical objectivism about bodies and turn philosophical (or is it "theoretical"?):

> Every kind of normal and abnormal phenomenon of nature and the human body, and their changes, are a response to and result of the opposed, interrooted, waxing and waning, balancing, and intertransformative mutuality of yin and yang qi. (Appendix)

This is phrased in exactly the same language as 1980s TCM, propounding a "dialectics of nature" vision, an approach that combines a very ancient yinyang worldview with the Marxist dialectics important in the early Reform period. But these Zhuang authors hasten to find in this cosmic dialectics a local specificity: "ZM emphasizes the guiding role of yang qi, holding that the traits of the lived body [*huoti* 活体] that have life are an expression of the existence and activity of yang qi." This bias toward one end of the yinyang polarity is not something we have found very often stated in the TCM literature. Moreover, a yinyang logic is impossible to grasp without understanding something about qi (气), so our authors add a ZM account of qi to their "particular medical reasoning":

> ZM calls qi "*xu*." Qi suffuses heaven and earth and the human body, being expressed as yang, motive power, energy, and as the life span that is the birth, growth, health, aging, and death of the human body; [this "*xu*"] depends on the qi of heaven and earth for its restraint and control. Human qi and the qi of heaven and earth intimately intermingle in their flow, they work in synchrony. Humans are the "magic" of the myriad things, they have a certain special agency in adapting to changes in the qi of heaven and earth. The human body is also a microcosm [*xiao tiandi* 小天地] such that the heaven, human, and earth qi sectors [called in ZM "the Three Qi"] inside the body must run in sync [*tongbu yunxing* 同步运行] and thereby mutually control the generation and transformation processes in the interest of maintaining a healthy condition. The significance of the "synchrony of the Three Qi" lies in "synchronizing," which means harmonizing movements and mutually controlling them in order to preserve a dynamic equilibrium between yin and yang. (Appendix)

Why do we quote this paragraph on qi, or *xu*, in full? Because it is here that the "theory" begins to help us make sense of the ZM clinical experience to which we will soon turn. This is a body of flow, a human body that participates in the currents of "heaven and earth," yet has a certain bounded integrity subject to "restraint and control."

As the Huang and Rong essay continues, it develops more Zhuang specificity and a better understanding of through-flow: the Three Ways and Two Roads, for example, are like routes of flow. These are categories that one does not encounter in either TCM or biomedicine. The Three Ways (*sandao* 三道) are the Grain Way, the Water Way, and the Qi Way, governing, respectively, alimentation, hydration, and respiration (though as can be seen in reading the appendix, the Zhuang authors don't adopt a human biology language of this generalizing kind). All these processes are specific forms of passage, passage of food, water, and breath through the human being, and they have complex relationships among their networks of passageways. Symptoms can be understood as belonging to one of these Ways, though it is probably more common for symptoms to reflect some problem in the relationship between two or more Ways, or between a Way and a Road.

Parallel with the Three Ways are the Two Roads (*lianglu* 两路), the Dragon Road and the Fire Road. The Dragon Road moistens and nourishes all parts of the body with blood and other body fluids, and the Fire Road—analogous to the central nervous system—"transmits information . . . in all directions" (but still in the body interior). These are pathways, or reticular networks, or hydraulic systems, or functional sectors of lived bodies. The Huang and Rong essay tends to describe them as dynamic, living configurations of physiological activity. The Three Ways and the Two Roads are as difficult to pin down as yin and yang, however; it is no accident that we have proliferated terms for such things—pathways, networks, sectors, configurations—adding even more metaphors to the conventional images of "way" and "road." Expert ZM doctors do not, we suspect, need to have these metaphorical ambiguities reduced to definitional clarity—which would settle on one word for one thing, one signifier for one signified—as they work with these bodily entities. They are able to address symptoms and adopt therapies on the basis of a fuzzy logic and a conventional vision of the body, as Zhuang medicine authorities have taught. The Three Ways and the Two Roads help doctors sort phenomena into correlated and differentiated groups, and they also propose a form of activity, a dynamic, that has real implications for the effective management of illness.[28]

SPATIALITY AND A BODY OF FLOWS

The Zhuang body of interpenetrating networks of activity "extending in all directions," mobilizing the pathways where entities flow, has effects both internal to the human frame and resonating through heaven and earth. But we think this body is not unique to the Zhuang nationality of Guangxi. Some of the analytics, diseases, and techniques discussed in the Huang and Rong essay no doubt are specifically Zhuang, and so too—it would appear—are a ZM emphasis on yang qi, on the Three Qi of heaven, earth, and the human, and on bodily Ways and Roads.[29] But much of this vision of a microcosmic body of through-flow, or *tong* (通), is shared across the south, as our observations of therapy in various areas have convinced us.[30] There is a complex spatiality that can be seen in the body manipulations typical of the nationality medicines we studied: practitioners need to know where on the body's surface to tweak collateral channels (and experts often told us that different nationalities recognize different circulation tracks, and thus work with acupoints that are not entirely identical to those known to TCM). Skin scraping (*guasha* 刮痧) follows lines on the surface that mirror the deeper pathways that organize the through-flow of (e.g.) heat and damp wind. Medicated thread cautery (mentioned in chapter 1) is applied at Zhuang medicine-specific points as well. And the medicated bamboo tubes used by both Yao and Zhuang clinicians are not attached just anywhere, they must be placed where they can access regular pathways and improve *tong*, or through-ness. And knowing how to improve flow with a therapy, how to connect a human microcosm with the macrocosmic processes of the world in a wholesome way—this takes experience and observant wisdom.

We were fortunate during our visits to ZM institutions and experts in Nanning, Guangxi, to have several long talks with Huang Jinming. Along with Huang Hanru, an author of the essay in the appendix, Huang Jinming has been a leader in salvaging and sorting, systematizing and elevating, as well as institutionalizing, Zhuang medicine since the 1980s. He is widely respected for his clinical experience and his grasp of the basic principles of healing in ZM. One evening in his private clinic, we asked him to give us some background on several posters we saw on the wall. These were diagrams of ZM-specific circulation tracks and acupoints. He affirmed that the tracks and points depicted were different from those used in TCM and said that in his research among ZM practitioners he had found them to be rather widely recognized. But then he went on to explain, with a rapidly sketched diagram, a key aspect of the spatial configuration of body that he manages in his own practice.

Organic System Affiliations

points on the navel's inner and outer circle

Heaven Sector
Brain, Heart

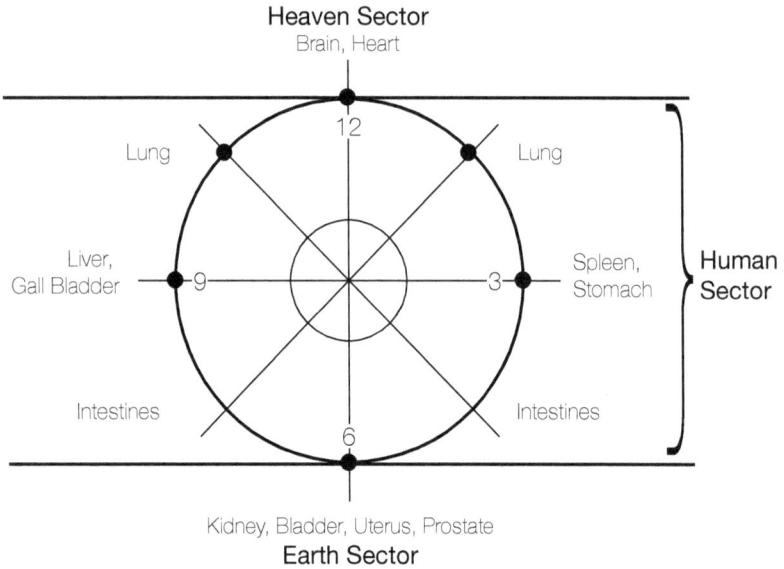

Lung   12   Lung

Liver,   Spleen,   Human
Gall Bladder   9   3   Stomach   Sector

Intestines   6   Intestines

Kidney, Bladder, Uterus, Prostate
Earth Sector

Figure 3. Courtesy of Jenny Addison, adapted from a sketch
made by Dr. Huang Jinming during an interview.

Grabbing a blank prescription form from his desk, he drew two nested circles, with six heavily emphasized acupoints (*xue* 穴) symmetrically located around the outer circle. These circles were labeled "points on the navel's inner and outer circles." He drew straight lines through these two circles. Two horizontal lines demarcated the space above both circles as "the heaven sector," and the space below both circles was labeled as "the earth sector." A bracket on the side marked the circles themselves as belonging to the "human sector." These labels began to persuade us, as we listened to his explanation, that he was not just giving us an explication of a few key acupoints in the abdomen, but rather diagramming the Zhuang medicine body in full.

We were not entirely surprised when Dr. Huang went on to fill in other names for things in the spaces his diagram proposed: Adding a general title, "Organ System Affiliations," he sorted the upper and lower, right- and left-sided organs, or visceral systems, in relation to the navel circles and the sectors of the Three Qi, or the heaven-human-earth triad. Heart and brain appear above the upper horizontal line, in the heaven sector, and kidney (not marked as two), bladder, uterus, and prostate are found at the bottom of the page, in the earth sector. The two lungs (one on each side) appear toward the top of the "human sector," close to the navel circles; liver and gall bladder are on the left of the center line, and spleen and stomach on the right; and the large and small intestines appear twice, on both sides of the circle, above the earth sector line of demarcation.

The circles in this diagram could be thought of as a picture of an actual site on the physical body, the navel, with useful acupoints distributed around it and available for direct needling on the body of a patient. But the straight lines passing through the circles, which form a star with vertical, horizontal and two diagonal lines, have to be understood as more conceptual. They are, after all, sorting the functional affiliations of the major visceral systems. Moreover, the star-shaped lines seem to be present mainly to allow a technical quantification. The points where these lines cross the curve of the navel's outer circle are both *xue* acupoints and positions in a regular twelve-degree sequence of divisions around the circle, like that of a clock face. The topmost point is labeled twelve, the lowest is six, and the right and left extremes along the curve are three and nine, respectively. We suppose this numerical division helps the practitioner to find the right acupoint on actual bodies, but there may be more abstract technical implications, a kind of numerology, that Dr. Huang did not bother to explain.

We all knew we were looking at a diagram referring to a body, but we still think it is refreshing that that body was neither bounded—it was open to heaven and earth—nor anatomical (a list of organs/visceral systems is not an anatomy); nor was it claiming to be the whole story. This was no comprehensive representation of the human organism Dr. Huang treated with his version of Zhuang medicine. The diagram doesn't even include any reference to the Three Ways and the Two Roads, much less bones or muscles.

Given that he was able to spatialize the affiliations of many important body parts with this diagram of some points around the human navel, we wonder if Dr. Huang routinely confines his needling to these few points. They seem to provide access to most of the body, after all, by way of the interpenetrating and spreading networks we have seen discussed in the textbooks. Presumably he could address disorders in the spleen-stomach visceral system by manipulating the *xue* at degree 3 along the curve, or achieve better through-flow for the intestines with the *xue* at degree 6. We think, though, that this model of affiliations is only one part of the conceptual and technical toolkit an experienced clinician like Dr. Huang knows how to use. After all, in TCM there are other microcosmic surfaces on the body—the ear homunculus, the soles of the feet—which are useful for acupuncture and massage, but only a crackpot would rely upon them completely.[31] And of course there is the whole world of herbal medicine—Dr. Huang's private clinic had a beautiful pharmacy with many local herbals displayed in large glass jars—in which each medicinal substance has its own organ affiliations and yinyang ways of nudging the microcosmic processes of life. If, as Marta Hanson's disease geography shows well, there are "southern diseases"—local heteropathies (*xie qi* 邪气, *du*-toxins 毒, *gu*-parasites 蛊, and so on) affecting bodies in the south—then it would not be surprising for Dr. Huang, as a cosmopolitan healer with a complex toolkit, to have more than one model of (at least!) "organ system affiliations."

We liked to think, though, as we carefully preserved Dr. Huang's diagram sketched on a flimsy clinic form, that we had been given an especially authoritative representation of *the* Zhuang medicine body, even though the "Zhuang body" is always multiple. This observation is parallel with what Judith Farquhar argued in an early study: no singular noncontradictory Chinese medical body can be found, even in the most systematic textbook accounts of "foundations."[32] The modernist pretension of anatomy texts and Gunther von Hagens (impresario of the art and science fantasia of "Body Worlds" exhibitions) that the body is a structure and can be comprehensively described and represented disintegrates with careful reading. And if we turn to practice, as Annemarie Mol did in her field study of routine discursive usages in an Amsterdam cardiac clinic, we find that a number of distinct, even contradictory bodies come into pragmatic existence in the course of clinical work.[33]

But Dr. Huang's diagram, with its two small circles around the empirical bodily navel, which anchors relations among dispersed and spatially distinguishable organs, has a particular importance. This depiction of the "affiliations of the organ systems" shows how bodies can be the result of centering and condensing processes, the lived results of gathering and scattering qi. Those six heavily emphasized *xue* are places where connected forms of qi can be jolted into more productive motion, turned to make new links between particular parts of the body, encouraged or restrained, altered in quality, slowed down or speeded up. As any practitioner of qigong knows, the body's forces can be collected and condensed at the *dantian* (丹田), that "cinnabar field" only a few centimeters below the navel, to which it is wisest to return the flow of qi.

So there is probably an experiential dimension to Dr. Huang's diagram. Not only when undergoing acupuncture needling, even in everyday experience perhaps, sensations of embodiment pivot on condensed centers, from which core there is an outward dispersion. And this would be true not just for Zhuang doctors like Huang Jinming.

SHA-AFFLICTED BODIES

This chapter's aim has been, and continues to be, to work through nationality medicines to pluralize the body. Making forays into the technical knowledge of minority medicines, we are seeking to show that no single structural, or even structural and functional, description of human embodiment is available (everywhere, for everyone). This despite the fact that many moderns presume that knowledge of "the body" must ground the everyday practice of medicine. But Laborjoy Wei, who practices Zhuang medicine in the Nanning area, tried to help us find our way through the thicket of bodies he encounters in practice by reminding us that a clinician has to operate with some rather simple rules of thumb. In several visits—in his clinic, on a fieldwork road trip, and in Beijing—Dr. Wei showed us the ways he has synthesized (*zongjie* 总结) complex bodies of knowledge from several forms of medical practice, especially emphasizing the production of useful knowledge for clinical work. There are interesting ways of imagining the human body lurking in his medical conversation.

When we first visited Laborjoy Wei in his Zhuang Hospital clinic, where he mostly treated cases of infertility, he was administering a hands-on treatment to a female patient (after first prescribing an herbal medicine mixture to her husband). While she lay on her stomach with heat lamps trained on her lower back, Dr. Wei used a split wooden wand to lightly strike her leg muscles in a regular and repetitive way; then he tweaked points along her spine with needles, slightly drawing blood.[34] When we asked how he chose the points and surfaces for intervention, he said, "I think of the patient's body, especially her back, as a leaf, with its spreading ribs and veins." This is a rather simple organic image that impressed us at the time as a useful rule of thumb, even though, as far as we know, it appears in no Zhuang medicine textbooks.

In chapter 2 we considered Dr. Wei's way of knowing the body from its surfaces, especially focusing on procedures he had published for diagnosing varieties of *sha*-disease (痧). Recall from the previous chapter that he relied on subtle things like color changes in the "fine hairs" and on evaluations of the "roughness" of the skin surface. After we had returned from Guangxi to Beijing and Chicago and were no longer in frequent contact with our Zhuang medicine friends, it occurred to us to wonder how Dr. Wei thought about local bodies. It was clear to us that he had a lot of ideas about *sha* disorders, which are widely thought of as local to China's south. And his various approaches to diagnosing and managing *sha* might indicate what sort of a body he usually found himself handling. Lili had an opportunity to explore these subjects with him when he visited Beijing in December of 2018.

On that occasion he had a lot more to say about *sha*. In Beijing, Dr. Wei was sitting near our library of books about nationality medicine, referring to them occasionally, and he had recently read an article we had published, an exploration of Zhuang medical knowledge, that cited him. In this context, he was happy to point out how his clinical approach diverged from the information that can be found "sorted and synthesized" in Zhuang medicine textbooks. As Lili pressed him on the question of local biologies (trying to zero in on something about embodiment), he argued that *sha* was definable as a disorder stemming from overwork, especially agricultural labor, and it had a local and seasonal character because "Zhuang people like to work." Clinically, he saw most cases of "getting *sha*" during the busy times for farming, and mostly among people of middle age, i.e., those who are performing the bulk of the manual labor. Seizing her moment, Lili asked whether farmers in northern provinces, with a less hot and humid environment, also got *sha* when they worked too hard in seasonal labor. Dr. Wei allowed that they probably did, precisely because he was defining *sha* as nothing other than a disorder that comes on after heavy seasonal labor.

But his differential diagnosis of *sha* disorders was a little more complicated than this definition suggests. He was at pains to explain that *sha* is a self-diagnosed condition that is usually self-limiting. That is to say, the overworked "patient" notes *sha* discomforts after too much exertion. What he mainly needs is a rest, sometimes of only one night. The ideal treatment is a light meal, a *guasha* (skin-scraping) treatment, and a good night's rest. If the sufferer identifies herself as having *sha*, and if everyone knows that this minimal therapy will probably resolve the disorder, then this is *sha*. These criteria ensure that "getting *sha*" is not confused with being "hit by *du*-poison" or "hit by *gu*-parasites," both of which are more serious diseases. *Du*, for example, is not self-limiting, but it is curable with needling and medicine; the even more serious affliction of *gu* needs to be addressed both with medicine and with (unmentioned) extramedical means that "concern the whole family." (*Sha* is also, incidentally, not "chronic fatigue" or "subhealth" [*ya jiankang* 亚健康], he remarks; these are diseases invented for city people who sit at desks all day.)

Indirectly, perhaps, this differential analysis gives us an idea of the kind of body that so commonly suffers from *sha*. Wei is not the only Zhuang doctor who believes that *sha* is the most common complaint seen by local practitioners, and because it's so minor, most "cases" do not even appear in clinics or health stations. Let's review the eight types of *sha* recognized by Dr. Wei and his folk doctor teachers:[35] white hair *sha*, red hair *sha*, yellow hair (foreign hair) *sha*, black hair *sha*, fast snake *sha*, mahuang (ephedra) *sha*, tangled guts *sha*, and tangled threads *sha*. A motley list indeed, and it would be folly to assign disease meanings to these terms without a lot more guidance from Zhuang doctors. But we can see that half of these terms (at least) refer to observable changes on the surface of the body, i.e., the fine hairs. A few others seem to express changes in the body interior. Is there a surface and depth relation in this list? Dr. Wei will get there in a moment.

In chapter 2 we cited Dr. Wei's published descriptions of diagnostic techniques in which the changing colors of the fine hairs helped to determine the type of *sha* that had "erupted." But his agricultural-labor-centered and self-limiting-disorder characterization of *sha*, above, suggests that there's not much point in knowing what kind of *sha* is presenting in the body of the patient: red hair and black hair *sha* would, we guess, be treated (or not treated) the same. But in 2018 Dr. Wei said something quite interesting about the "inspection" techniques we saw him learning *in situ* from old Dr. National Treasure Fan (see chapter 2). He said, really, the inspection is the cure. Recall that inspection of the skin, especially on the patient's back (or so it appears to us after watching him work), involves a lot of pinching and poking, and even some scraping or *guasha* techniques, so this interesting combination of diagnosis and therapy makes practical sense. Here's how Dr. Wei elaborated on this idea:

> We [Zhuang practitioners] like to use our hands to knead [the body]: Where does a problem emerge? When you inspect, you can see the different routes of the channels. When you pinch it and the channel doesn't change, if it's elastic, that's good, there's no *sha*. The places that are pinched all have their very exactly measured [locations]. I have studied this with the old people, but I haven't finished learning from them. Of their eight kinds of *sha*, one kind is according to color [of the fine hairs], another kind is according to symptomatology.

So diagnosis is a pretty participatory exercise, it would seem. The diagnostician must elicit a response from "a place that is pinched," and it is the nature of that response (elasticity or pain) that tells him what's going on with the whole body. So this very hands-on inspection has therapeutic value, especially for a "light" disease like *sha*.

We were pleased to hear Dr. Wei say that "we like to use our hands to knead." Throughout our research travels in southern mountain China, we had been impressed with the commonness, even the centrality, of manual and tactile therapeutic techniques in all of the nationality medicines. Bonesetters (who do much more than set broken bones) are often consulted by patients in the counties and towns we visited, and the *guasha* (scraping) treatments of which Dr. Wei spoke are widely used even by nonexperts. Whatever these southern bodies are, in practice they seem to be comfortable with touching each other both diagnostically and therapeutically. Laborjoy Wei understood our interest in such haptic techniques, and our suspicion that they marked a difference with both Chinese medicine and biomedicine, and he theorized a bit for us:

> Biomimetic practice [the theoretical framework he was currently developing] is a butterfly effect. How do changes on the skin influence the inner parts? That we just don't understand. But the influence is for sure. For example, a person with tension in his back, after doing acupuncture with me, was relaxed, his information had gotten better. Either his psychic tension or some bad weather had made his muscles rigid, but I resolved the problem at the level of the skin. Information influences the skin from outside, and the skin in turn influences the interior. The skin is an organ, we could say, and I perform *guasha* at the level of the skin. The *Inner Canon* names twelve skin regions, and we use the twelve skin regions in *guasha*. The twelve channels are used to regulate the [whole] body. [Further, working with] the twelve muscle systems we use a *tuina* rectification method to resolve muscle and tendon problems.[36] The twelve skin regions, the twelve muscle systems, and the twelve channels are all used in *zhentiao* [needle tweaking]. So this is to say, the *Inner Canon* is really very great. Our biomimesis method is done only on the twelve skin regions, while Chen Jian's [his friend and colleague who specializes in] *zhentiao* is done on the twelve channels, and *tuina* massage is done on the twelve muscle systems. I just do microsurgery on the skin.

This is a complex excerpt from an informal interview transcript, and some of it is hard to grasp without knowing more context. "Information," for example, happens to be a keyword for Laborjoy Wei and his Zhuang practitioner father.[37] And Dr. Wei shows his eclectic and cosmopolitan interests also when he says that "the skin is an organ," and when he adapts a term for "bionics" (*fangshengxue* 仿生学) to mean something quite different (which we are translating as "biomimesis").

Most interesting in these comments, though, for our efforts to "see" a body through Dr. Wei's ways of managing *sha*, were his insistence that he works only at the level of the skin surface, with his "microsurgery," and his fascinating theory of biomimesis. Though he says that "we just don't understand" how actions taken on the body's surface influence any part of the interior, in fact he does propose a model: "Our biomimesis method is done only on the twelve skin regions, while Chen Jian's *zhentiao* is done on the twelve channels, and *tuina* massage is done on the twelve muscle systems." So here is an anatomy that envisions a single integrated skin surface, groupings of muscles and tendons, and the classical circulation tracks that traverse the whole body, linking skin, muscles, "jing-essence, qi and blood," and visceral organs. (He does not mention the Three Ways and Two Roads so richly theorized by other Zhuang medicine leaders.) He specifies one kind of *zhentiao* that, like classical TCM acupuncture, accesses the twelve channels; but the kind of *zhentiao* that he performs, and that he studies in his fieldwork with village healers, seems to us to be quite like a microsurgery working "at the level of the skin." He is agnostic about how his tweaking and scraping, tapping and heat lamp warming, pinching and massaging influence the hidden interiors of the bodies he treats. "But the influence is for sure."

And what about his vision of what he calls (possibly under the influence of anthropology) biomimetic practice? This is not just a source of metaphors that help him visualize what parts of an infertility patient's back he needs to stimulate. As part of his effort to explain how, exactly, local bodies are responsive to local conditions, he said more about the usefulness of bodies-like-leaves.

> When I later put [the eight kinds of *sha*] together with the [TCM] eight rubrics therapeutically, one is a matter of needling a bit shallowly, i.e. scattering, and one involves needling more, i.e., condensing. Inspection is very important, and you need to dispel qi more. Like a big tree leaf [of the kind found at the bottom of mountains], a moist tree leaf, flat and open, it can dispel qi more. But the tree leaves from high in the mountains don't care about dispelling much qi, these leaves are adapted to that cooler environment, the arrangement of the leaves overlaps. From the point of view of biomimesis, with lowland leaves, there's more qi dispelled, they are flat and open, requiring only shallow [insertion]; upland leaves expel less qi, the leaves overlap, so needling should scatter a bit, with deep [insertion]. I use these methods to arouse people's latent abilities [to self-heal]. Or to mimic the qi pores on a leaf's surface, or mimic the channels and collaterals—this is biomimesis.

This is not just a good clinician imagining, with a natural metaphor, the bodily field on which his haptic technologies will most successfully work, or elaborating a visual rule of thumb. It is a theory of human material life embedded in and responsive to the changes of nature, it is "heaven and earth acting as one" (*tianren heyi* 天人合一). To see the world through biomimesis is a way of noticing how all bodies (not just human, not even just animal)

fold the yin and yang qi, the cool and warm airs, the shade of the forest
and the light of the town, labor in fields and work at desks, into particular
habitual forms, prey to particular disorders, responsive to different treatments, differently embodied.[38]

We have once again dwelt at length here, as we did in chapter 2, on
Laborjoy Wei's somewhat idiosyncratic clinical and theoretical knowledge,
because we have learned from his research and healing practice. Perhaps he
cannot represent for us "the body" of a collectively "synthesized" Zhuang
medicine; Huang Hanru and Huang Jinming are perhaps better authorities
for a more official nationality medicine (though we saw above that Huang
Jinming had his own version of a ZM body, centered on the navel). But
Dr. Wei gave us an opportunity to witness his work of gathering healing
powers to himself from his encounters with wild bodies, both those of expert nomad healers like National Treasure Fan and the self-healing capacities of infertility patients and working people suffering from *sha*. Given the
nature of the sources he so enthusiastically seeks out, it would be a surprise
if his vision of the world and its bodies accorded exactly with what is in
the Zhuang medicine textbooks. He proposes more than one (but less than
many) *other* bodies for medicine to work with.[39]

PLASTERS AND PORES

Dr. Wei kindly articulated a certain theory of bodily activity for us, and
though his vision didn't resolve all mysteries, at least he offered a kind of
synthesis. At the beginning of this chapter we confessed that the manipulations so often preferred by southern medicine practitioners remain a little
strange to us, since we didn't really understand the mechanisms that make
them successful. Huang and Rong explain cupping, briefly, in the appendix,
and we have no reason to doubt them. But this is not the only haptic method
that puzzles us. As we watch nationality medicine practices of handling,
"kneading," needling, electrostimulating, and scraping bodies, our attention
is again and again directed to a reflexive examination of our own assumptions about bodies and how they work.

Take the ubiquitous herbal plasters used by bone-setters and herbalists,
for example. We often witnessed doctors preparing these thick mashes of
mixed herbals, smashing prepared plants together, adding a bit of water,
crushing drugs in a mortar, bundling up the mixture in a gauze envelope,
and securing the package to the affected part of a sufferer's body, placing
the side with the thinnest gauze against the skin or lesion. Dr. Sun, to whose
practice we will turn in a moment, distinguished two broad types of herbal
plasters, those useful for fresh injuries, which work to reduce pain and

swelling, and those suitable for old injuries, which work more to enliven blood and transform stasis. These are more superficial and more interior targets, respectively, for the efficacies of the bundled drugs. Often these injuries are not lesions but rather sites on the unbroken skin close to the discomfort. Among the instances of herbal plaster use we saw were a senior Achang doctor wrapping the sprained wrist of his son in a plaster prepared from his large pharmacy; a Christian minister-healer among the Lisu who prepared a fresh leg plaster weekly for a visitor who came rather a long distance for follow-up treatment of a now-knitted broken ankle; and an urban Qiang bone-setter with a private practice who was treating extensive but healing burns on the foot of a victim of a cooking accident.

In the last of these cases, the bad burn, as with similar treatments we saw of injuries that involved skin lesions, our understanding of how bodies and drugs work was not especially challenged. Presumably the "effective ingredients" of herbal drugs could directly reach (e.g., via the bloodstream) whatever internal-body elements contribute most to the healing of wounds, because skin was temporarily not in the way. We tend to think of skin, we realized, as a barrier to the spread of qualities from the outside world that could influence the insides of bodies. And we feel that our American friends who break bones or experience sprains might feel that a mash of herbs applied to the outside of the body, to the unbroken skin, while their injured bones and tendons are mending, would be kind of silly. What difference could this plaster possibly make, Americans might ask, given that the skin is self-evidently a barrier?

We think no such skeptical question is likely to occur to patients or practitioners of nationality medicines in southern China. Empirically, every experienced primary caregiver we have met in the nationality medicine world has no doubt that the right herbal mash applied in a plaster to an afflicted body part speeds healing and eases discomfort. Even in theory, we can see their confidence expressed. Recall that the most modernist/scientistic account of body structures we discussed from textbooks above, that of Tujia nationality systematizer Zhao Jinghua, listed the "numberless tiny sweat pores" as one of ten Tujia orifices. Though Zhao in his book notes only a one-way functional role for these pores, i.e. sweating, we think that Tujia practitioners, with their frequent use of herbal plasters, are presuming that those numberless tiny pores actually do connect the person to the world. And that the microscopic "collateral vessels" and "threads" populating the surface of the body are two-way streets for what Laborjoy Wei would probably call "information." This body is porous over its whole surface and thus dynamically connected to its environment. Indeed, when we consider the forms of "through-ness" we have learned about in more than one nationality medicine practice, we begin to wonder if a discrete body in a surrounding environment is the right vision for understanding embodiment, action, and material change in these settings. As our Zhuang, Qiang, Achang, and other minority nationality friends kept telling us, embodiment is about heaven and the human acting as one.

PATRIOT SUN AND TROOPER GUO

But in medicine, all is not harmony and ease, even when bodies are handled sensitively by a healer drawing on a rich tradition of effective drugs and manipulations. Perhaps the saddest patient we met was a young man named Trooper Guo who had been the victim of a near-fatal traffic accident more than a year before we visited the Qiang medical hospital in Maoxian, Sichuan. Paralyzed from the neck down immediately after the accident, his body was the most reduced we had seen. If we had shared with him our idea that "the body" is a condensation of practices rather than a physical structure, he might have bitterly laughed at us. Unable to stand on his own or use his hands and arms, and until recently confined fulltime to a hospital bed, he was living in a way that must have made the normal practice of daily embodiment look like a permanent impossibility.

We met Trooper Guo when we sought out the lively and crowded Qiang "bone-setting" clinic of Dr. Patriot Sun.[40] (We repeat here the local characterization of Dr. Sun as a bone-setter [zhenggujia 正骨家], but as the description below makes clear, he did a lot more than set broken bones.) Sun and Guo were from the same hometown. The doctor had long lived with a severe limp, his lame leg possibly a result of polio. After Guo had spent eight months in the provincial hospital with no improvement in his condition, he was discharged because "there was nothing more they could do," and he turned to Dr. Sun, renowned in the region for his "magic hands" (moshu zhi shou 魔术之手) and master of a wide variety of haptic technologies and physical therapies. Guo had been brought to Sun's clinic on a daily basis for the past six months, and many special techniques had been tried. It sounded as if the state of his body when he left the hospital had been unbearable. When we asked him, he said that when he turned to this Qiang medicine clinic, he had been experiencing extensive spasmodic cramping and flexion of his arms and legs, he could not lie flat on a bed, and he could not rest. He had no feeling below the neck.

Dr. Sun started him on a routine of massage, acupuncture, moxibustion, cupping, and other forms of physical therapy. The plan that had been in place for almost the past month was this: Guo would spend three hours, starting about 3:00 p.m., strapped into a specially made frame that held him vertically against the wall, facing into the main room of the busy clinic. This posture was meant to improve muscle tension and take advantage of the downward flow of qi and blood (which bodies experience in the afternoon) to return sensation to Guo's lower limbs. After three hours in the vertical frame, Sun or one of his associates would administer a long massage, especially using the technique of digging an elbow into the muscles at acupoints. This kind of massage reaches the inner parts of a channeled body: the treatment had already begun to normalize Guo's bowels, and his perception had improved enough that he had sensations when urinating and defecating. For a while, strong massage would be followed by heating the urinary bladder channel and points along the spine by burning gauze soaked in medicated wine just above the skin, but because of Guo's generally numb perception, they decided the risk of burning his skin would be too great and switched to a series of herbal plasters targeted to stimulate those channels with heat factors. Everybody would finally go home about 8:00 p.m.

Trooper Guo told us that he has regained some feeling in his feet and can now take a couple of steps with assistance. His ability to move his arms and shoulders above the lumbar vertebra is also coming back, and the muscles of his whole body are much more relaxed; he is no longer afflicted with constant cramping. Dr. Sun, his associates, and all the clinic's regular patients are happy to see progress in Guo's condition; it has been a long time coming. But Dr. Sun is well aware of continuing difficulties. He pointed out that Guo has been ill for so long, he not only still lacks strength in his lower back, he has chronic wind and cold factors blocking the fine hairs and pores of his body. Under these conditions it is difficult to achieve wholesome throughness (*tong* 通). Moreover, the spinal ligaments have long been affected by adhesions. Though he has treated cases of injury almost as bad as this in the past, Sun is not at all sure how much of a recovery can be achieved.

Clearly, Dr. Sun's magic hands have more than one therapeutic trick to use. In his explanation of Trooper Guo's history, he used concepts and tools from biomedicine (adhesions along the spine), TCM (cold wind, heat stimulus), and from local Qiang herbal medicine (custom-made plasters). This *ad hoc* eclecticism is familiar to us in both nationality medicine and many clinics of TCM; we have seen a lot of this kind of practical integration (*jiehe* 结合) over the years. Surely his magic was more than just a lucky mixture of methods from different traditions? We could speculate: perhaps his own old injury and resulting lameness gave Patriot Sun a special sympathy for the body of his young patient? Perhaps Sun's delightful personality and his way of running a collective physical therapy clinic full of stories and jokes were intrinsically therapeutic? Or maybe it was just his patience with illness, his and everyone's willingness to spend five hours a day, every day, doing little interventions that never had any dramatic effects.

We are inclined to see all of these things as significant. But perhaps even more impressive than this collection of magic tricks was Dr. Sun's admission that he really didn't know enough about Trooper Guo's body to hope for a full recovery. All he could do was keep working on the surfaces and the disposition of this badly reduced body, aiming to reach some basic processes deeper in the interior (the downward flow of qi and blood, using heat to drive out wind and cold) with his haptic techniques. We suspect his approach to this "unknown land" that is the body was similar to Laborjoy Wei's: "How do changes on the skin influence the inner parts? That we just don't understand. But the influence is for sure." These two nationality medicine specialists are agnostic about both anatomy and the "holistic" physiologies theorized by their textbook-writing colleagues. But they are intimately familiar with bodies, and they do not require that there be only one sort.

CONCLUSION

In the latter parts of this chapter we have attempted to read through medical practices—especially haptic techniques that perform "microsurgery" on surfaces—to discern a variety of ways in which the bodies of sufferers are imagined and addressed. Looking back from Patriot Sun's clinic, where Trooper Guo represents a minimal version of lived embodiment, at the chapter's other and more mobile examples, we are most impressed with the down-to-earth physicality of the southern bodies treated by nationality medicines. One could think of many metaphors that would illuminate aspects of the local practices and local knowledges we have presented here: not just lowland and mountaintop tree leaves, but irrigation hydraulics, perhaps, or a road network, with Three Ways and Two Roads. But metaphorical images, useful as they can be, are only partly helpful to the healers and writers we have considered in this chapter. There is no such thing as a comprehensive metaphor or allegory for "the human body."

The seasoned healers who explained things to us in our southern mountain field research were ultimately better at showing their curiosity and openness to novelty than they were at imagining figures that could exhaustively represent local bodies. In their clinics, storefront pharmacies, and farmhouses they coped with very concrete, familiar complaints and breakdowns in ever-new combinations. Practitioners of nationality medicines have a rich toolkit, they know how to knead and tweak skin and muscle, push and pull qi and blood so that a particular embodied life can go on a little improved, a little more vigorously. But they do not know bodies per se as discrete and autonomous organisms subsisting in an external environment. When "heaven and the human act as one," a healer needs to treat every "case" of illness as a unique gathering of forces, some internal, some at the skin surface, some external. This active locus is hard to know but rewarding to engage, with magic hands.

CHAPTER 4

Plants

In the third century BCE, the philosopher Zhuangzi breezily sketched out a curious natural history:

> The seeds of the myriad things are the most minute works. In the water the seeds become Break Vine, but on the shore they become Frog's Robe. If they grow on the hillside they become Hill Slippers; if Hill Slippers find good soil they become Crowsfoot. The roots of Crowsfoot turn into maggots and their leaves turn into butterflies. Soon the butterflies transform and turn into those insects that hatch under the stove: . . . they are called *Quduo*. After a thousand days, *Quduo* become birds, whose spit becomes *Simi* bugs; *Simi* are the bugs that eat wine dregs. *Yilu* bugs are born from those wine-eaters, *Huangkuang* bugs are born from *Jiuyou* bugs, and *Maorui* bugs are born from Rot Grubs. Sheep's Groom grass couples with old bamboo . . . , and this coupling gives birth to Green Serenity bugs. Serenity bugs give birth to leopards, leopards give birth to horses, horses give birth to humans; humans then return to the unfathomable works. The ten thousand things all come out of the works, and all return to the works. (*Zhuangzi zhuan* 18, "Perfect Happiness")[1]

This dizzying passage has long been seen as illegible. Even though the text is teeming with concrete things, and the relationships between these "ten thousand" things are stated clearly, it is confusing to moderns partly because the names of many of these plants, bugs, birds, and leaping animals are unknown to us—we have no idea what creatures these words denoted. Plus, all that "becoming," being "born from," and, finally "returning to the works" (what works?) is implausible. Zhuangzi (or the member of his school who wrote this rather apocryphal "outer chapter") could not have been stating facts about nature. Or could he?

Zhuangzi expresses, with his exuberant myriads—his creepie-crawlies, leopards, humans, and the mysterious "works"—a familiar kind of love for the spontaneous and ever-changing natural world. Natural historians around the world and in differing historical eras have been empiricist, instrumental, commercial, nationalist, and imperialist. But they have always been more than that. Their science has shown an excess of affect: the work of natural history has never been a dispassionate objective science, concerned only with classification and its "narrow, skimpy, quasi-monopolistic" imperatives.[2] Even stolid, nationalist classifier Carl Linnaeus in eighteenth-century northern Europe read the Great Book of Nature with a "naïve ecstasy," translating nature's language into a sermonizing taxonomic poetics and, comparing himself to Adam in the Garden of Eden, claiming to bestow the true names on living things.[3] Two hundred years earlier, in the agricultural heartland of China, Li Shizhen assembled his magisterial *Compendium of Materia Medica*, a now-classic work that expresses its author's fascination with both classification of natural things and transformations among them.[4] Equally fascinated by metamorphosis in nature, Maria Sibylla Merian (1647-1717), working in the seventeenth-century Netherlands, folded the spaces and times of plant and insect ecologies together in her early and gorgeously illustrated field entomology.[5] Henry David Thoreau was enchanted by the "fugitive vitality" of the plants he encountered as he hoed his garden and botanized in the partly wild forests of Mount Ktaaden.[6] Colonial-era British plant collectors explored the mountains of south China in search of flowers and shrubs for Victorian gardens (and some of them found their twenty-first-century poet in anthropologist Erik Mueggler).[7] A French East India Company functionary in Orissa cataloged and painted hundreds of South Asian plants with translations of their medicinal uses, attaching a humble disclaimer about the partiality of his knowledge compared with that of the local "fakirs."[8] All these observers of nature, both armchair classifiers and ramblers and trekkers in field and forest, added to natural historical knowledge as they gratified their love of nature.

Gathering medicines in the mountains (*shangshan caiyao* 上山采药) is China's old and new way of talking about and enacting natural-cultural networks. Like Linnaeus and Thoreau, Merian and Li Shizhen, and like the Yao nationality Granny Waterstreet mentioned in the preface, grassroots peddlers and herb collectors of southwest China travel to and through the forests. In doing so, they enjoy both a rough life in the wild and the "farm family joys" of local hospitality. Itinerant herbalists are fewer now than they were before China's rural areas were reorganized into agricultural communes and managed forests, but there are still plant lovers roaming the high forests, finding and learning nomad science from plants, animals, sun and rain, rivers, streams and landslides, and—not least—local healers.

The relationships of all these grassroots natural historians with what

Zhuangzi called the ten thousand things have been passionate and appreciative; they all flirted with notions of the natural, wilderness, excess, otherness, distance, and rarity. The practical manifestations of a love of plants, however, have been very down-to-earth. Modern botany and zoology have a laboratory life, but at heart they are field sciences. Knowing wild and natural things everywhere and every-when has been the work of many people, of hands and feet, eyes, noses, palates, stomachs, intestines, strong backs to carry collections, discerning senses to take note of tastes, smells, textures, an understanding of subtle changes in one's own body. Knowing wild things has also demanded the patience to observe life cycles and seasonal changes and to understand the behaviors of diverse actors in ecological networks.

But though these many forms of love and labor—in Europe and the Americas as in China—have all been practical and embodied, they have not been identical around the world. Far from it. Nature and its creatures are not the same thing to all these passionate collectors. We will show in this chapter that the relationships southern Chinese healers have with the forest products they collect are very local, in some cases extending not far beyond the bodies of users and lasting not much beyond the treatment of a single instance of illness. The skills involved in gathering natural medicines in the mountains are difficult to describe, almost impossible to render as history or knowledge. Despite this recalcitrance, we will here attempt to trace, in part, the love life of some healers and some forest things.

In what follows, we first provide brief examples of local practices of gathering medicines in the mountains in order to identify general features of southern mountain engagements with the myriad things of the forest. These local practices include both travel to learn and teach herbalist lore and hands-on management of drugs. We also return to our overall theme of *gathering*, asking Heidegger, among others, to propose a philosophical language (of things, of distance and distancelessness, of forms of action) that can accommodate the thickness and specificity of minority nationality healers' local passions for medicines. Those who gather medicines in the mountains are not only doing botany and natural history; they are folding the things of the forests into their own growing and changing lives. And they are doing so in ten thousand ways.

The bulk of the chapter, therefore, is devoted to the work and lives of four healers and their helpers in Qiang, Yao, Lisu, and Li areas. Each of these experts is famed for a different orientation to the powers of the ten thousand things to heal, a different local way of gathering a life in nationality medicine. The chapter distills and differentiates their styles of thought and approaches to healing, as they presented these complex kinds of experience to us in our visits to their homes and clinics. We conclude with a reflection on a natural drug brought to market from the wild forests, treating it as an emblem of the (net)work of gathering it embodies. Such objects, understood in practice, hold lessons for thinking about history, nature, and the social.

ITINERANT KNOWLEDGE

Itinerant herbalists (*caoyi* 草医) have traveled through the southwestern mountains for as long as anyone there can remember. The uplands of Sichuan, Hubei, Hunan, Guizhou, Yunnan, Guangxi, and Anhui are famous for the diverse plant resources and high-quality herbal medicines they yield. These lush forests, with their rough tracks and scattered farms, attract healers and pharmacists from far away. Such traveling herbalists are small businessmen who ramble on foot (*manbu* 漫步) in medicine-rich areas, then sell what they gather to doctors in towns and farmsteads. Even when they don't do much business, they gather knowledge. They collect medicinal plants in their assiduous field study, making both botanicals and information useful in a nomad medical practice.

Caoyi travel is important to the history of salvaging and sorting local nationality medicines. This kind of itinerancy facilitated knowledge exchange among practitioners both in and outside of schools, research institutions, textbook publishing, and public health information systems. Though there were probably many more traveling herb peddlers before the hegemonic establishment of the CCP-led state, it is still easy to collect stories from healers about their experience of "medical exchanges" (*yiyao jiaoliu* 医药交流) covering a wide area. In Hubei, for example, a retired village doctor we visited attributed his extensive knowledge of local wild drugs to the frequent visits of herbalists who came every summer from Sichuan, especially in the 1970s and 1980s. These *caoyi* taught him how to recognize, collect, and appreciate the powers of local wild herbals. Throughout southern rural China, street markets in every town include vendors offering medicinals in the form of dried or fresh whole plants; roots, fruits, and rhizomes; and dried, smoked, or powdered animal parts. These small entrepreneurs still travel to many markets in a region, offering their wares to all kinds of customers and—especially since market reforms began in the late 1970s—operating under the radar of market or public health regulatory agencies. Some vendors have only a few "especially effective" remedies for sale, like the "wild mountain bee's honey" we saw for sale in Hainan. Even those market vendors who have a wide selection of locally known herbal drugs for sale often specialize in one or two items that—they will explain—are of especially high quality and unique to their own collection.

Some larger towns and cities have permanent herb markets, open daily.

At the Shuijie (Water Street) Market in Nanning, the provincial capital of Guangxi, vendors with identified ethnicities and formal licenses sell a wide variety of medicines from permanent stalls. The Yao nationality healer befriended by our assistant Fang Meijian (see preface) had traveled throughout the south as an herbalist when she was young, and with her daughters (who work from other stalls in the same market), she still frequently returns to their rather distant home area to replenish her supplies of home-processed wild drugs. "Granny Waterstreet" had a wide reputation as an effective herbalist in Nanning City. Most market herbalists are not just market vendors, they also advise on illness and perform treatments. Some market suppliers, in Nanning sandwiched between vegetable markets and specialists in dried, chopped, powdered, and compounded herbals, offer fresh herbs along with cooking tips and advice about the mundane uses of their leafy wares in medicinal meals. In the Water Street herbals market, it is not unusual to see a client with part of his back bared and sterilized with medicinal wine sitting in a herbalist's stall receiving an acumoxa cupping treatment or having a little blood let with a local needling technique.

In Jinxiu town, the county seat of a Yao nationality region, streetside herbalists consult on illnesses and on how to use medicines at home, while also providing therapies such as massage, herbal plasters, and minor bloodletting. These hands-on services are offered in association with the sale of herbals collected in the wild; apparently they are not thought of as clinical medicine. During one of our first visits to Jinxiu we enjoyed a ceremonial lunch with the very dynamic and ambitious director of the county health bureau. As we noted in the preface, she was a supporter of Yao medicine salvaging and sorting initiatives, but much more concerned in practice with local people's access to quality biomedical health care. Even so, she recommended that we visit the herbal medicines street market to learn more about Yao medicine from the herbalists who had traveled there.

Of course it is not just itinerant specialists and traveling salesmen who gather medicines in the mountains. Almost every healer we spoke with in every region said that he or she ventured uphill to study and gather wild plants as often as possible, though some indicated that the press of clinical work, or physical problems of old age, or the receding forests, were making it impossible to go as often as they might wish. Not all expeditions to gather wild herbs are literally undertaken in mountains, and it is not even always necessary to go uphill from villages and farms to find good medicinal substances. Indeed, many valued wild drugs thrive best along the edges of fields and roads, places where people have cleared away trees and brush, opening sunny land not only for crops and traffic but also for vigorous and medically powerful weeds.[9] What is important in this often reiterated claim to have gone into the mountains to collect wild herbs, this ubiquitous reference to *shangshan caiyao*, is its authoritative image of *travel*: departing town life to enter a less cultured space where there is much to learn about the habits of natural substances, and many linkages to be made between the world of human needs and desires and the myriad qualities of wild things in the upland forests.

Though in some cases specialists' claims to be gatherers may have been little more than wishful thinking, some who were especially serious about their gathering—as a source of unique medical resources, and as a foundation of their healing authority and therapeutic efficacy—took long treks lasting a week or two, several times a year. On these expeditions, medicine collectors said that they identified remote locations where specially desired varieties of rare drugs flourished at particular seasons and under particular niche conditions. Some also said that they gathered carefully to ensure that the populations of natural things they were harvesting would be able to reproduce and flourish, guaranteeing a good supply in the future.

Many herbalists told us that in expeditions to gather in the wild, because it is necessary not only to recognize but to *taste* potential medicinal things, experts need to carry herbal antidotes to poisons along with them. A well-administered purgative, for example, could save an herbalist's life—even though it makes him ill—when he is far from home. In speaking of their history of gathering, healers emphasize that they taste to know: they get down and dirty with plants, taking unknown things into their own bodies and attentively noting the results. With these experiments on themselves, they think up ways to recruit the wild and the unknown into therapeutic procedures; their understanding of the powers of plants is in this very direct sense embodied.

Trusted healing expertise results from a kind of travel, the personal, physical activity of going up into the mountains (*shangshan*) to manually pluck herbs (*caiyao*). Contemporary herbalists seek to close the distance between the medicinal plants depicted in ethnobotany texts and their own and their patients' experience. They make an issue of drawing near to locally specific plants.[10] A little skeptical of book learning, herbalists care about authentic encounter and direct contact. Below, for example, we turn briefly to the work of one Mr. Wellness Qin, a herbalist who had many digital photographs on his laptop of the plants he had found in the forests around his Guangxi village home. He spent his weekends in the woods, catching mushrooms in the act of springing up from the forest floor or proliferating on tree trunks. Many other healers showed us how they consult botanical handbooks to check their observations and hunches about the plants they gather; but they are skeptical about published materials, which, they say, tend to inauthentically or unreliably represent medicines from afar and across a distance. In the itinerant work that gathers qualities and efficacies into therapeutically useful forms, healers and herbalists move through their home region, looking for recognizable or promising plants, animals, and minerals occurring in the wild. As they climb, examine, dig, and pluck, they draw near to plants: they observe characteristics, taste and smell and feel for qualities, test for efficacies, and evaluate ways to usefully place new things, and pieces of things, in existing and evolving meshworks of health practices.[11]

Traveling alone or with one or two trusted disciples, these local herbalists and healers cultivate a personal expertise that links the scattered growth of plants with the medical needs of human bodies. In this process, they not only assemble collections of natural medicines, they gather together a practice of healing organized around their own knowledgeable, experienced persons. No wonder those itinerant herbalists who travel through drug-rich regions are respected by locals for their nomad science. Their long and difficult experience of gathering medicines in the mountains makes them figures of an almost uncanny authority.

HANDS ON

As visiting anthropologists, we cannot fully imagine what any particular herbalist or healer knows or embodies after many years of trekking through nearby mountains to pluck herbs. We can, however, bear witness to a general fascination with natural medicines as things in themselves, a fascination shared by almost everyone we have met in the course of studying the development of nationality medicines in southern China. We met a rubber farmer in Hainan, for example, who collects dried herbals to help her pharmacy-student daughter. As she collects and carefully preserves leaves, roots, and flowers between sheets of newspaper, she denies knowing anything special about medicines. Yet as she was showing us what she had gathered, she had a lot to say about the use of these drugs to treat common ailments: "I am no expert, I just know what to give for indigestion or the sniffles."

Her collection reminded us of the botanicals that a senior doctor of Yao medicine, Carrier Li, showed us in his hospital's research unit. Ignoring the carefully labeled color pictures ranged along the wall, Dr. Li preferred to show us the plants themselves, paging slowly through his well-documented plant presses. He was, predictably enough, displaying the authentic collections to visiting researchers. But we were impressed with his loving reverence as he revealed one dried plant after another and recited their names. We have met other true experts who are devoted to plants as well. One Zhuang village doctor we visited had a small botanic garden on the rooftop of his private clinic. During our visit to him, a hospital pharmacist traveling with us was thrilled when he saw a medicinal plant he had only heard of but never seen. Our professional companion rubbed leaves, tasted, smelled, and photographed this potted plant for his own collection.

We have watched health department cadres in Yunnan clamber through streamside garbage to cut wild mint (*bohe* 薄荷, a digestive) to take home, even uprooting a little for transplantation into urban pots. Traveling in Hubei with a historian of Tujia medicine and his driver brother-in-law, we found that the driver's knowledge of and interest in plants was as deep as or deeper than the scholar's. The two of them often scrambled through roadside weeds to study an interesting plant they had spotted from the car. During our travels with local researchers, no street market could be passed without our companions stopping to discuss medicines with the sellers of herbs. What looked to us like featureless chunks of wood became treasured finds: in the course of a Guangxi road trip, our Zhuang clinician friend Laborjoy Wei bought a woody chunk of sargentodoxa cuneata (*da xue teng* 大血藤) and then carried it through all our visits for the rest of the day, pointing out its rarity and interesting features to everyone we met. Two Tujia medical historians, neither of them clinicians of "nationality medicine," display samples of important local herbs in their book-lined studies, happy to talk about the special qualities and efficacies congealed in these objects.

And Mr. Wellness Qin, a farmer in Zhuang country, goes uphill every weekend to gather herbs, carrying a camera to document plants *in situ* and adding the photographs to his laptop computer database. Not only does he see patients in his village, he contributes his collected observations to the medical practice of his friend, a storefront doctor in town, who often joins these weekend rambles and shares this collector's fascination with the plants themselves. The two of them specialize in combining Zhuang herbal medicines with divination and ritual treatment of attacks by magical parasites (*gu*-worms, 蛊). Qin's little gallery of family snapshots on the wall of his sitting room had more portraits of mushrooms than of people.

Wild things take part in settled human lives as sustenance, instruments, and partners; they collaborate in social networks alongside human devices and the activity of other nonhuman actors. Experts not only study them *in situ* and collect them but also sort, preserve, transplant, refine, dry, grind, boil, mix, and roast them. The powers of wild medicines are routinely enhanced and transformed by the skilled labor, the processing, of those who heal with natural drugs. These herbalists know a lot. But everyone, expert and amateur alike, talks about plants, the forests, and even the mountains as only partly known. The most experienced gatherers are well aware that plants and other forest things harbor secrets; the objects herbalists seek and use withdraw some of their properties and characteristics from human view. This is why everyone we met was still so immensely curious, so sure that he or she could always find (and taste, and test, and use) new efficacies in the mountains. As they touch and taste, disentangle vines and dig for roots among wild plants, herbalists and healers enhance their own dwelling in place and focus local powers toward their own very human ends, while acknowledging that the ten thousand things have ten thousand propensities of their own.[12]

THE GATHERING OF THINGS

In the personal stories we recount here, we privilege the work of those who heal with natural drugs: their deliberation, attentiveness, humility, and creativity. By attending to their practices of gathering—collecting not just herbal drugs, but also knowledge, teachers, disciples, patients, experiences, and selves—we also glimpse the world of the ten thousand (scattered) things in which they do their work. The healers who are our chief access to this scattered and gathering world incorporate a partial perspective on southern Chinese lived natures and cultures: partial because rooted in place, planted. In solidarity, then, with the passion for plants and concern to heal displayed by our southern mountain interlocutors (researchers and healers alike), this discussion tries to sustain a focus on things and actions together, or *things as actions*.

The specialist world of medicine in China is familiar with the notion of "the thing" as active. A senior doctor and philosophical polemicist in Beijing, Lu Guangxin, for example, has contributed to the "theoretical foundations" of Chinese medicine with a discussion of the entities recognized in medical practice.[13] He uses the word *duixiang* (对象) for objects like qi, circulation tracks, and the compound organ systems such as the Triple Burner (*sanjiao* 三焦) and the Life Gate (*mingmen* 命门). But *duixiang* is not a term that can refer to an anatomical structure or an inert and discrete chunk of material existence. It is more like an object of attention, a salient companion, a partner in action. A *duixiang* object is active in a network of social (but not solely human) relations.

Recent "speculative realist" philosophers, in similar efforts to resist the naturalization and universalization of self-evident and inert objects, have revived interest in Heidegger's key essay, "The Thing."[14] The essay distinguishes between *objects* (e.g., objects of attention, topics for scientific representation) and *things*, which "stand" and "act" but have "subterranean depths" that "never become present to view."[15] The thingness of the thing, *because it is active*, constantly escapes our grasp (rather like Lu Guangxin's *duixiang*). The object, however, appears to be present-at-hand and know-able, usually as a discrete individual entity (named by a noun).

In the same essay Heidegger worries about what he sees as a modern flattening of space and time, the "distancelessness" characteristic of our highly mediated world, which comes to us, as often as not, on a screen. "Nearness" and its corollary farness have been almost abolished, he suggests, in a regime of universal representation.[16] He writes: "Nearness, it seems, cannot be encountered directly. We succeed in reaching it rather by attending to what is near. Near to us are what we usually call things. But what is a thing?"[17] Perhaps Wellness Qin, the mushroom collector we spoke of above, answers questions like this in practice. Comfortable both with the flat digital catalog of plants he has built on his laptop and with the smell, feel, and loamy forest homes of mushrooms, he is a master of nearing (and "farring"). His *duixiang* fungi hold pride of place in his life, right alongside his family snapshots.

To think things as actions while writing in an English language that is strongly biased toward the noun is not a simple task. A certain "suspicion toward grammar" is required.[18] For one thing, we suspect the noun in English of performing a metaphysics that insistently reifies relations, processes, qualities, and all the other active things in the world to which words might be taken to—somehow or other—refer. The commonsense language ideologies of modern Anglophone materialism presume a one-to-one correspondence between words and items in the world, discourse and nondiscursive objects. Language *performs* a world for us in a thoroughly emergent way: if there is a word for it, we presume, the object referred to must exist, parked more or less stably somewhere accessible.[19] In this research on local medical practitioners and their foundational practices of gathering things for use against illness (going up the mountains to pluck herbs), however, we have not encountered things as self-evidently always-already existing.[20] Rather we have tried to trace the pathways through which things gather and are gathered into efficacious existence, and how they transform (as well as who they transform) in particular situations.

In this effort, Heidegger and his readers have helped to focus our anthropological attention. At one point working from an etymological discussion of old German and Latin words for things, and sharing our grammatical suspicion, Heidegger justifies his tendency to speak of "thinging" (rather than, for example, positing a Kantian thing-in-itself) with etymology: the word thing (or *Ding*) originally referred to a *gathering*.[21] The elaborated example of "the jug" in his essay is shown in several discussions to bring together certain properties, or, better, *acts* of standing, taking, keeping, and pouring or giving. The jug's *thinging* is not ultimately a matter of its own making or of

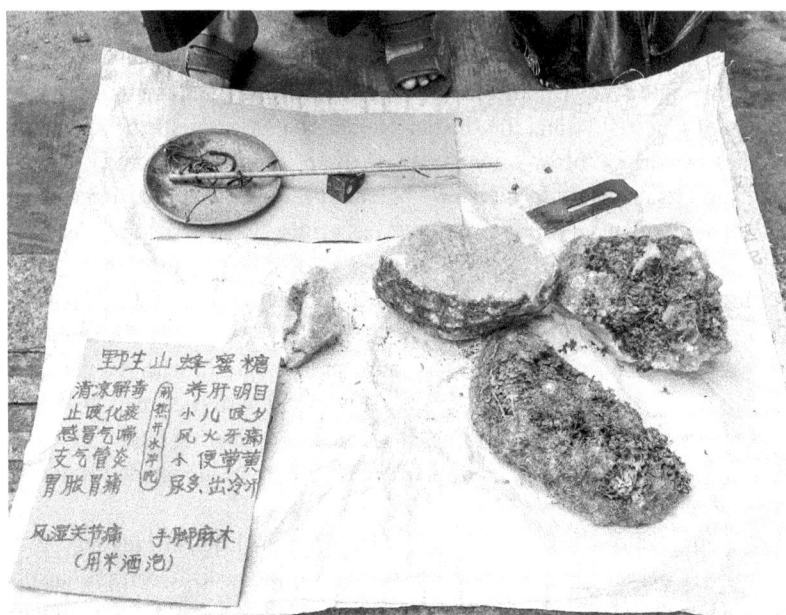

Figure 4. Wild mountain honey for sale in a street market, Hainan Island.

the materials from which it is made; rather it is the gathering of a void—the far-from-empty space gathered and held by the jug—that can stand, take, keep, and give, acting as a thing that things.[22]

This activity is responsive to situations, relative to present states of play among things. Again and again in the course of our itinerant field research, when members of our teams asked herbalists "what is this plant good for?" they replied, "it depends on the situation," or "it depends on the patient's illness." Consider, for example, the long list of efficacies advertised for the "wild mountain bee's honey" we found in Hainan: according to the hand-written sign provided with this medicine we saw for sale on a market street, it clears out cold pathology and breaks down heat poison (*jiedu* 解毒); stops coughing and breaks up phlegm; treats colds, bronchitis, and difficult breathing; reduces abdominal swelling and stomachache; nourishes liver system and improves eyesight; relieves wind-heat toothache; and treats rheumatic joint pain and numb extremities. This is not an unusually long list for a natural medicine, especially when it is being marketed on the street or incorporated in a comprehensive textbook. In any given case of illness, only a few of these healing powers would articulate with the patient's situation and thus become active in use. Doctors know how to narrow the range of claims made for any medicine they learn about from dealers or read about in books, but they also know about the flexibility and responsiveness of drugs to situations.[23] Much of their own gathered expertise has to do with their ability to play along with the affinities (*xi* 喜) and aversions (*wu* 恶) "natural" to plants and bodies in the encounter between a gathered medicine and a pathological situation.[24]

Medicinal plants—gathered and contingent as they are—are certainly things in Heidegger's dynamic sense, but we also witness them becoming, at times, objects in his sense.[25] That is, in healing they are objects of attention, present-at-hand tools for human actors, *duixiang*. The way in which things gather (drawn from an infinitely heterogeneous scatter), stand (each in its own particular and temporary way), and act as things for Heidegger, Lu, and Latour is quite similar to the active ways of healing we present in this chapter. In the more detailed healers' stories to which we now turn, we have witnessed the actions of thousands of herbal medicines, animals (like bees), organizations (like local health departments), texts (like textbooks and case notes), roads, fields, breezes, sunshine and rain showers, regulatory policies, research laboratories, and many differently positioned people (healers and patients, families and researchers). All these things circulate, connect, gather, live and die, each in its own way, and put down roots in China's southern mountains.

"SCIENCE IS LIMITLESS, AND SO ARE HERBS": VIRTUEFONT LI

In the short review of natural histories that opens this chapter, we emphasized the passions that have driven botanists and other field scientists in many places and times. In China's southern mountains, the daily life and medical practice of every herbalist we met offered evidence of a similarly concrete, personal nearness to natural drugs. Every healer is different, though, and each herbalist we met taught us something unique about nationality medical lives. To demonstrate, we now take up four distinct nationalities and idiosyncratic situations at greater length.

We begin with love of plants. It was one of our Qiang nationality hosts in the Wenchuan (Sichuan province) area, Virtuefont Li, who during our 2012 visit most forcefully showed us how intimately engaged a good healer should be with the mountains and the things that live there. We were introduced to Dr. Li and his son in a welcome dinner on our first visit to Mao County in postearthquake Sichuan.[26] Li and his son came to this gathering after work; he didn't eat much, but he drank and smoked a lot. Later he said to us that his daily clinical work in the county town exhausts him, and—perhaps in order to be sociable—he needs the stimulation from smoking. He tells us he started to smoke after the 2008 earthquake, which was when he was invited to open a clinic in the county hospital. In our visit the next day to his clinic, we encountered an anteroom full of patients who had come from all over the region to seek out Li's renowned Qiang nationality herbal medicine. He was obviously much in demand, and he told Zhang Dan, one of our researchers, that under this pressure of work he had a constant headache ever since he had "come down" from the uplands to this "urban clinic."[27]

Virtuefont Li turned into a completely different person when we accompanied him and his son to his house in the countryside, on the weekend. Like many others in Mao County, which was much damaged in the 2008 earthquake, he lives in a relatively new house, near a brother and his family, perched just below the stone ruins of his family's old extended family compound. In this mountainside site, where his family had lived for three generations, he was more talkative and obviously happier. He smoked only a couple of cigarettes during those two days, in comparison with his nonstop smoking in the county town. What struck us most, though, was his attention to and intimacy with the plants in and around his home, and the way he spoke in that setting of respecting nature, "the great self-so" (*da ziran* 大自然). One thing he constantly mentioned to our companion Zhang Jing, a Qiang medicine researcher trained in pharmacobotany, was "everything given to us by nature can be medicine."

Though he still goes farther up into the mountains regularly in search of wild herbs, Li has also planted about twenty different kinds of herbs in the hillside ruins of his grand old Qiang-style house. Leading us into this ruin-turned-herb garden, Li Lao was happy and relaxed. He told us that along with his transplanted varieties, there are also many different kinds of wild herbs in these partly reforested plots. "If you had come earlier, you would have seen masses of wildflowers blossoming from those herbs, it's breathtaking," he said. Zhang Jing noticed that he also planted wild herbs in pots in his courtyard to "test" the possibility of domestication. She described the scenario in a conference paper:

> While I was looking, amazed, at Li Lao's wonderful collection of herbs in his yard, he suddenly pointed to a plain-looking plant and asked me: what do you call this? I thought he was testing my knowledge, and I answered honestly: "I don't know." But with a smile, he said, in all humility: "I don't know, either." It turned out that this plant was a recent discovery in the mountains, and he had already shown it to be effective in certain illnesses in his clinical practice, so he gathered some more and brought it home to see if it would grow in his yard. Since I was here, an "herbal expert" from a Chinese medicine university,[28] he thought he'd take the opportunity to learn from me. His sincerity and humility greatly surprised me. As a re-

nowned Qiang medical doctor who has been practicing herbal medicine for many years, Dr. Li is nevertheless still actively pursuing knowledge of plants, not taking his mastery of herbs for granted. This also reminded me of the phrase he often said to me: science [*kexue* 科学] is limitless, and so are herbs.[29]

In this report from a field encounter, Zhang Jing emphasizes Dr. Li's "sincerity and humility" before the wonders and powers of the plant world. By reminding her that "science is limitless, and so are herbs," he was, perhaps, referring to his own scientific life as a doctor who deploys natural products as tools to intervene in human illness. All the working clinicians we meet in China are quick to point out that diseases are myriad, "doubtful and complex" (*yinan zabing* 疑难杂病), and therapies must be tailored to the particular illness situation if there is to be any hope of a cure. Dr. Li was not unique in his "sincere" appreciation of the manifold healing powers that "nature" makes available to the science of medicine.

In our conversations with him, though, not only was Li humble before nature, he was active in gathering for human purposes. He was always talking about medicinal plants: how to find them, how to dig them up, how to transplant and grow them from seeds, and how to assess the quality of herbs. From his childhood he had started to learn from his father how to recognize, pluck, and process herbal medicines, as they farmed and gathered in the area near their big house; now he not only uses herbs to treat illnesses but also shares a great interest in propagating herbs along with his three sons. He talked, for example, about panax notoginseng (*sanqi* 三七), a "precious species" from Yunnan, which he has been planting here as an experiment to see if it will thrive this far from its native environment.

When we first visited the Lis, Dr. Li's youngest son was practicing with him as his assistant and disciple in a clinic in the county hospital, and his second son was an herb farmer (*yaonong* 药农) working around their mountain home.[30] During the week, while Dr. Li and Li Junior are in their hospital clinic, the second son takes care of the herb gardens around the ruins and ventures further up into the forest looking for more elusive wild plants. He proudly showed us some fritillary bulbs (*beimu* 贝母) that he and his father had successfully cultivated from the wild plant. In fact, the Li family has entertained the idea of establishing an "herbal medicines base," where they could harvest their own herbs such as Chinese angelica (*danggui* 当归) and astragalus (*huangchi* 黄芪), two herbs that, like fritillary bulb, are commonly used in Chinese medicine. With an herbal medicine base, Li and his family would be able to both guarantee a supply of high-quality natural drugs and establish a base for their healing practice away from the onerous regulations of the county hospital. Dr. Li complains, for example, that many herbs purchased on the market and sold from the hospital pharmacy are speed-processed using sulfur. He considers this wrong, so he would rather plant near home and also process herbals on his own land in his own way.

The intimacy between Li and his plants is palpable. As Zhang Jing concludes in her essay cited above, not only did Li inherit an understanding of medicinal plants from his ancestors, who all grew up in the mountains and had been gathering and healing for years, but this sensibility was also built up day by day in an embodied practice. Dr. Li's often-voiced distrust of purchased herbs has even led him to avoid using the hospital pharmacy just down the hall from his weekday clinic. In his daily practice, he insists on using medicines "of our own," meaning gathered by him and his sons from the mountains, or planted in their own gardens.

Virtuefont Li's clinic imported some of the magic of gathering medicine in the mountains into an urban institutional setting. His consulting room was also his pharmacy, the walls lined with dried herbs and powders sorted into plastic tubs in large metal shelves. We estimate that more than two hundred different kinds of herbs were available there. Departing from the usual clinic practice of senior Chinese medicine doctors, who mainly diagnose patients and write a formula on a prescription form for a pharmacy located elsewhere, Li Lao after examining each patient turns around to look at the herbs on his shelves, mentally formulating his prescription in the process of seeing, contemplating, and assembling herbs. He then gathers what he needs by handfuls from the boxes and bins around the room. Unlike pharmacists of Chinese medicine, he doesn't use a scale to measure the dosage in grams. After Li Lao finishes assembling the herbs for one dose, with every ingredient displayed separately on a sheet of newspaper, Li Junior, his disciple, studies the "formula," quietly concentrating on the ingredients arrayed before him in piles. He learns their combination by heart, then proceeds to assemble the herbs for the second and third doses. Though the younger Dr. Li is a college graduate and quite literate in Chinese (his father is officially "illiterate"), he too gathers the herbs by hand without using a scale. Dr. Li said to us later: this is like cooking, you feel it in your own hands (*zhei jiu hao bizuo cai ma, ziji shouxia shi you ganjuede* 这就好比做菜嘛，自己手下是有感觉的).

Local people in Mao County refer to Li Lao as a "divine healer" (*shenyi* 神医), an appellation that refers mostly to the unusual effectiveness of his therapy. And Dr. Li is not above claiming near-magical powers as he discusses his history of discovering and applying local remedies. He told us that he had saved his own leg with herbal medicines after suffering a serious laceration far from home, amazing doctors a week later when he finally went to show them his healing wound. In that incident, his knowledge of how ritually charmed water (*huashui* 化水) can be used to treat wounds was a helpful added measure. Residents of a village near the county town all know how he brought a pancreatitis patient back from the edge of death with his amazingly effective treatments. Indeed, Li Junior drove us to this patient's house for a visit, hoping to impress on us the exceptional quality of his father's healing powers. And even Virtuefont Li's embodied person is known to have a special auspiciousness, or perhaps a special relationship to the mountains: some we talked to wanted to tell us how the old herbalist had nimbly dodged falling boulders and trees as a landslide took out the mountainside where he was gathering medicines alone. He emerged from the forests after the earthquake without a scratch, everyone said. Surely this incredible good luck and miraculous efficacy (*miaoshou huichun* 妙手回春) bespeak a special relationship with this place, his patients feel. But when we ask Virtuefont Li whether he is really a divine healer, he deflects the credit for his success to the herbs themselves: "Any doctor can do well, all he needs is herbs that can do well" (*yisheng dou neng xing, zhi yao yao de xing jiu de xing* 医生都得行, 只要药得行就得行). Once again we could appreciate Dr. Li's sincerity and humility before the diversities and powers of (what he calls) nature.

Virtuefont Li does not live in a world without distances. Perhaps especially because he seldom reads or writes Chinese, relatively little is mediated to him as a "world-picture."[31] He is acutely aware of the physical cost of his weekly treks up and down the mountain between his formal clinic and his home-based practice. He seemed to us never happier than when he was climbing slowly over the forested slopes near his old home, traversing nearness and farness, speaking to us of the even farther away (and farther uphill) sites where wilder plants grow, and handling natural medicines with an eye to their efficacies in the diseases he would be seeing in the near future. He still cares about his town-based clinical work, expressing his intention to serve the earthquake-traumatized population living around the county town.[32] In his presently rather too itinerant life, he draws near to both plants and people; he literally and manually puts drugs of the forest together with symptoms in bodies. The powers that are set in play as these two kinds of life are brought together, if they are to be wholesome rather than dangerous, require the gathered expertise of his whole lifetime of humbly making herbs useful in his (relatively) nomad science.

GATHERING AND CULTIVATING *LING*-EFFICACY: SPRING INCENSE FENG AND SELENA HUANG

One common term for speaking of efficacy in modern Chinese is *ling* (灵, agile, adept, flexible). The most common noun compound in use is *ling-*

yan (灵验), usually translated as "effective/ness." Especially powerful medicines are *lingxiao* (灵效), so *lingxiao* also means the specific efficacy (of a drug). Other word compounds refer to quick intelligence and responsiveness (*lingxing* 灵性, *lingmin* 灵敏), virtuoso abilities and ingenuity (*linghuo* 灵活, *lingqiao* 灵巧), nimbleness (*lingbian* 灵便, *lingkuai* 灵快), and inspiration (*linggan* 灵感, *lingji* 灵机). The special powers of respected gods are *ling*, and the most common word for the individual human "soul" is *linghun* (灵魂). The transition zones surrounding death and the funerary are often marked with compounds of the word *ling*.[33]

Most of the senior nationality doctors we met, like Virtuefont Li, were locally known for their *ling* powers. All had cultivated expertise and efficacy in their years of gathering medicines, techniques, and insights, both through their teachers and on their own. Some of them had worked mainly outside the public health institutions in which TCM and biomedical services were locally provided; some claimed a special relationship with the yin side of things and could combine ritual with drugs and manipulations. Ethnic healers garnered authority from a certain "wildness" while facing the increasing hassle of being slowly marginalized by the new royal institutions of nationality medicine. (See chapter 1.) But one retired couple we visited in Jinxiu county town demonstrated that it was possible to be a healer—even a "divine healer"—while living in close relation to official structures.

Dr. Selena Huang and Dr. Spring Incense Feng, a married couple who are retired county-level officials in Jinxiu (a Yao nationality autonomous county), told us charming stories of gathering herbs in the surrounding Great Yao Mountains. They both come from families who practiced medicine in that area for generations, and they saw patients clinically even when they were working in administrative jobs that had little to do with medicine. Dr. Huang had been the party secretary of a county administrative office, while her husband, Dr. Feng, was retired from the county public health bureau. Spring Incense Feng had been a leader in the institutionalization of Yao medicine for several decades, helping to shepherd a Yao ethnic medicine clinic and then a hospital into existence from an initial "herbal medicine base," a collective farm that cultivated local herbs for use in Han Chinese medicine (TCM). Dr. Huang's first job had been as a barefoot doctor, and in that position she received some basic training in biomedicine and TCM from the later 1960s into the 1970s.[34] Her mother had worked as a doctor in the county hospital, she told us. Counting her daughter-in-law, who runs a storefront clinic, and her herbalist granddaughter, who also trained as a nurse, in the family heritage, Huang said there are seven generations of medical practitioners in her family.[35]

Both Dr. Feng and Dr. Huang are critical of some of the new institutions of Yao medicine in Jinxiu County, especially of the way they "pander" to health department regulations that privilege biomedical services.[36] Dr. Huang irritably denounced the muddles and mixtures of therapies she believed were going on in the county's biggest Yao hospital, and she insisted that it was possible and preferable to treat patients with purely natural, purely Yao medicines. Her husband had retired, she said, when it became clear to him that the work on salvaging and sorting Yao medicine was moving away from local expertise and local priorities. (She sometimes referred to this locality as nationality, so her critique was partly challenging the claims of the instituters to be offering genuine "Yao nationality medicine.") Though these two retirees remained in touch with many who still pursued official medical careers, and they were proud of their long careers in government agencies, both had now turned to treating patients outside of formal medical institutions.

Like almost all the healers we met, Selena Huang had often climbed into the mountains with the elders in her family to "find herbs" (*zhao yao* 找药). In this process she was always required to taste the herbs: her elders would tell her how to correlate the taste of an herb with what symptoms it is used to treat. During our interviews, her granddaughter in her twenties, sitting beside Huang, added that she too had tasted almost every herb she gathered. She knew what herbs taste most terrible: "some even taste pungent" (*la* 辣, like chili peppers), she said with a smile, being amused herself at the variations in qualities one finds in the forests. Meanwhile her grandmother firmly stressed, "you've got to taste them all." Dr. Huang went on to explain that some medicinal plants look very similar, so they need to be tasted to tell the difference. Meanwhile, tasting can be dangerous. Dr. Huang herself had been rendered unconscious for three days after testing an unfamiliar herbal medicine. She said, "Herbal drugs, after all, they're closely connected to human life. You must aim for perfecting [your knowledge], you can't have even the least bit of hesitation. If you're going to use this herb, you absolutely must have tasted it with your own mouth. That is to say, you must have tested it on yourself."[37]

In this connection Dr. Feng wanted to explain to us that the process of gathering herbs involved careful discriminations to maximize the *ling*-efficacy of even the most well-known plants. Taking the example of a famous poisonous herb, yellow jessamine (*duanchang cao* 断肠草),[38] he said,

> [Suppose] you see an herb growing nicely in the wild—whether it is a tonic or any other kind of [wholesome] drug, if you see *duanchang cao* nearby, you can only dig up the herb you want if it grows more than one meter away from that poisonous plant. The only exception is, if your herb

has grown about 1/3 to 2/3 of a meter higher than the *duanchang cao*, [you can gather it]. But if it is growing lower, you must forgo it, even if that herb is really flourishing [at that place]. So! Gathering herbs in the mountains requires particular care. You must discriminate carefully!

Dr. Huang then added that "for a severely sick person, we have a particular rule: that is, the very first digging of the herbal plant for the treatment must go without a hitch. If we see worms in the soil during the digging, we will give up on this patient." We asked, "Does this indicate that your treatment won't work?" "Maybe other doctors can treat the patient," she said, "but we can't." Noting our puzzlement, the granddaughter said: "In such cases, we don't have a predestined relationship [*yuan* 缘] [with the patient], that's what my grandmother meant." Affinities and aversions, in other words, are part of the very makeup of the herbal and clinical object, and of the practitioner as well. A gathered substance or subject is not inert, not neutral toward the world. Drugs and people (and all other things) have their fated, inbuilt likes and dislikes, tendencies and leanings, and these affect how they will work in combination with other things.

Dr. Huang was arguing that the particular efficacy of drugs and treatments lies in the contingent doctor-patient relationship, as inflected by time (when to dig the herb), space (where to dig the herb), and even the foreboding agency of the worms. Efficacy is also inseparable from the teacher-disciple relationship, as manifested through relations with herbs. Dr. Huang told us that if a disciple betrayed his teacher in social relations, the herbs learned from the teacher would no longer be as efficacious in that student's practice; they would no longer be *ling*. Smiling at our dubious looks, she said,

> Our Yao medicine is that miraculous. You must apply [its knowledge] with sincerity. If you don't, the herb won't be as effective as it was when your teacher taught it to you. Not to mention, the process of selecting a disciple is crucial. Whoever comes to serve an apprenticeship must be faithful to her teacher. If s/he ceases to be faithful, then whatever herbs [s/he learned from the teacher] would thereafter stop taking effect on the patients [*Ta bianxinle, jiu bulingle* 她变心了，就不灵的].

Her husband, Dr. Feng, hearing this, added with a smile, "There are lots of tricks!" (*mingtang hen duo* 名堂很多).

In our second visit to the household of these two doctors, we asked more explicitly about ritual means of curing. As soon as we broached the subject,

Selena Huang laughingly pointed to Dr. Feng and said, "he knows how." She warmly praised her husband for his mastery of Daoist techniques. She told us, by way of example, about a child who would not stop crying at bedtime; treated by Dr. Feng with a few gentle pats, the child stopped crying immediately, without the use of drugs. Even on a later return visit, the child was still well. In another case, a woman who had been undiagnosable at the hospital came to Dr. Feng for help. He "drove out a ghost" for her, first rubbing her body and then squatting and flinging the ghost away; "it ran right out the door," Dr. Huang assured us. She relished telling these stories of successful curing using ritual means, but she was reluctant to claim much expertise of this kind herself—her reticence in this respect reminded us, indeed, of how severely "superstition" had been criticized in the years that these two worked in government agencies. But in the course of praising her husband's powers, she also says, "That hospital director said, these sorts of things are hard to explain, and anyway they are not observable. This is still thought of as 'superstition,' and whatever it is, nobody can explain it." But she certainly wanted to emphasize to us that these methods—which would certainly be called *ling*—clearly are effective.

In our experience throughout the south, in fact, casual conversations among medical people often turned to suffering caused by ghosts, witchcraft, and magical parasites (*gu*-worms), and ways of treating these afflictions. The concepts named with the word *ling* 灵 seamlessly combine practical effectiveness and healing magic. The retired Yao doctors Feng and Huang made this particularly clear—living as they did in the always magical Great Yao Mountains—but they were not alone in this. Storytellers in many places enjoyed surprising us, their urban visitors, with inexplicable events and strange apparitions; some even liked to boast of having mastered love magic and ritual antidotes. When State Follower Wang, for example, whom we visited in Lisu country (northwestern Yunnan), spoke of the healing talents of his village shaman (see chapter 1), our health department handler, Mr. Zhou, sighed and said, "Ah, there's so much that science cannot explain!" At first, this kind of remark from educated officials surprised us more than did the existence of ghosts. Later we began to expect to hear such agnostic attitudes toward "the supernatural."

Spring Incense Feng is not alone among Yao healers in combining Daoist ritual techniques with herbal therapies. His longtime colleague in Yao medicine development work, Carrier Li, liked to recount to us his systematic collecting of botanicals and his clinical career in government hospitals and clinics. Though he impressed us as a rather spiritual (if playful) person, with us he downplayed his ritual skills and experience. But he always carries with him a written amulet (a *lingfu* 灵符), and in private he had much advice for a local friend of ours about magically protecting herself from the hostility of an enemy.

Selena Huang speaks little about her own approach to ritual and magical healing, but one could count as magical her very intimate relationship with the powers of plant medicines. Her ordinary and domestic participation in the world of healing powers seemed to us to be of a piece with her hospitable and convivial ways of opening her home to visitors, feeding us, and inviting us to taste her homemade wine. She is a town-dweller living in an apartment, but like so many healers we met, she has a garden of commonly used herbals from the mountains transplanted into pots. They fill a corner of the paved courtyard behind her apartment building. The neighbors and her own grandchildren help themselves to these simples, she says, when they have a cold or aches and pains.

But what she really specializes in now is medicinal wines. Blending, bottling, packaging, and shipping medicinal rice wine even to some very remote parts of China, Dr. Huang is proud of her herbal products, which are good both as food and as medicine. She says she has gotten too old to spend time rambling the Yao mountains looking for wild herbals herself; but her home is only a short walk from the Jinxiu herbal medicines market street, where "herb farmers" (i.e., collectors, *yaonong*) offer many forest products and a few therapies of their own. We imagine some of these street merchants also sell Selena Huang's aged and bottled wine.

After we had sampled her wine made with *lingzhi* fungus (good tasting, and good for tonifying liver and kidney functions, supplementing germinal essence, calming the spirits, settling spleen functions, and more) and admired her attractive bottles of wine made up for sale, Dr. Huang showed us her small extra kitchen that functions as a lab, where she steeps natural products in alcohol. In addition to her large vats of medicinal wine for oral use, she also makes up bottles of alcohol-infused herbals for external use. One vat of wine (for drinking) was full of dead bees and ants floating in rice liquor, very good, she said, for rheumatic complaints. The bottles of medicine for external use were also for rheumatisms, but they were carefully labeled as "external use only." No doubt they included some drugs that were so effective as to be poisonous when ingested by mouth.

We think of Dr. Huang's pots and bottles of herbal-flavored alcohol as emblematic of the *ling* powers that experienced Yao medicine practitioners—in homes, on the market street, and in public institutions—have cultivated throughout their lives as healers. Recognizing, choosing, tasting, and even occasionally risking one's own life and health in coming to terms with wild plants; learning how to combine herbs (and insects and minerals) into useful medicines for common complaints; taking advantage of the enhanced *ling*-efficacy that rice wine can add to forest products (even when they are bought from dealers); building and maintaining family, community, and even official networks in which healing powers can be circulated as service to the people—these acts of cultivation produce experts and tools of a kind specific to the Yao Mountains. Like the steeping, fermentation, distillation, and aging processes Dr. Huang controls in her kitchen-lab, and not unlike the cosmic attunement her husband Dr. Feng expresses in his use of Daoist ritual healing, medical lives and liveliness are gathered in this place in a local Yao way.

But not just any gathering produces *ling*-efficacy. If this were the case, to hear Dr. Huang tell it, the conscientious and experienced doctors running the Yao Hospital would be much more *ling*. In her eyes most of these experts, with their biomedically compromised muddles of "impure" "non-Yao" medicine, have betrayed and vitiated the powers that can be assembled here. She and her husband, on the other hand, have gathered not only drugs and techniques, not only knowledge and skill, but a magical excess. Like the rice wine (a commercial product) in which Dr. Huang soaks wild ingredients that she (nowadays) buys from dealers, the experience, courage, and connections of these senior doctors have purified and intensified the *ling*-efficacy of Yao Mountains medicines into a local essence, the power of which can circulate in bottles far beyond Jinxiu County.

Dr. Huang thus had all sorts of ways of refining and purifying wild things into products that have *ling*-efficacy. However domestic, mundane, and comfortable her methods and her life seemed to be, there was a kind of magic in play in her household and family. Perhaps especially in the Great Yao Mountains, there is a taken-for-granted slippage between ordinary daylight effectiveness and social relations with gods, ghosts and ancestors. Wherever *ling*-efficacy is claimed or sought, the powers of those intimates who occupy the yin world of the shades are not far away.

We were reminded of this rather general principle, which is a staple of Chinese religious studies, by a nonmedical friend in Hubei. Chen Jie, the wife of a historian, was always full of stories of the uncanny that could interrupt work and travel and life in general. She invited us for lunch one day with her large tea-farming rural family. After we had arrived at her family farmhouse that morning, she took us up the hill behind the hamlet to see her grandmother's grave. "Make a wish, Lili," she said. "I often ask Nainai for a favor, and she is very *ling*, she always helps." This was not a ghost story. It was a remarking of some well-known *ling* powers of place. Families and their dwelling places too, almost unnoticed, gather extraordinary powers.

YINYANG EMBODIMENT: LASTING LOYALTY SU

In Yunnan province, across the Erhai (洱海) from the city of Dali, we visited a Lisu nationality healer who lived and worked in his farmhouse on the slopes of Chicken Foot Mountain. Lasting Loyalty Su considers himself to be a pretty successful Lisu doctor. Seven or eight patients a week navigate the rather terrible roads to come see him at his house. He tells us that he charges no fees for his services, and he never buys drugs, only gathering them in the mountains around his home and processing them himself. Like the other doctors we have discussed, he always "tastes" the drugs he gathers as he decides what they are good for. He subjects his body to their qualities and powers before he works them into his medical practice.

Su Lao's isolated farmhouse is very pleasant, with folk art motifs painted on the walls and plenty of orderly space, both indoors and in a large courtyard, for all sorts of farming activities. Once a year, the Su family hosts a birthday celebration for the Medicine King god, identified by a nephew as the historic doctor Sun Simiao.[39] There is a small and smoke-darkened shrine to the Medicine King over the stove, positioned just below the shrine of the God of Heaven and Earth (*tiandi shen* 天地神), with family ancestors in lower and smaller spots nearby. The one-day god's birthday party was reported to us as a very "hot and noisy" (*renao* 热闹) event. Sixty or seventy people, both former patients and relative strangers seeking treatment, navigate the rutted and partly unpaved mountain roads to come, bringing chickens, rice, wine, and other gifts. The day is devoted to kowtowing to the god and to Su Lao, feasting, and "playing." Though this is certainly a special occasion, combining eating, healing, and ritual, some form of respect for the Medicine King is maintained in this household year round. The rituals involved are an integral part of Su Lao's practice, and he avoids sharing them with other healers.

He told us that he had been practicing for only "six or seven years," since his father, also a healer, died. Su Lao was the ninth of eleven children, and the only one to take up his father's healing path. He thinks of this choice as "fated" (*yuanfende* 缘分的), but he only really started down this road as a result of his father's deathbed request. Before that, he never especially paid attention to the knowledge that was involved in his father's work, though he admits that just being around in the same household all those years, he probably picked up a few commonsense things. But when his father died, and the patients kept coming, he had to do something, so he started going out into the forest and up into the mountains to see what medicines he could find. He began to figure out his own system of healing practice through exploratory experience. As he put it, in the mountains he would "think and think and then pluck [the herb]." Tramping through the forested mountains near his house, "thinking on the one hand and gathering on the other," he came to embody a good understanding of the natural things, with all their affinities and aversions, that can address human illnesses.

Around the time of his father's death, and working to his father's deathbed specifications, he constructed an herbal medicine storage system for the pharmacy room of the house. This wall-mounted system of pockets, currently made of pink synthetic silk, held both single drugs and mixtures. Each pocket was labeled in magic marker with an idiosyncratic term. Seven pockets were simply "women's medicine" (1 through 7); others were named by their function: "stomach medicine," "cooling," "opening bones," and the very general "greater blood" and "lesser blood" medicines. A few terms were charming but could have functioned only as personal mnemonics: "field wildflowers," "summer wildflowers," "women's medicine flower pollen," and "cliff fruit." Faced with such generic and nonbotanical labels, the researchers in our team were fascinated; they wanted to identify the things themselves, if possible translating this collection into their known pharmacobotanical names. Su Lao welcomed them to handle and taste the dried herbs in any of the pockets, but when we left we were all still puzzled about what sort of herbal medicine, exactly, he had been practicing. Everyone believed that he was too uneducated to learn to use the standard names—all on his own out in the mountains as he was—and some felt strongly that he was "keeping secrets" from us. The pink satin pockets system was, however, a perfectly mundane and practical way to classify and name the things he used in his work with patients, and he was in no way hesitant to show it to us. The problem for our researchers was that he "spoke" a personal and thoroughly local therapeutic "language."[40] His coding of ingredients and functions was realized and named (and, presumably, practiced) in a way that left the botanists unable to read the language of his practice. For the experts, it was not possible to connect his words with things, his signs with referents, even though we were able to hold the drugs in our hands.

As we talked, Su Lao insisted again and again, in many ways, that no one had directly taught him his medical knowledge; rather, he had "just thought it up." As we pushed him on his history, we began to see that his use of the word "think" (*xiangqilai* 想起来, *xiangyixiang* 想一想) included a lot of processes: memory, hearsay, observation, tasting, classifying, analyzing, imagining, testing, and so on. Even the physical exertion of going up the mountains to pluck herbs, a process that he emphasized had helped him draw near to plants growing in only a few places, and one that had made it possible for him to observe how wild animals and birds benefit from a life lived in close association with wild plants, was part of his "thinking up medicine." In other words, in becoming a healer he had had a lot of help. But very little of it was direct teaching or information transfer: after their deaths, his father and grandfather[41] sometimes came to him in dreams to help him decide what drugs would work best against what illnesses. When they did so, it was because he was facing a particularly knotty clinical problem, and his ghostly teachers helped out by entering his sleep to convey their own useful thinking.

Like Virtuefont Li, Dr. Huang and Dr. Feng above, and like so many other healers we interviewed, he also spoke of a direct communion with the plants themselves, a sort of fellowship that he experienced through tasting and testing. He didn't know (or need) the names of the things he collected, but he had a special "fated" gift for understanding and using natural medicines. "I know through my own feelings" (*wo ziji ganjue* 我自己感觉), he told us. Actually, his whole career as a healer was fated. He was the only one among eleven siblings to follow his father's path as a healer, and there was even some doubt about whether his father had realized, before his death, that Su Lao had what it takes to develop a special relationship with the worlds of plants and other powerful agents. But he certainly claimed a special relationship now, and his powers also seemed to be acknowledged by his friends, relatives, and neighbors.

Su Lao, even as he shielded his special herbal knowledge with his illegible body, as it were, was willing to admit that he knows a thing or two about divination and ritual healing. His nephew explained that he hesitates to talk about it because of the "bad name" such things have gotten. Though he was certain that such techniques should never be shared, perhaps not even with one's own disciples, at least in life, he was willing to generalize about ritualized relations with gods and ancestors. All his medical skill and understanding, he said, is *yinchuande* (阴传的)—brought from the shadows, or handed on by the shades, having its source in that *yin* other side that is inevitably paired with the well-lighted *yang* world of the living, the public, and the explicitly named.

This made immediate sense to us when he said it, as we talked with him and his nephew, as we took pictures and scribbled notes in his sunny courtyard. Everything he had told us about how he had become a doctor, and how he continued to gather and deploy healing powers, was in some sense private, or kept just out of view, even though he had answered all our questions more or less willingly. His curing skill, his selection by "fate" for a life of healing, his accumulated knowledge gained from trekking and plucking in the mountains, his father's and grandfather's nighttime help, even his unfamiliar filing and naming system for dried herbs—all these occupied a kind of interior of things, illegible to our curious researchers. Indeed, it was not just we who were kept at a distance: Su Lao's powers as a healer were not conveyed in detail even to his nearest family members.

The ability to gain understanding and healing power from the yin side thus seems to fate its possessor to rather solitary work. Su Lao had no interest at all in "scholarly medical exchange," either with state agents (like us) or with other Lisu medicine practitioners. Nor did he seem anxious to recruit the abilities of his clever nephew or educated daughters as his disciples,[42] so they could learn (and perhaps convey to others) the embodied skills and habituated judgments of healing work. He claimed that no one presently accompanies him on his tramps in the uplands to gather herbs. His dreaming relationship with deceased teachers takes place in the yin hours, in the dark. His very carnal process of thinking is organized through the illegible and private patterns of his own practical life. When he performs rituals of respect to the ancestors and the Medicine God, these invoke the yin side of the world. And even his personal system of classifying and labeling his stored herbals is impossible to translate into the terms of the yang world of nationally known medicines. The drugs themselves hide in the light of explicit but unshared labels.[43]

It would be reasonable to see Su Lao as a very typical folk healer, one for whom local or Lisu nationality knowledge and power are naturally embodied. Even he sees himself as operating at a remove from official published knowledge and as inventing in practice his own system, which only he knows, materializing it with his whole life and putting it to work in the service of his neighbors near and far. We are sure that his patients, and the guests who come to his birthday celebration for the Medicine King, see him as incorporating healing power in his very body, able to transmit the *ling* efficacies of "women's medicine flower pollen" and "cliff fruit" through his personal collecting and handling of these things, which remain in the shade for us.

But as Judith Butler has suggested in her book *Bodies That Matter*, materiality itself is socially and historically constructed.[44] We—researchers from far away—had sought out Su Lao with the expectation that his medical expertise would be secreted in the solidity of his body, his house, and the forests around him. We were guilty of finding exactly what we expected to find, and Su Lao—it could be argued—knew just what to perform for us. We were all taking (nationality) bodies to be the very essence of materiality, and presuming that this materiality—the opaqueness to us of Su Lao's medical practice—was the foundation of his healing legitimacy. In other words, why did Su Lao encode what he knows and what he does in such impenetrably embodied but practical terms, and, especially, why did he perform this embodiment on the occasion of a visit from highly educated, official researchers? Ultimately, we do not think his refusal of conventional discourse is a cynical manipulation of our team's expectations of the "nature" of "the folk." (Indeed, he showed few signs of even being interested in what our group knew about Lisu or any other kind of medicine.) Nor is his practical orientation a mere performance of healing charisma intended merely to draw in credulous patients. Rather than see Su Lao as an "embodied" exemplar of Lisu or Chinese mountain healing power, a clear "other" to the "salvaged and sorted" formal knowledge that is being rationalized into new institutions and publications in China (as discussed in chapter 2), we prefer to learn from him a certain cosmological stance.

Recall Su Lao's own vision of his expert power: it is brought into the yang sunlight from the shady and hidden side of his world. What he knows and does is transmitted from the yin. The yinyang dynamic by which a yang stimulus produces a yin state of completion is, as scholars of Chinese medicine and premodern science have argued, fundamentally temporal.[45] Emergence is yang, and it is always followed by a yin phase of consolidation; yang is an action that makes a difference, its yin result falling into the background as an achieved and conservative state (which nevertheless harbors the seeds of yang emergence). In the context of this chapter, we like to think of yang as naming the "equipment," or relation, or transformation that is present-at-hand, and yin as the domain of the unnoticed, "out there," but always ready-to-hand.[46]

As Judith has previously argued in connection with the logics of the clinical encounter in Chinese medicine, a yinyang dynamic makes the classification and correlation of things possible.[47] Thus, the domain of death and the invisible world of gods and ancestors is classified yin, not merely because it is dark and cool, but also because it is a phase of transition between the open, warm, yang initiatives of the living and between successive yang states of overt activity. The yin and yang worlds cannot be divided from each other, or bounded like territories, because their things—which are always relations, and always decomposable into other yinyang processes—shift in the course of a day, a season, or a year, like sun and shadow on a hillside. As transformations between active and passive, stimulus and response emerge, some things are occluded, or put in the shade, even as others come to light. Seen as a formation of time, yinyang is common sense, as clear as day and night, winter and spring, or the hand of the potter and the stoneware jug it makes.

The fated affinities and *ling* skills transmitted from the yin side into Su Lao's mind and farmhouse, emerging in meshworks of plants and patients, kin and household altars, do not suggest that bodies or drugs, ancestors or gods, are massy things-in-themselves. But the healing powers that come to light in Su Lao's work are not especially mysterious, nor are they really secret. He may deliberately, or even polemically, present his tools and learning as embodied, and he may hope that we will not be able to translate his expertise into a "Lisu medicine" that can be taught—and profited from—far away. But his reliance on the yin side of life makes for a practice that is concrete and material beyond the body proper, one in which the play of light and shadow in the world can be worked with to increase the nimbleness of his gathering powers.

NEARING PLACE AND POWER: PRECIOUS CASSIA WANG

Heidegger opens his essay on "The Thing" with a denunciation of a certain flat "distancelessness" that he especially associates with a highly mediated modernity. We are familiar with this notion under different names: rapid globalization, information technologies that eliminate time, empire, a universalizing neoliberalism.[48] Perhaps the critical concern is an increasingly common form of experience that seems to dematerialize or virtualize everything, as "the world" comes to us on screens, as a world picture. "The Thing" proposes a resistant understanding of lived spacetime, focusing on processes of thinging and—just as important for us—nearing.

When we look at healing in the southern mountains from the point of view of modernist anxieties about materiality, movement, and gathering, the experience of going up the mountains to pluck herbs by hand seems particularly significant. There is hardly a healer in these parts who does not claim to assemble his/her authority and efficacy through personal movement, across rugged distances, to establish and maintain relationships with medical things—including, for many, other healers—both near and far.

Precious Cassia Wang (whom we addressed as an older sister) is a Li nationality healer who practices herbal medicine in Hainan Island with her daughter-in-law disciple. Like so many others we met, she has traveled around her home province, often with others interested in herbal medicines. She is well-known to locals as a person who knows herbs. Her life is a good example of the complex intertwining of a mediated or "distanceless" world, which has become plausible throughout China, with a practical activity that does not collapse near and far and that resists reducing the herbal thing to an image, or picture, or item of information.

Sister Wang and her daughter-in-law work both from their home and from an open-air "Farm Family Joys" (*nongjiale* 农家乐) restaurant they have established nearby, next to the parking lot of one of Wuzhi Mountain's

tourist hiking trails. The restaurant serves meals featuring the wild vegetables the family gathers, and there is plenty of space under its canopy for a
well-stocked and carefully labeled pharmacy as well. At the family house,
there's also a pharmacy where the washing, sun-drying, and packaging of
the herbs that both women gather on the mountain are done. Sister Wang
spoke of her excellent recipes for medicinal versions of congee (rice gruel),
and at the house we saw her stores of medicinal wine, which is not only
drunk but also used as an external medicine in the bone-setting part of her
practice.

At the restaurant we were invited to admire a large framed color photograph of Sister Wang meeting with then-premier Zhu Rongji on the occasion of his "inspection and survey" visit to Wuzhi Shan in 2002. The picture shows her elaborately dressed in Li nationality costume, surrounded
by smiling neighbors, shaking both hands with Premier Zhu, who is pressing a "red envelope" containing (she told us) 600 RMB into her hand.[49] The
caption reflects her rather sudden national recognition as a "Li nationality
folk herbal medicine specialist," but it also emphasizes that this was a personal, even physical meeting (*qinqie jiejian* 亲切接见) with a central national
leader, one who had come a great distance to visit a remote village.[50] More
recently, in 2005, Sister Wang was respectfully visited and interviewed by
Beijing's leading intellectual in the field of minority nationality medicines,
Professor Zhu Guoben.[51]

Wang's local reputation is much thicker, however. She is known in Hainan as a true healer, an "herbals king" (*yaowang* 药王), and a local authority on medicinal plants. Indeed, we found her with the help of two sisters named Yang who are among the very few educated authorities to have
published on the characteristics of Li nationality herbal medicine. The Yang
sisters' main book is an illustrated guide to Hainan's medicinal plants and
their uses in local Li nationality medicine.[52] Like many other local and regional herbal medicine handbooks—a genre that was revived into national
importance in the 1970s and 1980s—this handbook, *Collected Specimens of
Li Nationality Folk Herbal Medicines*, gathers photographs, names, and identifying information for several hundred Hainan plants, arrayed one or two
to a page over 150-plus pages. This kind of reference work is a particular historical intervention in minority nationality knowledge, with a complex relationship to the practical knowledge embodied by Sister Wang. One part
of this relationship is very direct: In our two visits to Wang's place in Wuzhi
Shan, and after several visits to the Yang sisters' clinic in the county town,
we began to realize that Sister Wang had been a very important consulting
resource for the two textbook-writing sisters.

We were thus surprised to hear Sister Wang say that she was illiterate. We found this a little hard to believe, especially as we admired her very orderly and well-labeled shelves full of herbals, both in the restaurant and at her home. She said that her son and daughter-in-law help her keep these stores in order and do the labels; and at one point, too, she indicated that the Yang sisters had taught her some procedures for running a pharmacy of natural medicines. On another occasion, though, she said her (also uneducated) father had taught her everything important about herbal pharmacy work.

Yet there is a deeper story about this family's literacy. As we asked Sister Wang about her own history of learning and teaching medicine, she wanted to explain why she, and her father before her, had never received even a minimal formal education. With some bitterness, she suggested that her family had once been local elites (and thus highly literate), in her grandfather's generation and before. But in Maoist times "we weren't allowed to learn," and because it was impossible to practice herbal medicine privately in those times, because farming was controlled by the collectives, and because there was just no money around, "we even had nothing to eat." This story imparted (to say the least) some greater significance to the menu of "wild vegetables" displayed in the restaurant—Wuzhi Shan's natural vegetable life must have helped to sustain the family for many of the "hard years" of the famine (about 1959–61) and during the time of the agricultural communes.[53]

What kind of knowledge does an "illiterate" local woman like Sister Wang command? To us, it seemed uniquely tied to this place, which seemed remote even with its nearby tourist traffic. We noticed, for example, that local usage in Hainan tended not to refer to medical work as *kanbing* (看病), looking at illness, in the usual Chinese way; rather, experts spoke of "finding medicines" to match the illness situations they must address. Wang said, "When a patient comes, I find the medicine then" (*bingren lai wo jiu zhao yao* 病人来我就找药). This mundane usage, replacing a cognitive contemplation of an illness object, or *kanbing*, with an embodied project of searching for good tools, *zhao yao*, departs from modern protocol-driven practice in both Western and Chinese medicine. Sister Wang, though she was helpful with us and willing to work through a language barrier to talk about her practice, no doubt felt that we would never understand just what this searching and finding really involved. Indeed, she has little confidence in anybody's ability to "understand" plants and illnesses, flavors and efficacies in her special way. Like other healers we have met, she used the word "understand" to distinguish between those who can really *find*, *see*, and *use* powers and those who just have language and images for plants and diseases.

Seeking to get a sense of how Wang had been sharing her expertise over many years, our colleague Dai Shuiping, a TCM herbal medicine specialist, sat down with her to go through the Yang sisters' pharmacobotany text. Looking at the pictures, Sister Wang confidently rattled off useful information about every item. At times she wanted to argue with the text, pointing out, for example, that the drawing for a certain plant was wrong or misleading. We could easily see what a great resource she must have been to the formally trained and rather scientifically oriented Yang sisters. She spoke of spending many days with them in past years, wandering in the mountains, identifying, photographing, gathering, and discussing plants. Though nowadays she spends little time in town at their clinic, her contribution to the province-wide movement to develop Li nationality medicine is long-standing.

But as hinted above, Sister Wang's understanding of local herbals is of a particular kind, rather different from what ended up in the only full-blown textbook. She was not able, for example, to identify or provide a rationale for the "characteristics" (*xingneng* 性能) or "nature and flavor" (*xingwei* 性味) of the plants, which are the properties supplied with each item classified in the book.[54] These terms identifying each drug's "character" had been provided by the authors of the book, and in fact we still want to know by what means the Yang sisters and their editorial colleagues decided on the proper functional properties and classifications of all these previously unreported entities. We do know something about how Sister Wang comes to understand the character of these local drugs, however. She tastes them.

She tastes them fresh, while gathering them, and teaches her daughter-in-law as they go to recognize particular types of plants and degrees of efficacy within each type; she compares herbals by taste, classing together things whose similar qualities and efficacies she infers in this process. Having done so, she can then substitute one plant for another, depending on availability, as she composes prescriptions. And she understands (without explaining to us, or perhaps even to her disciple) how certain flavors reach and match certain disorders and discomforts in human bodies. When we ask her to compare her process of recognizing and classifying drugs with that of the Yang sisters, she says, "When it comes to treatments and recipes, they just don't understand."

This is not to say that the Yang sisters are bad doctors when they use local medicines (though Sister Wang seems to have had reasons to imply that they are). Visiting the Yangs' clinic and talking especially with the older sister (like Wang, a former barefoot doctor) and people who were waiting around, we could see that she is respected as an especially sensitive and even rather prescient doctor. Moreover, she too tastes the drugs: during one of our visits she was recovering from a rather serious gastritis that had resulted from her taste-testing an unfamiliar drug, more toxic than she expected. Though she seemed physically fragile, she is, like Sister Wang, proud of her long history of wandering Hainan's mountains to find medicines.

Sister Wang has had similar experiences of incorporating the powers of medicines, putting her own body and health on the line as she finds herbs for the illnesses that come to her for treatment. Taste for her seems to be literal; having so little use of writing, she seemingly must bypass the standardized classifications of drug properties to keep possibly idiosyncratic classification tables in her head, as it were. With regard to Wang's practice of tasting medicine, she seemed to us quite like a good cook: when she assembles a medical prescription, she doesn't weigh or otherwise quantify the amounts: "just grab some in your hand, that's good enough" (*zhuazhua duoshao jiu xing* 抓抓多少就行), she advised us.

Sister Wang's home village is now in an ecotourist area, with signs at the parking lot base area near her restaurant identifying the place as the "Wuzhi Shan tropical rainforest scenic district." Hainan Island as a whole is a popular tourist destination, known for its beaches, a few remaining high tropical forests, and superb seafood and fresh fruit. Though Wang has made a place of business among the food vendors and boat rental companies who serve the daypack-toting crowds that are disgorged by the tour buses, she also draws a local clientele who appreciate her as a different sort of natural resource. As she claims to have told Premier Zhu Rongji, "Li people from all over who don't want to go to the hospital show up on my doorstep looking for treatment."[55] Especially effective in cases of kidney stones, acute nephritis, uremia, arthritis, cirrhosis of the liver, and hepatitis—these are the biomedical terms supplied by a reporter interviewing her—her herbals also assist her successful bone-setting practice. Thus her carefully collected and stored medicines, some of them "secret formulas," are powerful enough to reach and alter the interiors of sufferers' bodies, bringing the natural *ling*-efficacies of the plants she has been studying since she was a girl near to the human symptoms they can alleviate.

The restaurant where we met Sister Wang and her daughter-in-law is just across the river from their home, which itself is just at the edge of a small Li nationality hamlet. Despite all her botanical sophistication, and her background of consulting with the nationally known herbalists, the Yang sisters, Sister Wang impressed us as especially planted in this beautiful spot. These days, her patients tend to come to her. Her consulting for Hainan's only comprehensive herbal pharmaceutical guide is now finished, and she seldom goes to the county town a long bus ride away.[56] Her most cosmopolitan moment, the meeting with Premier Zhu, just seemed to deepen this sense of local rootedness: she was, after all, wearing Li ethnic clothing for the occasion that was photographed, and she was "representing" her community for the premier's "inspection tour." Yet her continuing mobility—gathering medicines in the mountains, for example—and her way of staying in place are linked. Unlike the tourists who trek through Wuzhi Shan looking at the scenery with their eyes and cameras, Wang Jie engages eyes, mouth, feet, digestive tract, and hands in finding, drying, tasting, identifying, and combining medicine. She draws near to healing things with her whole body. But however much healers like her may play with titles like "herbals king," they would never claim comprehensive knowledge of the plants in the mountains. Indeed, they often believe that a lifetime of going up the mountains to pluck, and coming back down to offer gathered healing things to people, is required if they are to be intimate with some essentials about life.

CONCLUSION

In a 2012 visit to Achang communities in Yunnan province, we met a high party cadre running a "legal affairs" office in the county government building. As we noted about Evertrue Zhou in the introduction, he identifies as a member of the Achang national minority, and he talked at length about his and others' activism in developing ethnic culture, medicine, and history in the area. In his urbane and rather administrative manner, he is not much like the rural senior healers we have discussed in this chapter, though he shares with them a deep enthusiasm for local things. He spoke also of developing his own research, and when we asked what that would be, he said, "I'm interested in bees." This seemed odd to us at first, until we recalled the small beehives we had seen attached to the walls of many farmhouses and thought of the medicinal claims made for bee products in small-town markets and big-city boutiques. Perhaps from this cadre's perspective, Yunnan bee culture is as broad and deep a topic as Chinese tea culture might be for others.

We have several times mentioned "wild mountain bee's honey" in this chapter. In its very materiality and thingness it speaks to all our themes: gathered local powers, the agency of things, the cultivation of unique healing expertise in long lives of engagement with the forest. Honey from the forests congeals a great deal of mobility by a great many agents into what looks to the customer in the market like a solid, stable lump. But this wild product has been consummately gathered. Bees wander the mountains, gathering pollen from plants that thrive in deep forests and along the edges of cultivated and cleared areas. The plants on which bees draw to make honey exist because of the flight of seeds and spores in the wind, they grow upward above rhizomes tunneling underground, they ramify branches and unfold leaves toward the sun, and, especially, they flower. Great collectives of bees accumulate plant pollen in hives, where it is refined and combined and purified—gathered, our philosophers would say—into a thing we can carve out as honey.

In the same way, itinerant herbalists and village-dwelling healers go up the mountains to pluck medicines, tasting, collecting, transplanting, and piling plants into their homes and clinics (as Virtuefont Li and Precious Cassia Wang do). It is in these workplaces that almost all "natural" medicines are processed—at least with culling and sun-drying—to enhance their efficacy and improve their combinatory affinities. The natural substances thus gradually gathered, with the addition of much human thinking (à la Su Lao), experimentation, and labor (like Selena Huang's wine-making), are very often assembled in human collectives (like hives) and into herbal assemblages (*yaofang* 药方, formulas).[57]

Yet like the lump of wild mountain bee's honey reposing in a market stall with its qualifications as a drug listed alongside, herbal things are decomposable, and more knowable, in use. In the market stall where we saw this wild mountain bee's honey, the vendor had a scale handy for weighing small amounts and a strong hand-blade for breaking off useful pieces. Small broken-off pieces of wild honey, put to use in a customer's home, with her own wine or boiled water, dissolve to manifest this drug's efficacy as a sort of partner to other qualities. Its powers to soften the discomforts of rheumatism or to settle coughing with its sweet nature (*xing* 性) unfold in practice, as a lumpy yin-forest thing reorganizes into a yang-active drug, in human homes and human bodies.

Honey is not one of the more powerful drugs in use in southern China. The list of efficacies listed alongside the lump of honey could be seen as a little too long; experts tend to be suspicious of "cure-all" claims made by sellers. But customers want to know what kind of *ling*-efficacy might come into play as they themselves use it. We don't imagine they are surprised to find that it folds itself around their own circumstances, not curing everything, but lightening some particular burdens. The diverse minor powers of this honey, as listed, can be seen as a gathering of collective healing experiences—the people who have discovered that wild mountain bee's honey is good for bronchitis or rheumatism, coughing or swelling, have contributed their successes to local lore about drugs.

And it is local, the bees have seen to that. Their nomadic labors congeal and materialize *place* in this object. No honey I could get at a North Carolina farmers market would be likely to have this same set of efficacies (though it might have others). We think of the many strands of activity that brought this lump of honey into existence, took it to market, and have made it an issue in this chapter as a process of drawing near to the wild. Patients with rheumatism or a cough, a stomachache or numb feet, apply a wild thing, a bee-and-plant-and-human-gathered medicine, to their condition. This kind of canny healing action brings the unknowable wild to bear on uncontrollable symptoms. The proliferating changes of the ten thousand things, the *shengsheng huahua* (生生化化) of the world, may be myriad, but they are not chaotic. Zhuangzi, the ancient natural historian cited at the beginning, also said: *Human life is a gathering of qi: when it gathers, this is life; when it scatters, this is death*. Healers who gather medicines in the mountains learn over a lifetime how to play the changes to benefit human lives. But these trekkers and tasters, peddlers and compounders, also know their place in nature. Neither humans nor bees are fully in charge of the scatter of natural powers and hazards. Rather, everything is always gathering, like seeds from the unfathomable works, drawing things together to serve for a time as human medicine within the unknowable scatter of the myriad things.

CHAPTER 5

Encounters

"Give me one matter of concern, and I will show you the whole earth and heavens that have to be gathered to hold it firmly in place." This is Bruno Latour adopting—with his "whole earth and heavens"—an idiom quite like that of an ancient Greek or Chinese philosopher.[1] The reference to Archimedes' pivot that can move the world is clear, of course. But we also note in Latour's mention of gathering a similarity to the metaphysics of Zhuangzi: "Human life is a gathering of qi: when it gathers, this is life; when it scatters, this is death."[2] Human life is certainly one matter of concern in both anthropology and medicine, and our challenge—if we follow the philosophers—is to find better ways to witness the vital gathering, and more effective means to help "hold it firmly in place."

Yet the earth and heavens that can be observed at work, realizing and stabilizing things and knowledge and institutions and even bodies, can never be seen or shown as a whole.[3] The contemporary agents of the Chinese state, with whom we have pursued a number of questions in these pages, know that their findings as they conduct surveys of folk medicines are always partial. So do rural healers in nationality areas as they keep returning to the mountains to gather medicines, from which natural things they continue to learn. Anthropology might multiply the points of view from which the salvaging and sorting of traditional medicines can be perceived and described, thereby assembling a broader view of a contemporary social landscape. But it cannot offer a comprehensive account of any "whole earth and heavens" we might hope to grasp in the act of gathering.

No wholes, then. But the parts remain fascinating, and they lead us to the fringes of the knowable. Looking back over the chapters of this book, full as they are of stories from "the field," we want to show again how important these experiences were and are for us, and how they remain at the same time mysterious. We don't know if we truly understand the lives that have been shared with us in southern China. We don't know if the generalizations we have drawn out of them adequately account for this historical moment of nation and knowledge in China. Rather than generate a series of generalizing abstractions, then, in which we would finally have little faith, we turn now to recount and reflect upon some of the concrete encounters we were part of, in China's mountain south.

Anthropology research in practice is not much more than a series of encounters: meetings between diverse people, things, discursive traditions, matters of concern, socially constructed macro-agents (like healing gods or the Ministry of Public Health), language worlds, forms of expertise, and the mute infrastructures that give form to everyday life. It has been rather classic to characterize anthropology as the encounter between "Self" and "Other," and though we reject the cultural essentialism and individualist psychology implied in this model, we nevertheless hope to present here a further landscape of scattered "others."[4] Encounters of the everyday kind are full of surprises. Recalled as such, encounters are intrinsically unexpected, they are little accidents from which we learn something new, however trivial, however hard to articulate. When field research is understood as a historical scatter of unexpected meetings, anthropologists like Lili and Judith are easily decentered from these encounters. People and things are always coming up against the unexpected and the novel, even in the midst of their settled routines, and generally responding in interesting ways. In this chapter we seek to appreciate the richness and diversity of minority nationality medicines' everyday life of knowing practices.

In what follows we present a number of encounters (*xiangyu* 相遇) as we witnessed them and heard about them in the course of our fieldwork. By thinking in terms of encounters—rather than culture, or structure, or meaning—we are constantly reminded of the heterogeneity of experience as it gathers into events and actors.[5] In our efforts to talk with local healers, nationality activists, and cadres at several levels of government, we were often reminded of the distances that could still be maintained between the parties gathered in encounter. We perceived embodied identities facing each other, discrete and stable objects going back and forth, puzzles and mysteries complicated by irreducible distances—in other words, frictions and lacunae of all kinds.[6] The difficulty of working, orally at least, in many different local languages and dialects—a task at which Lili excelled but Judith despaired of mastering—is only the most obviously frictional dimension of the encounters we gathered in the course of research.

Perhaps the trope of encounter is particularly useful because we originally set out to study the relationship in practice of the Chinese central government and all manner of local agencies: It is rather classic to speak of how the modern state encounters the people, and certain questions that arise when one analytically divides "the state" from its people have inhabited this project from the beginning.[7] The very notion of a grassroots level of Chinese life—a phrasing that we have tried to avoid throughout this study—presumes that there is some superordinate agency, a macro-actor that can see and attempt to manage all the gathering and scattering micro-actors "on the ground."[8] But we also think that it is in encounter that agencies and institutions become perceptible as separate and objective, not to mention as large or small, weak or powerful. And it is in encounter that we discover all the ways that historically constituted actors are unable to dissolve into each other because of their stubbornly different natures.[9] Yet when forces gather, when actors meet, when communication (*goutong* 沟通) is hoped for, unexpected transformations occur on all sides. Insofar as an encounter is an event, participants whose lives swerve together for a time don't have the option of returning to a prior self afterward, or of restoring an earlier situation before any swerves happened.[10] An ethnography can observe and join in these changes. In this chapter, then, we conclude this study with a catalog of some productive encounters we witnessed, participated in, and had narrated to us while gathering medicines in the mountains.

TUJIA FRICTIONS

Herbalist Daybreak Li runs a well-stocked herbal pharmacy from his shop-front house in Qingshui, a small town in Hubei. When we visited in 2012, large bottles of herbal wine and dusty collections of woody roots, twigs, and rhizomes, mixed in with a few still-fresh leaves, were arrayed on tables next to the printed banner that serves as his advertising. Next to photographs of classically famous herbals and an artist's drawing of Li Shizhen (the seventeenth-century father of Chinese systematic pharmacy), the banner announced that here a customer would find "secret family heritage formulas" and could be confident that "when the medicine arrives the illness leaves." The sign listed the following specialties:

We mainly treat:
Mouth twisted after a stroke; sciatica; rheumatic numbness; stomachache and stomach ulcers.
For males: Gonorrhea, sexual exhaustion, inflamed glans penis, reopened wounds, joint pains.
For females: Excessive bleeding and discharge; infertility; menstrual discomforts; extending life and improving old age.

This list does not include everything usually encountered in a rural medical practice, and with the exception of rheumatic disorders—very prominent in the practices of southern mountain medicines—it doesn't even emphasize most of the illnesses we were beginning to see as usual. (One would have expected more emphasis on poisons, for example.) Right across the street from Dr. Li's shopfront is a government-regulated pharmacy offering "Chinese Medicines" and "Western Medicines," which sells a rather comprehensive stock of useful drugs. But Li Lao ("Old Li," as he was called by everyone) seems to do a good business despite the competition. Perhaps there's a niche market, even in a small town, for strongly gendered herbal medicine? But Li Lao was also advertising a special relationship with esoteric drug lore: in one corner of his commercially printed banner he had pasted a drawing of a botanical that only he offers for therapeutic use. This message was at least as attractive as his other announced specialties, along with the other note included on his sign: Medical consultation free of charge.

We visited this old herbalist several times in the course of the research. Our Tujia medicine collaborator Brightness Yang (a professor at the medical college of the Hubei College of Nationalities in Enshi City) found him particularly interesting and wanted us to have an opportunity to learn from Li Lao about his ways of gathering and using drugs and his herbal discoveries made in a long life of local practice. When we visited in 2012 (Lili's second encounter with him and Judith's first), we first spent some time studying his collections—during which he helped us by comparing his herbals with entries in decades-old botanical field guides for Enshi and Guizhou—and then we followed him up into the weedy slopes behind the row of shops to gather herbs. We followed almost invisible footpaths leading steeply up to fields where tea bushes were growing in orderly rows, with a few elaborate graves scattered among them. As we climbed, Li Lao pointed out a number of plants with medicinal value, growing wild in sunny places. He showed us where he had planted the popular drug *danggui* (当归, Chinese angelica) along the edges of the fields. We made our way through rows of tea bushes and then slipped and slid downward again on an invisible path, entering a glade shaded by large trees and full of wild plants.

Li Lao wanted to show us several rare plants that he had brought here from the higher forests and transplanted, chief among them a plant called *qiangdao cao* (强盗草, "bandit grass"). Brightness Yang's attention was fully engaged by this prospect. He told us this plant, good for stopping bleeding from wounds, was in the literature but thought to be nearly extinct. We began to suspect that he had brought us here for a repeat visit only because he believed that Li Lao would be sharing a sample of this drug with him and educating him about its virtues as a medicine. Professor Yang was anxious to receive this esoteric wisdom. Perhaps if he hadn't come back several times he would not have been trusted with this nomad science. Indeed,

Li Lao pointed out that he purposely made it difficult to reach this hidden corner of a (mostly cultivated) part of the town's edge. The paths were not obvious and hard to negotiate, he said, precisely to prevent other herbalists (like us, we presume) from knowing where this rare plant could be found "in the wild."

Drugs like bandit grass are the kind of secrets and discoveries that motivate many nationality medicine researchers throughout China. And such esoteric lore very much interested Professor Yang. He had told us in 2011 that he was the principal investigator on a large grant from the State Administration of Chinese Medicine (SATCM), the explicit goal of which was to "disseminate effective nationality medicine drugs and techniques." SATCM researchers had already identified a technique, common to a number of nationality groups, involving tapping patients' bodies with a sturdy piece of wood cut from a tree branch. This was supposed to be good for kidney problems and lower back pain, and the government agency had awarded Yang's group 300,000 RMB to persuade clinics and hospitals around the province to adopt the technique.

We were a little skeptical about this general approach, seeing the quest for effective therapies as, at best, piecemeal. And we also had lots of evidence that nationality practitioners were reluctant to share their idiosyncratic knowledge and skills—the sort of special powers that brought them local fame and clients—with researchers from outside. Meanwhile, Brightness Yang, despite his years of studying and cataloging Tujia medicines, was not able to satisfactorily answer our questions about the principles and tendencies characteristic of "Tujia medicine." As with this rather arbitrary and miscellaneous ethnic category itself,[11] it was hard to tell what characteristics set Tujia medicine apart from traditional Chinese medicine (TCM) or neighboring traditions like Miao or Dong nationality medicine.

Indeed, it turned out that Professor Yang didn't make many distinctions about nationality types of practice. This despite the fact that he was employed teaching history and practice of Tujia medicine at the Hubei Nationalities College and had been urged to collaborate with us by his medical school dean, who—the dean told us over a good meal in Enshi—hoped to establish a Tujia school of medicine partly based on Yang's research. Eventually Professor Yang admitted to us that he didn't understand our interest in "minority nationality medicines" very well. He thought perhaps we just wanted to see some countryside and meet some herbalists, and he himself was a little uncertain about who among his folk medicine acquaintances was identified as Tujia. Apparently he hadn't often asked that question.

Li Lao, we discovered from him, was not identified as Tujia at all—he said he was Miao. Professor Yang introduced us to a few practitioners who were proudly Tujia, but it was more common to see herbalists using what seemed to be rather hybrid forms of therapy. Frustrated with Yang's approach to nationality medicine research, Judith wrote this in her field notes after complaining to Lili:

> Lili feels that Brightness Yang is in one sense just trying to respond as a scholar and teacher to the national demand for "development" in ethnic traditional medicines, though he doesn't really see anything much that is specific to Tujia. She doesn't think this is entirely cynical, even though he doesn't require or even seek a group "cultural essence" or important difference with Chinese medicine. This is a kind of eclecticism, perhaps, that doesn't think to challenge itself toward greater systematicity. It continues to appear that the real focus of Yang's interest is the local herbs themselves, insofar as they are thus far unrecognized in CM, and the "secret recipes" and techniques that might be salvaged for government-supported product development.

Even though his recent research career, partly supported by Beijing, was nominally dedicated to Tujia medicine, then, clearly Professor Yang thought of any local practice in that part of Hubei as within the purview of his research. It didn't trouble him that medicine on the ground in this region is mixed among at least Han, Tujia, and Miao practitioners.

This kind of hybridity (accompanied by a great concern with the most local of all medical things, the drugs themselves) had already impressed us in our visit to the Enshi area in 2011. That summer, Brightness Yang took us to see Dr. Brilliance Zhang in a county hospital of TCM. As we talked with Dr. Zhang, it became clear that he was one of the nationality medicine authorities on whom Professor Yang and some other published scholars had depended for much of their information. Zhang hauled out book after book on the subject of Tujia medicine, pointing out which parts he had substantially authored. At one point, when we jokingly suggested that he should go to Enshi city and help Professor Yang to teach his classes, Dr. Zhang laughed: "No need, I'm already teaching his classes! Every time he has a question, he calls me up and I tell him what to teach his students."

But even Dr. Zhang was not very committed to the idea that the medicine he knows and practices is characteristically Tujia. The hospital clinic where he worked (which drew dozens of patients daily) was called "State Specialty Clinic of Nationality Medicine," and the major sign over the entrance, as well as the shingle for his own clinic, advertised "Rheumatic Disease Specialist of Miao Medicine and Tujia Medicine."[12] Though he appeared to enjoy talking with us about the social and technical characteristics of what he referred to as "our Tujia medicine," among the books he showed us, with his name listed as sole author, were two textbooks on Miao medicine (one on drugs for rheumatism and one on women's medicine). But he also gave us his single-authored book on "Tujia women's medicine." In speaking of the latter book, he noted that some of the old Tujia authorities he consulted relied heavily on *tima* (shamanic) ritual methods, such as writing magical characters, burning paper money, and transforming water. Naturally, he could not write about these methods because they were all part of a ritualist culture (*tima wenhua* is the local term he used for such techniques). But he hastened to add: "Don't think this is superstitious! These methods work!"

Zhang was originally trained in Chinese medicine. As early as 2000 he was recruited to join a nationally funded research project that would begin the work of salvaging and sorting Tujia medicine. Even so, according to him (speaking in 2011), Tujia medicine is ultimately little more than everyday knowledge, common to every household, about how to use wild herbs. But he did differentiate between Tujia medicine and Chinese medicine, making acute hepatitis his example: "our herbal medicine works faster than TCM in treating hepatitis." But he also said: "Any doctor in China, whether he is Tujia, Miao, or Han, is a Chinese medicine doctor. I myself think it's only a difference of naming and interpretation, we are one great nationality, sharing common experiences. Given the great culture we all share, all human medicine should belong to one common system." Lili pressed him on this: asked if he mixes Chinese, Tujia, and Miao medicine in his prescriptions, he said that he does. Eventually he confessed to us that he himself is a mixture of Tujia and Miao: his mother is Miao, and he learned everyday herbal medicine at her side from childhood. In this respect, he says, "my background is a mixture. My main aim is to heal people's diseases, no matter what methods I need to employ."

Judith and Lili stubbornly kept pushing Brightness Yang to help them find Tujia medicine at work in the hands of Tujia healers. He tried to oblige by asking a friend, township doctor Lin, to introduce us to local healers. Lin took us to see a very elderly couple who first impressed us as unlikely to be very forthcoming. But the seventy-five-year-old wife, Granny Du, who had a local reputation for bone-setting and herbal medicine expertise, turned out to be very lively and informative.

She and her husband are both identified as Tujia, but because Mr. Pan had been in the army for many years, they had traveled. They had also lived in the Beijing area off and on to help care for grandchildren. Their house suggested a kind of generalized "Chinese" nationality to us: there were patriotic posters in places of honor in their sitting room, including one of Chairman Mao with the familiar red sun rising behind him; and Old Pan was wearing his army cap and blue "Mao jacket," neatly buttoned up, for our final photograph. These patriotic gestures are not unusual in Hubei, but they were particularly emphatic in this house.

As a young woman, Granny Du had studied with a local herbalist and bone-setter (her teacher was referred to as a "master," and he might have been more Daoist adept than medical man); and she had successfully treated a child in Professor Yang's wife's family. Even though elderly, Granny Du was still climbing into nearby forests to collect the six or seven medicines she knew. Her husband, though he said he really knew nothing about herbals, accompanied her to help carry their collections. Their bedroom was stuffed with herbs, some of them considered unusual by Dr. Lin and Professor Yang.

Also in the bedroom was an old edition of the *Barefoot Doctors' Manual*, open to the herbal medicines listings. This was a slight surprise because everyone had told us that Granny Du is "illiterate" (*wenmang* 文盲). We asked, and the old couple told us that Old Pan reads out entries to his wife while she compares her own recognitions and classifications with those of this official (1970s) national source. Clearly, she was a serious herbalist who sustained continued learning about natural medicines.

But she was not only an herbalist. We noted above that the family of Professor Yang's wife, Ms. Chen, had benefited from Granny Du's expertise. Unlike her highly educated husband, Brightness Yang, Ms. Chen made no effort to confine her conversation to the secular realm of scientific pharmacy and botany. When we traveled together, she often told us about ghosts and other uncanny things, and part of her appreciation of Granny Du had to do with the old lady's mystical skills. Ms. Chen told us, for example, that Granny Du sometimes used divination techniques to determine whether an illness on which she was consulted was treatable or hopeless. Warned to expect some ritual expertise on Du's part, we asked if she used the "egg marking" (*hua jidan* 画鸡蛋) technique to treat colic in children. She did. And she demonstrated for us.

The technique is simple, it's just a matter of rubbing the abdomen with an egg that has been marked with a magical character (like a *lingfu* 灵符, amulet). She carefully inscribed in Lili's notebook—several times, with somewhat divergent results—the character she used. To us it looked rather like the character for spring (the season), but everyone insisted that because Granny Du is illiterate, it could not be any normal Chinese character. We were happy to agree that both the character and the technique were magically efficacious (or *ling* 灵), especially since everyone insisted that this method almost always worked to relieve a child's stomachache.

Old Pan maintained a stoic demeanor throughout our encounter with his wife and her Tujia medical practice. Only when we particularly asked what nationality they belonged to did he perk up and venture some thoughts of his own. "We're Tujia," he said, "but really, it's a made-up category. We lived here for years and nobody worried about being Tujia or Miao or Han or anything else, and there were always people from many places coming here to live. Then Enshi Metropolitan District became a Tujia/Miao autonomous prefecture, and suddenly we all have to be Tujia." He thought it was really silly, this "Tujia" stuff. He is an old Maoist, by the look of him, and in the collectivist times of his younger years there was little by way of multiculturalism, only solidarity among the workers of the world.

Our visits to a few healers near Enshi in 2011 and 2012 were not our only effort to come to terms with Tujia medicine. We later traveled through Tujia territory in Xiangxi, Hunan province, with the assistance of a very different authority on nationality medicines, Dr. Chinasong Tian, and his research collaborators. The results of that later work were markedly different from what we gleaned while traveling with Brightness Yang and his friends and family.[13] At the time we found the parts of our field research that followed Professor Yang's government-directed quest for marketable drugs and techniques quite unsatisfying. Our expectation had been, after seeing so many specialized works in print about Tujia medicine, that we might find a unique nationality medicine operating from storefronts and township clinics in the highlands around Enshi. We had been naively hopeful that an acknowledged authority on this nationality like Professor Yang would be able to lead us to local experts who could articulate local knowledge with thoughtfulness and depth. (This was not an entirely idiotic expectation; see below for accounts of field relationships that were more satisfying.) And Professor Yang was, after all, a teacher of Tujia medicine. Perhaps it was unrealistic of us to expect that he would have been able to sort Tujia medicine out from its matrix of folk practices, other nationalities, and landscapes full of diverse herbal medicines. After all, none of his friends were even troubled by the confusing mixtures of ethnicities coloring the medicines of this southern region.

Looking back a few years later, as we write about our encounters with Daybreak Li, Brilliance Zhang, and Granny Du, we find a hard lesson lying beneath the surface frictions we once found so frustrating. These three healers were quite different from each other, and, more important, they asked us to acknowledge real local things that we had not expected. Most fundamental perhaps was every healer's claim to some form of magical efficacy. Li Lao, with his promise that "when the medicine arrives the illness leaves," was implicitly embodying a kind of guaranteed natural efficacy beyond the reach of scientific pharmacy. Dr. Brilliance Zhang, a much-published local authority and a hospital clinician, noted that Tujia medicine was partly set apart by its (as yet unpublished) use of ritual interventions (though he never forgot local herbals, either). And Granny Du made no distinction between her mystically marked egg and the wild medicinal herbs she gathered and dispensed from her bedroom.

Our encounters with these healers could only persuade us that at least in Hubei and Hunan, locality is a lot more important than nationality recognition. We had to face the possibility that "Tujia" is just one among several labels that refer, very loosely, to these forested mountains, these small towns, these farmers, these mountain gatherers, and, of course, these drugs. As we argued in chapter 4, herbal medicines are not just a superficial list of tools added to more foundational medical methods and theories. Especially for local medicines like Tujia and Miao that have grown up, been learned, practiced, and handed down in these botanically very diverse mountains, the drugs themselves are really the center of medicine.

PRESENT AND ABSENT ACTORS

We opened this chapter with the story of our encounter with some (putative) Tujia doctors partly because these visits left Lili and Judith so frustrated. Though we didn't always admit it to ourselves, all these things challenged us to try to cross a divide, to *understand* despite social, linguistic, and historical differences. We don't feel at all certain that we saw Hubei and Hunan Tujia and Miao practices accurately. But we still rehearse between us the events of our meetings, perhaps because they were complicated, and also because stubborn differences continued to be an issue for our overall project.

Such encounters are always complex. There were many kinds of meetings taking place just during a few hours spent in Qingshui town. In addition to encounters between a folk healer, a government researcher, and some esoteric plants, there was our own somewhat different stance, that of a social science from much further away. At issue was not only what "the state" could see but also what anthropology could learn and, facing us, the knowledge and practice of a local medicine that was only partly manifested. Parts of the encounter could not be directly witnessed by us: Li Lao's discoveries and experiments with transplants and wild herbs on his solitary rambles above the town; Granny Du's divination methods and ways of using the Barefoot Doctors' Manual; Brilliance Zhang's rich understanding of ritual healing techniques that he "could not write" in his Tujia women's medicine book. Even the embodied expertise Dr. Zhang and presumably the other practitioners we met had acquired in family kitchens over many years was inaccessible to us. Depending on how one identifies the things or actors (micro-

or macro-) that might be brought to "face" each other in an encounter, we could also list meetings between global science and indigenous knowledge, urban and rural networks, the yin world of an occulted cosmos (allowing divination and *tima*) and the yang world of visitors with name cards and notebooks. Even Judith's and Lili's ways of relating to each other, as field-workers, writers, and friends, was not far from our minds. The encounters in question, then, were many, all unfolding in the same time and place.

WHY ENCOUNTER?

Perhaps every encounter, like this one in Hubei, is a complex mixture of gathering and scattering, frustration and enjoyment, past presences and present absences. In the rest of this chapter we will recount and analyze a few other field encounters, attempting to hear and see again and afresh the multitudes of human and nonhuman personages and things we met. But first we reflect on the value of an anthropology of the encounter, with the example of those 2012 visits to Prof. Brightness Yang's "Tujia" acquaintances in mind. Though as collaborating ethnographers we naturally treasure our own direct experience in the field, we want to argue that every encounter extends far beyond the face-to-face activity of anthropologists and other embodied human interlocutors.

Every encounter is an *event*, full of historical specificity. Events take form from a specific past and, at least in a minor way, alter the future of the many specific actors involved in them. The mere fact of the visit of anthropologists and a government researcher from far away, for example, was doubtless more important to Li Lao and Granny Du than any quaint cultural principles or deep structures we anthropologists might seek to interpret out of this event. Writing a proper history of either healer's medical practice would not be easy. But it could be done. As in other "history from below" projects, though, there would be ambiguities: When does "an encounter" begin, and when does it end? What is the relationship between what Granny Du chose to show us and the more "natural" everyday life she leads when there are no visitors? How does Li Lao keep track of his experimental uses of the herbals only he really understands? What "really" happened when Brightness Yang's brother-in-law drove through a ghost's body one night in the forest? Why do patients prefer Brilliance Zhang's rheumatism medicine to that of TCM? Questions like this keep ethnography happily embroiled in the concrete and in the event.

Encounter is perhaps especially attractive as a frame for the research of the *Gathering Medicines* project. Because Lili and Judith decided very early not to attempt a classic village study based on long residence in one small place, we think of encounters—by contrast—as happening along an *itinerary*. Writing about events from a mobile (or even nomad) point of view, an itinerant ethnography can track the lines of narrative and influence, and the circulations of things, that make field encounters consequential. Speculations about linked past and future events that might gather to contribute to the storylines of a history are part of the pleasure deriving from a mobile anthropology. Thus, by turning our attention away from deep cultural structures and instead seeking to connect the events of a local history, we feel we are making ethnography yield significance in fresh ways.

In telling the story of these 2011 and 2012 visits to Tujia country, we tried to provide glimpses of the many kinds of personages and things active in these frustrating encounters. In keeping with both Latour's and Zhuangzi's visions, mentioned at the beginning of the chapter, no process of gathering that might interest us would be a simple meeting between two human beings.[14] Every encounter involves a whole earth and heavens, all kinds of lives. And not every actor in an encounter event is immediately audible or observable. The whole earth and heavens that made Brilliance Zhang the thoroughly "mixed" man and healer that he was, and presumably still is, not to mention the actor-networks constructing the anthropologists, health researchers, and textbook authors who rely on him, are irreducibly plural. Though our ears are not equipped to hear everything remembered, everything imagined, and everything trying to speak, we are certain, in an anthropology of encounter, that there is, and has been, a cacophony of voices at work. The openness of encounter encourages ethnography to draw in, to gather together, as many actors—and their actions—as possible.

Though as anthropologists we hope that something of broad value can be learned from even itinerant encounters, part of the charm of these events is that they cannot be exhaustively explained with reference to general principles. Ultimately, only a particular history explains the complexity of any specific contemporary situation. Li Lao's gendered herbalist practice, and his personally unprecedented willingness to show us some secret places in the forest, is not a "case" of some known set of sociological principles or historical forces. His situation, which we now realize we were lucky to encounter, is a life, always under construction, that addresses the challenges of natural-cultural worlds in variously successful ways. Armed with a method that appreciates the creativity and contingency of every specific form of life, we lose interest in system, structure, and the generalizable.[15]

By the time they end up as part of a chapter in a book, encounters have taken the form of a useful fable. Like Aesop's fables, stories told by ethnographers have "a moral of the story." But these are usually implicit. For us, as we reflect on our encounters in several houses in Qingshui town, one major finding is our realization that we had to recenter the medicinals themselves, at least if we were to understand nationality medicine in Hubei. Li Lao's bandit grass and Granny Du's marked egg are nonhuman actors of a very quotidian kind, but they are undeniably important. We were required to give up on an abstract category, "Tujia," before we could appreciate their importance.

In 2012 we were experiencing frictions with Professor Yang partly because he seemed to us to be charting an easy route among practitioners he knew well who were never too far from a decent restaurant. Possibly we were yearning to meet wild mountain healers harboring trade secrets, like Lisu healer Dr. Su whom we discussed in chapter 4, with his highly idiosyncratic way of naming and storing herbal medicines. In some respects, we were blind to the little mysteries around which the lives of mundane healing in Hubei circled.

This is a *mea culpa*, then. Having been troubled by the ways Chinese history is sometimes told, in very accessible and even sentimentally touching stories, we worry that when human lives are placed into the grand modernist master narratives of the individual, of life and death, of freedom, and of self-expression, everything specific about encounters with "things Chinese" is lost. Stories should be surprising, we feel, they should not be easy to follow, the translations between worlds should never be *too* successful, there should be frictions.

At the same time, it is in the very nature of anthropological fables to propose a human common ground and travel across it. The surprising story, the intervention of a nonhuman agent, the narrated event that opens our eyes to some previously unsuspected undercurrents of everyday life, still pose the perennial problem of grasping uniqueness. Rather than resolve that "problem" in favor of either specificity or generality, perhaps it is in the nature of anthropology to just live with it. Our frictions are generative.

SURVEY (*DIAOCHA*) AS ENCOUNTER

And speaking of frictions, in our Hubei travels with Professor Yang, we two anthropologists were part of an all-too-present officialdom, in force. In the course of our research we witnessed many similar encounters between the official world of legitimate knowledge and more local, "earthbound," forms of medicine.[16] But these were not usually confrontations between discrete personages, or unevenly matched meetings between total strangers. Rather, we were in a position to observe government and institutional *engagement* in the everyday life of nationality medicines, as it existed in several formal or informal arrangements. This witnessing often led us to ask, what histories gathered these "official" and "informal" actors together, what contingencies produced a partial common ground for them? What earth and heavens converged on these sites of encounter between local healers and the knowledge-producing state?

One of the most complex answers to these questions is offered by the several encounters of our local collaborator in Yunnan, Academy Director Resolution Ma, with a few healers of the Achang nationality. In 2011 and 2012 we were privileged to follow Director Ma's research in the field. At the time he was the research director of the Yunnan Academy of TCM. He is a veteran field researcher on public health issues who has worked at the Yunnan Academy for many years; his survey research (*diaocha* 调查) has taken him to many parts of rural western Yunnan.[17] When the State Administration of TCM announced a new research initiative for salvaging and sorting nationality medicines, shortly after 2001, Director Ma led the way to organize projects with other academy researchers to excavate and publish the local medical knowledge of some nationality groups in Yunnan province. He himself decided to concentrate on the small and scattered group known as the Achang. This group, we were told, had no written language, and they have not been assigned any self-governing counties, townships, or villages.

By the time we were able to accompany Director Ma and members of his research team to an Achang-majority village in Caojian township (western Yunnan), in August 2011, he and several other researchers had visited and interviewed medical practitioners there several times. Eight months earlier, Lili had been part of the team that did preliminary interviews in the Caojian area. By August, the kinship and discipleship relations of the various medical practitioners in this area were still being worked out, but it had become clear that there were only two senior, dominant doctors of Achang medicine with active home clinics in the area. Both lived in the same spread-out Achang village. Despite the small-scale character of this local medicine, Academy Director Ma was confident that in establishing connections to these two men and their families, he had begun to salvage a genuine nationality medicine of great public health interest.[18]

The evening before we arrived in the village, Director Ma convened a planning meeting in his Caojian hotel room for the whole team.[19] He needed to divide up the work for the next day, assigning responsibilities to different members of the group for framing interview questions and keeping notes on various topics (history, pharmacology, diagnosis and therapeutics, and heritage transmission and dissemination). But he also wanted to instruct us on the proper methods for this kind of research. He told everyone that they were fortunate to have real anthropologists on this trip and that he hoped Lili and Judith would demonstrate to academy researchers the true and proper way to conduct an ethnographic interview. And he cautioned everyone on research ethics: we needed to respect the intellectual property rights of these medical practitioners, using no pressure in asking for access to case records and formulary books. And we were to tactfully yield time with the doctor to any patients who might visit. He himself took charge of obtaining informed consent for the whole project. And though we two anthropologists expressed worries about the unwieldy size of our visiting group, he argued that the doctors we were interviewing might see some benefit from the outside attention their skills had obviously drawn. Through the rumor mill, patients might feel even more confident about the powers of an Achang medicine that had been scientifically recognized in this way.

In this evening meeting Director Ma repeated a point he had been making more privately to us, and on other occasions to his research staff: Nationality medicines have a lot of *yao* (药, pharmacy) but sometimes it's difficult to find the *yi* (医, medicine) in all this plant lore. He was hoping our well-orchestrated group visit could begin to reach a deeper level with the Achang doctors. Perhaps with the proper tactful/anthropological approach (one that did not overemphasize the collection of formulas or local pharmaceuticals for market development), these experienced healers would yield up their "theory," explaining to us the medical principles that governed their specialized use of natural drugs. This would be a way of drawing closer to the principled medicine of the Achang and achieving a contribution beyond the mere collection of interesting drugs.

With this background, we were surprised at the openness expressed by the older of the two senior practitioners, Literary Luster Zhu, whom we visited on that trip. Though we had been warned that he was probably "keeping secrets," and would not want to share his formulary book, he did fetch this fabled volume out from its drawer and allow us to have a look. (In Judith's reading what he had recorded there used a lot of TCM vocabulary, but because we were just being given a brief look, there was no time to analyze his cases or his recipes.)[20] Moreover, he encouraged us to follow his daughter upstairs to the pharmacy as she assembled a complex order of drugs for a waiting patient.

This highly competent disciple of her father ran a very orderly and well-stocked pharmacy. She climbed over large shelves and piled-up sacks of dried herbals and weighed out the specified amounts of each component drug, making neat packets labeled for use in a sequence (the patient would not be able to return for some weeks). She also had quite a few powdered herbal drugs; these also had to be combined proportionally and wrapped in very small packets for dissolving in hot water. Our team was fascinated and took a great many documentary photographs. We were especially impressed with the instructions for preparation and use marked on each of the packets. We were happy to witness the competent work of a female disciple who was obviously much trusted by her teacher. But more important, with so much information recorded in our cameras and notes about how drugs were being used, it might be possible—with Dr. Zhu's continued cooperation—to find the "medicine" guiding the deployment of herbal *medicines*. This, at least, was the hope of Director Ma and his colleagues in the team.

In the end, when we packed up the video camera and our notes, after the several Achang informants had signed on the dotted line for their interview fees, and as we faced the prospect of coordinating our six or seven different sets of notes and records, Director Ma remained unsatisfied. His role for several days of fieldwork had been to listen in to the interviews, to quietly advise the rest of us, on the fly, about how to improve our work, and to maintain good relations with various local health department cadres who visited the project. He headed back to Kunming still complaining that Doctors Literary Luster Zhu and Greatwave Li—the other important practitioner in the Caojian area—had not handed over the essential "theories" of Achang medicine.

We really enjoyed engaging with him over this ambition and this dissatisfaction.[21] For us, the Academy-led field project was a precious opportunity to learn more about the "salvaging and sorting" process in nationality China, as we tried to better understand Director Ma's canny and critical approach to *diaocha*, or field investigation. During strolls through Caojian town, over meals on the road, in long backseat conversations in the van, we engaged in a form of scholarly encounter that Judith and Lili and Director Ma enjoyed, even though it tended to bore the other members of the team.

Our friend—somewhat disingenuously, because he knew quite a lot already—kept asking us to explain anthropological method to him. On one occasion Judith told him that she thinks contemporary anthropology is distinguished by its grounding in a concept of practice (rather than, for example, structure or culture). Hoping to clarify what we mean by practice, Judith invoked Mao Zedong's 1937 essay "On Practice." Director Ma was surprised and pleased (as was Judith, in turn). He considers himself an heir and practitioner of Maoist practice theory and argued that the philosophical and methodological essays of the early Mao (such as "Report on an Investigation of the Peasant Movement in Hunan") had, very early, modeled the proper "mass line" form of *diaocha* for rural China.[22] In his own practice, decades after Mao Zedong Thought in China had been superseded by a global, liberal social science, Director Ma still sought to live up to the ideals of a form of research that was fully engaged with the grassroots and its people's movements.

As part of this engaged methodological orientation, Judith recalls (and Lili doesn't) a little speech Director Ma made in Dr. Greatwave Li's court-yard as we were leaving. Perhaps at the time this aspect of our encounter with Achang culture and medicine was unmemorable to us because it was not unexpected: Director Ma had told us earlier some of his opinions about how "the Achang" were falling down on the job of nationality development. In his emphatic remarks to some village elders, he argued that if Achang nationality leaders wanted to develop local culture for the benefit of all their fellow Achang, medicine, not "culture," was their main hope.[23]

We had learned that at least a few medical families near Caojian had significantly increased their family income by making their medical skills known. When asked about the special characteristics of Achang medicine, we were told first of a specific diagnostics—focusing on facial physiognomy and pulse-taking at both wrists and feet—and then given a list of Achang medical specialties: kidney disorders, traumatic injuries, and "breaking up [kidney and gall] stones." Director Ma was anxious to publish a textbook explaining these specialties of Achang medicine (and, of course, detailing the theoretical foundations of the system, if he could learn them), and he was in talks with Caojian health department officials about transforming a township hospital into an Achang medical center. All of this would have fallen under the head of local development for leaders like Ma and his pub-lic health colleagues.

Director Ma's ambition for "the Achang" and his concern to push them toward collective and institutional development (or more aggressive insti-tuting), possibly quite against the will of practitioners who were doing well as competitive individuals, made a lot more sense after our conversations about Maoist *diaocha*. Insofar as field investigation is a foundation of the "mass line" approach to the responsibility of the party-state, investigators should be discovering the wants and needs of the people at the grassroots, and then turning these demands into higher-level policy and broader im-plementation of service programs. Though there was sometimes a slightly imperious tone in the communications of government officials with nation-ality healers and local experts, professional *diaocha* knowledge producers like Director Ma also persuaded us that, for many conscientious leaders, genuine service to the people (with all their presumed "cultural" character-istics) was still the goal of social research.

Reflecting on our visits to Achang territory in western Yunnan with the work group from the Academy of TCM, we could list numerous significant encounters that took place. For example: Senior healers running home clin-ics were asked to cooperate with the public health agenda of a developmen-tally inclined local government. Academy scientists were faced with unfamiliar bodies of local knowledge they were not certain of understanding. Achang activists seeking to excavate and represent "culture" found anthropological interlocutors (though we were, in the end, not much help). But the encounters that remain of greatest value to us are our warm and stimulating exchanges with Academy Director Resolution Ma.

After visits to Caojian with him in 2011 and 2012, Director Ma continued to advise our project by participating in the *Gathering Medicines* working group training meetings, sometimes also meeting with one or both of us for lively conversations when he had business in Beijing. (He has retired now, and we see less of him.) We often talked with him about how anthropological research could work better under Chinese conditions, analyzing our experiences in the field from our three somewhat different points of view. Judith and Lili gained respect for the engaged and state-led research methods of the *diaocha* approach, just as Director Ma critically evaluated his ethical protocols and the power of his investigative methods to excavate hidden cultural principles.[24] We admired both his honest self-scrutiny and his willingness to push a national collective agenda with local experts. On occasions when Judith and Lili step back to consider the nationwide (or at least southern Chinese) minority medicine movement in the second decade of the new millennium, we increasingly credit a few individuals with having done the most to bring minority medicine to the fore and salvage fascinating areas of expertise, even to enrich the healing environment of China. Director Ma was one of these leaders.

SO MANY TIGERS: NOMENCLATURE AND STANDARDIZATION

In the course of a working meeting on nomenclature standardization among leaders in Yao medicine development, senior doctor Goldstamp Huang burst out in exasperation: "the guy who made this list of Yao medicine's so-called 'Five Tigers and Nine Oxen' drugs didn't ask us for our opinion! Yao medicine has so many tigers, how can he say there are only five?"[25] Dr. Huang had been simmering resentfully for most of the afternoon, and he was not the only one among his clinician colleagues to resist the working draft of a standard list of drug names that they had before them. Their discomfort was understandable: though everyone acknowledged that Dr. Huang embodied genuine Yao medicine better than anyone, efforts to translate his local expertise into formal medical knowledge had not yet been particularly impressive. This old Yao healer was losing patience.

In late July 2013 the medical staff of the Jinxiu (Guangxi) Yao Medicine

Hospital was convened for this workshop by several leading researchers and administrators visiting from the provincial capital of Nanning. Their task was to decide on standard names for many of the drugs in local use, some of them not listed in previously published sources. One of the prestigious visitors, Professor Elegance Dai, along with his plant-chemist wife, Dr. Qiu, who was also present at this meeting, had already published rather extensively on Yao medicinals. Now Dai, along with another visitor from Nanning, Dr. Vermilion Li, was under pressure of a deadline to complete a new pharmacopoeia for Yao medicine. Their usages in the new list needed to be at least partly consistent with previously published materials. But both of these Han nationality researchers were also anxious to make Guangxi's *materia medica* usage more fully reflective of Yao clinical practice.[26] Dai, acknowledging that his earlier catalogs had been incomplete, and also contained mistakes, was hoping to solicit authoritative decisions on names and categories from the real experts, the doctors working in the key Yao homeland of Jinxiu, amidst the Great Yao Mountains.[27]

Professor Dai and Dr. Li were not unwelcome in Jinxiu. Clinicians in modern institutional settings, even though they can be conservative in sticking to their own lifelong and local habits of work, also realize that collective standardization must be taken seriously. We saw evidence of this concern early in the afternoon of the nomenclature meeting. As researchers, administrators, anthropologists, and doctors were assembling in the hospital conference room, Professor Dai was showing a few of us a fresh plant he had collected just that morning. He called it "white *zuan*" (白钻). Dr. Zhao, the hospital vice-director said, "But I don't recognize this plant; I have never used it." Dr. Pang, who runs the hospital's small botanicals archive, told Dr. Dai, "What you've got here isn't the right thing, we've just collected something similar, I'll show you." Fetching the already dried and pressed comparison plant from his rooms downstairs, Dr. Pang with Dr. Zhao and Professor Dai carefully compared the two samples. They found that the stalk of Dai's plant was round, while that of the hospital sample was squared. The former is white *zuan* and the latter is yellow *zuan* (黄钻), everyone decided. Moreover, it is yellow *zuan* that is most used clinically. Professor Dai directed his graduate student assistant to take careful pictures of the hospital sample, perhaps to be used in a future textbook. We suspect the clinicians felt that with this encounter between two plants and several experts, they had prevented the inappropriate use, in some faraway clinic in the future, of a textbook drug from the Yao Mountains.

It was a long and hot afternoon of paperwork in that conference room in July, sometimes irritating, sometimes hilarious. After everyone had decided that time would not permit discussion of disease nomenclature (an ever-troubled issue in the relationship between global biomedicine and traditional medicines),[28] the group turned to the work of sorting drugs. Professor Dai and Dr. Li had brought a draft table of drugs with the following column structure:

0. <u>Rank-ordered usual name</u> 收录排名 (each drug numbered in order, the list being ranked according to the frequency of appearance in earlier sources)
1. <u>Recorded Yao drug name</u> 经典瑶名 (common names in Yao usage for the first 104 items [recorded in Chinese], followed by alternate names, "often used" and drawn from books)
2. <u>Name in Yao language</u> 瑶文名 (using phonetic/alphabetic Yao writing and Chinese characters chosen for their phonetics)
3. <u>Character/flavor/circulation</u> 性味归属
4. <u>Plant (or animal) source</u> 植物(动物)来源 (Latin and Chinese botanical and zoological names)
5. <u>Body part affected</u> 入药部位
6. <u>Already standardized?</u> 有标准? (yes or no)
7. <u>Notes</u>

Dai and Li were not naïve about the difficulty of getting all these columned cells properly filled in for all the complex medicines known to Jinxiu practitioners. There were a lot of blanks in the draft list. And a number of problems were brought up at the outset of the meeting. The languages in play, for example, were multiple: there were common names in relatively easy Chinese for most of the well-known drugs (column 1), but Yao speakers often did not know the drug in question by that name—there were not, in other words, only "five tigers" in use, though an earlier scholar (not present on this occasion) apparently had decided there were. So the rank-ordered names in columns 0 and 1 were highly provisional. They needed to be replaced in many instances with a more widely (Yao) recognized name. But should that official name be recorded in the (new, and little used) Yao language alphabetic system, or using Chinese characters? If the latter, should the Chinese characters of the official name be chosen for their sound or their meaning?

These general policy matters of translation and standardization could not be finally settled at this meeting, but decisions had to be made anyway. At one point Dr. Li made a little speech that claimed for this group a weighty epistemological authority. He said, "This list has been the model for the stabilization of Yao pharmacy. However it was that all sources wrote it down before, that was how 'outsiders' knew it. Now, we'd better just do these tasks, and later we can slowly revise, if necessary. The responsibility for integrating [*tongyi* 统一] the names of Yao medicinals rests with the exact group here today."

As the work got under way, it was clear that each proper name and its translations and alternatives would be decided on an ad hoc basis, one by one. Everyone's best intention, it seemed, was to register a name that would be widely understood, accepted, and correctly used in Yao medicine and pharmacy work. But this was not a comfortable process. Sometimes even the clinical co-workers—three eminent Yao medicine healers, all belonging to the Pan Yao subgroup—disagreed, and often they had to decide, in the interest of time, who would defer to whom.[29] And there were many discomforts with what was *not* presented by the master list—how could a conscientious expert make room in the grid for variants, debates, uncertainties, and potentials? At the same time, the authoritative local experts seemed to enjoy translating Yao names into sometimes foolish-sounding Chinese equivalents. These senior doctors would chew over a few sounds, first in Yao and then in Mandarin, joke about mismatched meanings, and gleefully reject some earlier proposed equivalents presently on the list.

As the afternoon wore on, a shared sense of arbitrariness grew. Lili wrote in her field notes: "The words most often heard from the three senior Yao doctors were, 'okay, more or less' and 'whatever.'" Judith noted everyone's increasing alienation from the seriousness of this task with the following note: "Dr. Li pushed and pushed and, quite late, got through all 150 drugs on the list. He came to sound like an auctioneer or Bingo caller. '87! 87? Okay? More or less? Okay! 88! 88?' and so on we went." Eventually, driven on by a more or less shared categorical imperative, our group made some kind of decision about each of the Yao and Chinese drug names on the draft list. We suspect, however, that few in the group went away with a sense of scientific accomplishment, and we doubt if they saw the results of their work as helpful to clinical practice.

Though the afternoon meeting wound up late, our working group could not adjourn without gathering for a group photograph. As we were organizing our pose for the camera, Vermilion Li also asked everyone (including Lili and Judith, Professor Dai's graduate student, Dr. Qiu the chemist, Yang Jian [a junior doctor in the hospital also working with the *Gathering Medicines* project], and Yang Jian's administrator husband) to sign a register of those present. He insisted that today had been a "historic moment" and a "historic meeting." We guess that he took this list of signatures (which also included our work units, ages, and phone numbers) back to Nanning to stand as support for his forthcoming official pharmacopoeia.

BEYOND THE ARBITRARINESS OF THE SIGN
(OR DRUG NAME)

Riding with the visitors in the Yao Hospital's ambulance van to a late din-ner, Judith and Lili were able to ask visitors Dr. Li and Professor Dai how they assessed the meeting. Both feared that the rendering of local Yao lan-guage names for medicines in Chinese characters imposed a foreign episte-mology, and they could see problems developing down the road. Outsiders would come to the Great Yao Mountains, for example, asking for certain medicines published in the pharmacopoeia, and possibly no one at the Jin-xiu Hospital or Outpatient Department would know what they were talk-ing about. Dr. Huang's and Dr. Pang's trainees, working in the same hos-pital, might use the same name for different plants or (even more likely) different names for the same plant. How would ambiguities and mistakes in clinical work be avoided? How would pharmacies function and manage their inventories and records? Possibly thinking of his brief lesson on white and yellow *zuan* earlier in the day, Professor Dai—who had gathered many herbals himself in quite a few mountains—expressed his concern that any new authoritative nomenclature would still be unable to help practitioners distinguish between "the real and the fake." And though Professor Dai and Dr. Li were encountering a few frictions in their collaboration on standard-izing the things of Yao medicine, they were at least in accord in predicting that the upcoming work on disease nomenclature was going to be an even worse nightmare.

The meeting described here, boring, tense, and funny all at once, was a complex encounter among people both senior and junior, Yao and Han, local and visiting, expert and novice. Of course, there were plants, documents, and technology also gathered in the room, all these nonhumans making their particular contribution. We cannot leave this working meeting, how-ever, as a mere record of everything that happened to be physically present one afternoon in a hospital conference room in 2013. Rather, because we are aware of many of the conditions that informed this meeting, making it indeed a "historic moment," we need to draw near to some other influential presences, not quite in the room, but important nevertheless.

One of these near presences was, in a sense, the state, or one instituted agent of it. We have argued that the Chinese national project for salvaging and sorting minority nationality medicines has been a rationalizing process, in several senses. Some nationality groups have been able to build brick-and-mortar institutions like clinics, hospitals, and training centers. And all minority medicine activists have sought to develop a rational "system of knowledge" that could be taught and studied by various kinds of researchers. Recall Director Ma's anxiety, described above, to fill out the "medicine" of the Achang nationality for his Yunnan province research project. The Achang and Tujia, Zhuang, Qiang, Li, and Yao nationality initiatives, partly supported by the State Administration of Traditional Chinese Medicine, all of which sought to "salvage and sort, synthesize and elevate" local minority medical systems, were a form of formal knowledge production sponsored and closely watched by the state. In the Guangxi Zhuang Autonomous Region, there was a lot of province-level funding for nationality medicine research, but the surveys, the collections of records, the research projects, and the resulting institutional programs were regulated by the central government, as it channeled Ministry of Public Health demands through the SATCM.

Thus, in the Yao medicine standardization meeting, part of the rationalizing pressure to generate a better pharmacopoeia was coming from rather far above. In conversation with us, the visiting leaders Professor Dai and Dr. Li sometimes referred to the interest of historian Huang Hanru in this process; indeed, it was Professor Huang who had set the deadline they were trying to meet. Huang Hanru—a crucial founder of Zhuang medicine and a leading researcher in Guangxi and nationally since the early 1980s (see chapters 1 and 2)—was managing in turn a rather extensive research network combining the work of a number of scholarly, scientific, and clinical experts. However, the part of this project devoted to Yao nationality research was not as advanced in the rationalization process as the long-standing project on Zhuang medicine was. The standardization meeting is thus a reflection of the fact that, in 2013, Yao medicine was still in an early "sorting" (*zhengli* 整理) stage. The state was demanding an authoritative list of Yao drug names and an agreed-upon nosology of diseases. But if our experience in Jinxiu that July is any indication, the SATCM may have to wait a while before they have a full complement of "salvaged, sorted, and synthesized" sources on Yao medicine.

Why was this standardization meeting so important? Why were the authoritative old practitioners willing to endure the indignity of "more or less" formally (re)naming their intimately known local medicines? Yao medicine practitioners and activists, as they seek a more public and institutional future for their specialty in Guangxi, are anxious to produce a next (and a next) generation to replace the aging "traditional" healers, many of whom are retiring (and some of whom are going into private practice).[30] We were constantly reminded of this problem of "passing the medicine down" as we talked with nationality medicine activists. The dilemma of transmission was deeply felt by some, but not all, practitioners of these local healing modalities.

The group of Zhuang medicine developers we came to know in Nanning, under the long-standing leadership of Huang Hanru, has "elevated" (*tigao* 提高) Zhuang medicine to a very notable institutional existence, at least in southern Guangxi. Any such "elevation" demands that serious effort be devoted to the other three keywords of nationality medicine-gathering: what is elevated (*tigao*) to formal authority must first be synthesized or made systematic (*zongjie*), what is synthesized must first be sorted and classified (*zhengli*), and what is sorted and classified must first be found "on the ground" and salvaged (*fajue*) from extinction or disappearance.

The Yao Hospital group had no problem with salvaging; they had been gathering and using medicines all their lives. And they saw those Great Yao Mountains herbals as unproblematically "Yao": local herbs were truly a salvaged nationality heritage. The hospital experts were willing, albeit somewhat sarcastically, to sort herbals by name into a list of discrete entities with properties.[31] But thus far the leadership had spared them the task of systematizing (*zongjie*) Yao medical "theory." (Elevating is another matter. The hospital pharmacy had developed a successful product line of eight different herbal baths that could be shipped anywhere in attractive boxes. For some nationality medicine movements, to "elevate" means to scientize and establish clinical protocols, but perhaps another sense of the term "elevate" for activists can be to commoditize in a way that spreads Chinese minority nationality medicine to the world.)

The premise of the standardization meeting was that the "medicine" that can be passed on as the old experts pass away, that can be practiced into the future in meaningful careers and made available for the benefit of patients, is not a transmissible thing until it is gathered and crafted, made rational and coherent, and (endlessly) tested in practice. The mundane and irritating work of standardizing the names of drugs, with all their local variations, was taken to be an unavoidable moment in building the future system, which will be rational, no longer nomad, Yao medicine. (Though one wonders whether Yao medicine, with its reputation for magical efficacy, could ever truly join the ranks of the royal medicines recognized by the SATCM.)

Systems are hard work to maintain, and they do not guarantee a rational future. Consider the Jinxiu Yao Medicine Hospital where the standardization meeting took place. This hospital was being held together and expanded by Director Liang in the face of rather considerable difficulties.[32] With only a few senior Yao clinicians,[33] and a complement of younger medical residents who had not yet been fully trained in (a still emergent) Yao medicine, the hospital needed to recruit and retain formally trained and certified medical staff in accordance with Department of Health regulations. Ideally, these interns and residents would have studied either biomedicine or Chinese medicine, as well as Yao medicine (the last mostly in Nanning). After a period of training at the hospital, they should be able to pass a Yao medicine licensing exam. Of course, persuading educated urban youth to make a career in a sleepy rural town like Jinxiu was probably not easy, either.

A specialized hospital with professional medical and support staff can succeed (or even be established) only if it is fed by a great many other institutions. The infrastructure that must be in place for practitioners of a minority medicine to be professionally certified is complicated and expensive. Medical education (including classrooms, faculty, a curriculum, textbooks, and the research base from which teaching materials are derived) must be provided and accredited. Clinics and hospitals must be available for internship training and practicums. The senior supervisors who teach while serving in wards and seeing outpatients must be willing to devote time to training. And stipends are required for trainees who must develop their careers far from their homes. At the very least.

OTHER AGENTS

Reflecting on the larger salvaging and sorting undertaking led from Nanning, and with Dr. Vermilion Li's declaration of a historic moment echoing through these pages, we want to point out that the drugs list itself was an important agent in the task at hand. This catalog of Yao medicines had been laboriously assembled from rather miscellaneous earlier sources, but those who were involved in that project were less impressed with its resulting character as a tidy database than with its many lacunae and problems. Yet Professor Dai and his co-workers, as they culled historical materials for a draft pharmacopoeia, knew that they could not succeed if they tried to start from scratch. Better to be embarrassed by Dr. Huang's complaint—so many tigers had been missed!—than to try to get an adequate list *de novo* from working clinicians like him.

Like everyone else, Vermilion Li got a little testy when faced with difficult-to-resolve matters of overlapping names, impossible gaps in pronunciations, and unknown provenances. But even as chair of the meeting, like the others present he was driven by the list. The order of the items on the list (as seen in column o noted above) began to constrain what could be done with any one item occurring later in the list. Let us explain: Once a Chinese language transcription for a particular Yao language phoneme had been agreed upon for one drug, higher up on the list, the logical thing to do was to use that same Chinese sound/character for all similar Yao language sounds as we moved down the list. But sounds are not meanings. Use of the same Chinese character in two phonetically similar names implied a semantic kinship that might not exist between the drugs. Thus the very order of the list—so reflective of a history of collective work—made the group less and less satisfied with the names available to them for the drugs appearing later, after certain conventions had begun to emerge. The names themselves gained in arbitrariness as the list dragged us onward, increasingly appearing as mere conventional compromises far from the living pharmacobotanical collections deployed every day in the clinic by these experts.[34]

And what about that living world of effective natural drugs? This was another active nonhuman near-presence exerting pressure on the standardization meeting. Drugs were a kind of agent that, while we were in Yao country, we were never allowed to forget. Every clinical story we heard invoked the powers of the *materia medica* of the Great Yao Mountains. Dr. Goldstamp Huang famously took to the hills himself to find rare drugs needed by nearly incurable patients. We had witnessed him insisting on preparing, with his own plastic-gloved hands, a herbal plaster "with high toxicity" for a lymphoma patient in the hospital. A retired senior clinician, Vitality Pan, enthusiastically took us to the hospital's two-room herbals research unit both to show us his careful collection and preservation techniques and to impress us with the number of local drugs documented there. In these rooms, he lovingly paged through big storage folios made of archival paper, telling stories about this or that drug as if they were old friends. And the extensive hospital pharmacy, full of nonstandard herbals, was run with pride by a senior herbalist who kept in close touch with both the clinical staff and market vendors of natural drugs.

Thus as we think back on that July afternoon in 2013, an occasion when the enframing database,[35] or the information imperative of official botanical knowledge, was making such demands on the flexible expertise and local commitments of a group of nonstandard healers, the first thing we think of is plants themselves. Those samples of yellow and white *zuan* handled so attentively and with such investigative zeal by seasoned collectors, and the herbal medicines archive one floor down from that conference room with its many lovingly preserved samples, also exerted a certain authoritative weight in the struggle over nomenclature.[36] Perhaps, in other words, it would have been acceptable to simply arrive at a series of discrete names and range those names alongside a series of plant and animal substances in common Yao clinical use. The connection between name and thing would have been arbitrary; but presumably everyone had encountered data of that kind before.

But we think that everyone there (and some who were not, like Huang Hanru) felt responsible to the plants themselves. The lively variability and the quirky powers of the medicinal substances to be found in the Great Yao Mountains made demands of their own on the mere mortals sincerely trying to craft a reasonable and reliable catalog for future practitioners of Yao medicine. Those yet to be identified younger healers (present as a potential only) would learn to be frustrated by the list, they would begin to see that there were a lot more actual tigers in those hills to be known. Perhaps the list and the herbs it standardized, under sometimes ridiculous names, will lead these next generations to more tigers and oxen than today's elders can even imagine.

KNOWING PRACTICE, EMBODIED HISTORY

We witnessed the Yao Hospital standardization meeting as a condensed node of thickly layered local actors/actants (including local plants, doctors, researchers at all levels, and lists resulting from earlier efforts at sorting), all of us encountering several state agents, with their databases, who were seeking to standardize and institutionalize Yao medicine. We have argued above that every encounter is an event, one that—like the Yao Hospital nomenclature workshop—gathers many threads of past encounters while at the same time promising to alter the futures of those present, and of some who are just nearby. In the various fields of minority nationality medicine we visited, there are different ways of envisioning the future, and different degrees of importance accorded to building nationality medicine for a future. But we also found that in some respects, the *past* of nationality medicine is held even more in common, as a shared memory, by many nationality doctors.

In the summer of 2014, when we spent a few weeks in the Nujiang Gorge (western Yunnan), several of the healers we visited impressed us with the depth of their feelings about how they had been trained, decades ago, to be health care workers. After hearing a few of these memories, we felt we were encountering an important part of the history of the PRC that is now seldom remembered. But it is embodied.

The Nu River (Nujiang, or Salween River) is located in western Yunnan province, running along the border with Myanmar. Nujiang Prefecture's terrain is striking, with the rapid, deep, and nonnavigable river carving one of the world's longest deep gorges, with dramatic high mountains hugging both sides. One main road follows the river from Liuku in the south to Gongshan in the north, and there are few other towns. Many of the Lisu, Nu, Tibetan, Naxi, and Dulong people who live along the Nujiang maintain farmsteads in small hamlets scattered high on the steep slopes above the river, connected only by footpaths. Indeed, the region has a reputation for being "wild" and inaccessible.[37] Arriving there as anthropologists, we felt this was an excellent place to test James Scott's assertion that "the state does not climb mountains."[38] Since we have devoted much of our research effort to "catching the state in the act" of producing formal knowledge and regulating and domesticating bodies, even rather "remote" ones, this mountainous strip of southwestern China interested us particularly. Would we find a shortage of government institutions and services, a general ignorance of "Chinese" culture, history, and modernity? Would there be radical non-modern difference here?

We didn't really think we were encountering the wild, but we had long been told that "the Lisu," one of the seven groups on which this project has focused, were not well organized in relation to the task of salvaging and sorting, synthesizing and elevating their minority nationality medical heritage. Experts in Beijing and other big cities said that Lisu healers were scattered and unwilling to band together to develop an effective form of local knowledge that could be transmitted in institutions. The image was one of rugged individualists, jealously guarding secrets in forested redoubts. We received a somewhat different picture, however, from our encounters in Nujiang with local senior doctors in their late sixties and seventies.

The first doctor we met was a friend of our Lisu-speaking research assistant, Lina.[39] Dr. Benefits Hu and his wife were staying with their eldest son's family in an apartment in Fugong county town, helping to take care of their granddaughter. Their own home (*laojia* 老家) was in Puluo village of Pihe township, along the river's edge. Dr. Hu was seventy-seven, and rather deaf, when we visited him in his son's apartment. But he is fond of Li Na, and he could hear her translations of our questions into Lisu language better than he could hear us. Though he warned us that he had been retired from active health work for a long time (twenty-six years) and "had forgotten everything," he surprised us with his rich memories.[40]

We were excited, for example, to learn that he and his wife had just come back from a health school class reunion in Lijiang City, a day's journey away. The reunion gathered many graduates, those who were still alive, from a class of forty who had received two and a half years of training in a provincial health school (*weixiao* 卫校), graduating in 1973. Memories still fresh, Dr. Hu showed us a group picture entitled "Forty-Year Anniversary of Classmates Reunion, No. 14 Class of Lijiang Health School (Chinese Medical Assistants)." The classmates with their gray hair posed in front of a statue of Mao Zedong, some wearing 1970s-style hats.

Most of the forty original classmates, Dr. Hu told us, had already been practicing as medical assistants (*weishengyuan* 卫生员) before they were offered the opportunity to study in the regionally important city of Lijiang. The Lijiang Health School was more advanced than their prior basic health education. The students studied medical theory and technical procedures in courses like traditional Chinese medicine, diagnostics of Chinese medicine, gross anatomy, and formulas of Chinese medicine. Hu had fond memories of students exchanging knowledge of medicinal herbs among themselves.

As we urged him to tell us more about his education and youthful practice, he explained that like many of his classmates, he had been through several kinds of medical training before going to Lijiang. Benefits Hu was a village accountant before he was selected to be the village health assistant in 1963. Soon after that, he said he "encountered an opportunity" to study in Liuku, the Nujiang prefectural capital, for a three-month training course. This training course, as we discovered later, was a most memorable experience for a whole generation of village doctors in this area.

According to Hu, every village of each township was asked to select one health assistant to attend a Chinese herbal medicine training class (*zhong-caoyao xunlian ban* 中草药训练班) in Liuku. All four counties of Nujiang Prefecture sent health assistants to the training class, so it was divided into two sessions, in 1965 and 1966, serving the youth of two counties each time. This training was a step up for health assistants, most of whom became barefoot doctors with more responsibility in their home villages and townships after their three months of training.[41] The retired head of the Fugong County Bureau of Health, Dr. Everlasting Mu, later told us that even the vendors, whom we had seen selling vials of processed herbs on the streets on market days, were mostly trained barefoot doctors and quite likely products of the 1965–66 Liuku training classes.

Benefits Hu attended the training held in 1965, which ran from October to December. He recalled fondly the two senior doctors who taught hands-on knowledge of local medicinal herbs. These teachers, named Li and Huang, usually took the students into the mountains during the daytime to gather herbs, with on-the-spot explanations of the medicinal functions specific to each herb, along with talks about ways to recognize the right plant, select the proper parts to harvest, and determine when to gather it. At night the teachers would lay out the samples gathered during the day to test the students' newly gained knowledge. Dr. Hu also remarked how serious Teachers Li and Huang were about finding the exact right herb. He said sometimes their group would trek in the mountains for a whole day or more, just to find one important herbal medicine. This three-month training course taught its young students how to find locally available herbs, memorize their medicinal functions, process the plants they had gathered, and combine different herbs to compose formulas for common diseases. The trainees also studied some basic techniques of bone-setting. Indeed, this class in the prefectural capital, taught by two senior experts in herbal medicine, equipped its students with everything they might need to practice primary health care using local resources.[42]

EMBODIED HISTORIES: SHIMMER ZHANG

When we were talking with Dr. Benefits Hu, we didn't fully realize the local importance of the Liuku Herbal Medicine Health Training, though we were impressed with how fondly he spoke of that experience. It was a couple of days later, after we had met village doctor Shimmer Zhang and made our way to his house far up the slopes above Pihe, that we understood better the impact that health schools like this had. Dr. Zhang was like his older friend Dr. Hu in his affection for the old herbalists who had been his teachers in Liuku. (By the time we left Nujiang we had met at least five practitioners who also felt this way about their health school experience in the prefecture.) Dr. Hu had a group photograph to remind him of the past, the era when local medicine was actively practiced and propagated in the mountains, by the river. Dr. Zhang, we discovered, had a little Liuku archive of notes and textbooks that he still consulted in the course of his village practice.

We were introduced to Shimmer Zhang by a Liuku ethnobotanist who had engaged in herbal medicine field surveys in the area and who respected Dr. Zhang's healing skills.[43] We arranged to meet Dr. Zhang on the next market day after our arrival in the county town of Fugong.[44] Patients apparently knew to look for him in the market; it was easier to see him there than to make the trek to his house, especially for those with injuries. He immediately impressed us with his bone-setting skills,[45] treating three patients in quick succession on this market day. Zhang set the broken arm of a tearful and frightened little boy in a small group gathered in front of a China Mobile retail store. He told the parents to go to the hospital to make sure of the realignment with an X-ray, then went to see a woman patient who had crushed a toe in a landslide on her way back from migrant labor in Myanmar. This was Dr. Zhang's third visit to her, so his chief task was to change the medicinal plaster he had applied last time. The formula, he told us, was based on what he had learned in the 1965 Liuku training class.

A third patient who sought him out on the street had a compound humeral fracture with malpositioning. She had gone to the hospital already, but upon being told that the hospital treatment would include surgery and metal pins, she and her family decided to pursue a more traditional medical procedure, and they sought out Dr. Zhang, the locally famous bone-setter.[46]

When we saw him in Fugong in July 2014, he estimated that he had treated more than sixty bone-fracture patients just that year so far. He compounds his own herbal plasters for external use, with functions varying from stopping bleeding and reducing inflammation to invigorating circulation, resolving blood stasis, and alleviating pain. Working with more than bone-setting techniques, he uses herbal formulas for oral medicines that he learned in Liuku to treat lower back pain, urinary problems, kidney and bladder stones, and more. He also said he combined these methods with what he had learned in the Kunming and Lijiang health schools to deal with the complaints commonly encountered in the work of an uplands village doctor.

No wonder Mr. Zhou the ethnobotanist respected Dr. Zhang's skills! He must have been one of the better-educated village doctors we met in western Yunnan. Shimmer Zhang's educational history is a good example of local engagements with the socialist state. Now in his early seventies, he had been appointed as health assistant for his village in 1960 (he was a teenager in fourth grade then) and doubtless received the rather minimal training in hygiene and triage provided by the health department and mandated by the Ministry of Public Health. Five years later he was enrolled in the same Liuku training class for herbal medicine that Benefits Hu had so appreciated. Only two years after that he was able to take another three-month course in herbal medicine, in Lijiang. In 1968 his biomedical education was advanced further thanks to a long visit from a health department medical team focused on typhoid prevention and infectious disease control. And not much later (1969) he was able to attend a one-month herbal medicine class taught by experts from all over China, convened in the provincial capital of Kunming.

Still working as a barefoot doctor in 1974, he went for his longest period of training at that time to the Bijiang county health school.[47] This precious opportunity was a one-and-a-half-year training in Western medicine, including anatomy, physiology, pharmacology, microbiology, and parasitology. Among all these trainings, however, Dr. Zhang said he benefited the most from the Liuku training class, especially the on-the-spot teaching offered as the young classmates were all gathering medicines in the mountains. Here is where he also learned bone-setting medicine, so important in dealing with injuries from hard labor in field and forest.

Seeking to understand more about his practice as a village doctor, and still curious about any specifically "Lisu" character his work might have, we visited Dr. Zhang in his house high above the riverside road. We were able to have a long conversation about his clinical practice and his life experiences, and he told us a little more about the 1965 Liuku herbal medicines school. He spoke fondly of his two teachers from the 1965 training class, especially

Dr. Li Shengtang. But then he surprised us: digging in his storage room, he fetched out his treasured book collection to show us.

By far the most precious items in Dr. Zhang's small archive were his mimeographed teaching materials and personal class notes from the training in Liuku in 1965. We could see that the textbooks and Zhang's notebook were much thumbed and the worse for wear, the paper and binding suffering in a damp climate and an overstuffed farmhouse storeroom. But they were lovingly preserved and, Dr. Zhang assured us, still very much in use.

The textbook was handwritten by the two doctors in elegant Chinese script. Clearly, Dr. Li and Dr. Huang were educated men, but not necessarily Lisu (no one we talked to knew their "ethnicity," and minority nationality status would have meant something quite different in those days anyway). The book is structured as a straightforward list of (mostly) botanicals with a clear focus on medicinal drugs. For example, the entry for a drug named *Yizhijian* 一支箭 (literal translation, "an arrow") reads like this:

- Locality of growth: halfway up the hill, across the Nujiang area
- Gathering and processing methods: the roots are the part to be used as medicine, should be gathered in winter, grind the root and cook over a slow fire with egg
- Character and flavor: bitter, cold
- Dosage: 5–10 grams

Almost all the entries for drugs are like this, concise, ordered, and useful for the working practitioner. The format is similar to that of other published pharmacopoeias, with the difference that these teaching materials list only the drugs that can be found locally in the Nujiang area. Interestingly, there were quite a few items added expressly for the training by Drs. Li and Huang. Presumably these had not appeared in previous listings of local natural medicines; those entries are noted with the teachers' name beside them—*Yizhijian* is one such new entry. If a medicinal plant can be found only in a specific area in Nujiang, this is also carefully noted: "halfway up the hill, Lushui county, Nujiang," "tropical areas of Nujiang," or "on big trees and stones across the Nujiang area" are examples.

Dr. Zhang's personal notebook, despite some water marks and fifty years of wear, has survived rather well inside its dark-red rubber cover. The first page shows the date: October 10, 1965. Most of the notes are written in phonetic Lisu language, but the drug names are written in Chinese. From the notebook it is clear that the class started with medicinal plants and then went on to formulas. For example, a page dated late in the three-month term (December 20, 1965) is headed "Rheumatic Disease: Prescription."

We left Shimmer Zhang's farmhouse very impressed with him and his life. At age seventy-one he was still working as the village doctor and making house (or street) calls for ailing friends in Fugong on market days. (He told us he had tried to find a family member to serve as village doctor, but that didn't work out and he is still required to do this difficult job.) Despite his relatively inaccessible (for urbanites) location in a high part of the Nujiang gorge, he had been thoroughly engaged with modern medical knowledge from an early age. Clearly, the health department organizers of trainings saw him from the beginning as talented and well worth training for medical public service. Most fascinating to us was Dr. Zhang's continuing reliance on herbal medicine teaching materials that had been developed by local experts for the advancement of local health work fifty years earlier. Far from being obsolete, this deeply local and therapeutically useful knowledge was both precious and in great danger of being completely forgotten.

That day in July we said goodbye to Dr. Zhang and his family, threaded our way on narrow paths to the gravel road that ran nearby, and started to walk the long distance downhill—we estimated more than ten kilometers—to the riverside township of Pihe where we could get three-wheeled motorcycle rides back to Fugong. We had worries about the feasibility of this plan, though they were lightened by the knowledge that Dr. Zhang, no longer young, still made this journey every market day. But we were lucky—a Nujiang Prefecture forestry department truck happened along, coming from even higher up, and invited us all to cram in and ride down to the river. Lili and Judith laughed: who says the state cannot climb mountains?

ENCOUNTERING HISTORY

Drs. Hu and Zhang were far from being the only veteran servants of the people that we met in western Yunnan. Other doctors there frequently reminded us how important health department training courses had been in shaping their lives in primary care work. One of these interesting practitioners was Dr. Literary Lore Yang. We met him in Weixi, a Lisu autonomous county located over a high mountain ridge to the east of Nujiang, a very long and circuitous bus ride away. Dr. Yang, after participating in several local health schools and being disciple to an old Tibetan healer, had been picked to study medicine in Kunming in a course lasting more than two years. He showed us a volume of training materials used in that course, entitled *Conference on Exchange of Scholarly Experiences by Senior Chinese Doctors in Yunnan Province: Selected Materials* (云南省老中医学术经验交流会—资料选编). The preface says the book, published in 1973, resulted from a meeting that gathered senior Chinese medicine doctors and pharmaceutical workers, minority medicine doctors, recently trained Chinese medicine doctors, and Western medicine doctors, all of them coming together to exchange their experiences of using Chinese medicine and drugs to prevent and treat diseases. This was clearly a meeting of some historical importance, and it is interesting that it took place in the supposedly "anti-expert" cultural revolution period!

Flipping through the worn pages of this collection, we could see that books like this were rich resources for training and practice: it included 35 academic papers, 48 case studies, excerpts from treatment experience with 28 common diseases, and a listing of 245 clinically proven prescriptions used by health professionals all over Yunnan province. The emphasis on herbal medicine and locally available natural medicines in such sources is notable. Especially in the period before the formal beginning of the barefoot doctor program (about 1968),[48] there was a national policy emphasis on using "the great treasure house" of Chinese medical expertise, especially herbal medicine. But another friend still practicing as a village doctor in Weixi County also reminded us that there were long periods when he simply could not get Western medical drugs—though they were in demand—and he and the villagers had no choice but to rely on herbals that he gathered himself in the mountains.

The many health school trainings provided by the state in the collectivist era were hardly unique to the Nujiang and Lijiang area. A historical review by Susan Rifkin that surveys health care policies for all of rural China from 1950 to 1969 found that both biomedicine and indigenous knowledges were important components in the development of rural healthcare expertise, albeit in shifting forms and at different times.[49] Health teams "sent down" from higher administrative levels began the work of increasing health services and hygiene work in the rural areas as early as the Great Leap period (beginning in 1958). Rifkin notes that short course health schools constituted an important state program for improving public health services in China's vast and underserved rural areas. Folded into the barefoot doctor programs around 1968,[50] such rural health schools continued to support local health care delivery at least through the 1970s.

Driven to seek out the scanty literature on the 1960s and 1970s health schools by our encounters with the embodied histories of health workers in Nujiang, we were led to reflect on our own good fortune in meeting some of the original public health trainees from the collectivist era. Our several encounters with herbalist Benefits Hu and village doctor Shimmer Zhang were not the most dramatic events of our 2014 fieldwork, nor were these two doctors the most "different" practitioners of a "nationality" medicine we met. But we still love to reflect on the life stories of these two men. We imagine the historical moment of the early 1960s when a national public health system seized upon these enthusiastic and kindhearted men when they were mere boys, each with only a few years of primary education. Gradually providing them with the basic information and tools they needed to practice primary care medicine in their home communities, health schools at various levels helped them to embody effective skills and make use of unique local knowledge. Dr. Zhang and Dr. Hu were both gathered into the socialist state, and in return they spent decades gathering experience and refining their skills for the sake of local people. By the time we met them, their embodied histories showed us how global, national, and regional medical worlds could be gathered into local forms of medical service.

During our time in Nujiang Prefecture and Weixi Lisu Autonomous County, we saw so much very particular and historically situated medical work, like that of these two health school classmates, that the idea of the local (*bendi* 本地, or *tu* 土) began to be filled with special meaning for us. Becoming ever more comfortable with thinking of the minority nationality as just another word for a *local* gathering of things and practices, as in our discussion of Tujia above, we only occasionally remembered to ask about "Lisu nationality medicine." One person we asked, though, confirmed some of our long-standing suspicions about the significance of nationality in the medical domain.

Dr. Everlasting Mu was the former head of the Fugong County health department. When we asked him how he would define Lisu medicine, he said, "the herbal medicine practiced in Lisu areas is called Lisu medicine, just like the medicine practiced in China is called Chinese medicine. This term, Chinese medicine, is a general one, it is not limited to the Han Chinese." Dr. Mu clearly did not think it was necessary to mark out a Lisu medicine distinct from Chinese medicine, yet he acknowledged geographic specificities. It is significant that he spoke of the *herbal* medicine practiced in Lisu areas. Indeed, he constantly employed the term "Chinese herbal medicine" (*zhongcaoyao* 中草药) to talk about the practices we had come to study. And he was another among our acquaintances in the area who especially respected the herbal medicine knowledge—the deep understanding of the powers and qualities of the natural medicines of the Nujiang gorge—that had been gathered and taught in the 1965-66 Liuku Health School. This may not have been "minority nationality" knowledge, but it was this knowledge that, for medical people, defined the local—which was only, at best, partly Lisu.

Lisu doctor Benefits Hu had been retired for twenty-six years when we met him in 2014, and he told us right away that he had forgotten all the medicine he ever knew. Yet as we asked him about his career and experiences, he began to enjoy introducing us to local herbs and formulas. He was proud of having had a long career practicing medicine in the county hospital, where he had encountered many interesting cases and often trained younger health workers. Throughout his career he had also found time to gather medicines in the mountains, an activity he loved. He told Lili, "I forgot I knew all this stuff, but when you come here asking questions, I find I can actually remember a lot."

Dr. Hu generously invited us to visit his home and pharmacy in Puluo village. Divided from the street by heavy wooden doors, the little shopfront was dusty but orderly. The adjoining porch was stacked with drying whole plants, and the balance scale for weighing out drugs was at the ready. Dr. Hu happily opened drawers to show us some of his more treasured medicines, and he pointed out that a big red wooden pharmacy storage chest he had there was brought down from the old county seat of Bijiang when the county seat moved and the hospital closed. Asked whether he still saw patients in this township dispensary, he said yes, there were a few who still best liked to come there for their medicine. And though he is much slowed down in his retirement, clearly he still found ways to gather.

CONCLUSION

In this chapter we have told of encounters that took place along an itinerary through China's southern mountains over a period of more than five years. Our research travels, as we reflect on them, recall for us the ancient and multifaceted metaphor of the path or Way (the Dao 道). We have made no effort to exhaustively record or recount that itinerary; after all, the Way that can be spoken of is not the constant Way.[51] It is, we suppose, rather akin to the nomad itineraries of "traditional" healing. We have resisted the temptation of drawing a map of our route, or detailing a chronology of encounters, or listing a cast of characters. We promise no illusion of comprehensiveness in either space or time. After all, the paths we authors took, sometimes together and sometimes apart, through the emerging terrain of nationality medicines were constantly cross-cut by other roads, other projects, other people's agendas, and our own vacillating attentions. Chinese government policy and administration apart, the development of minority nationality medicines was of central importance to just a few of us as we met along this road. To everyone else, the nationality medicine development project might have been quite invisible; minority nationality medicine may not have been much of a thing for many people.

Our storytelling has sought to preserve the event quality of some field encounters in our research. We have described medical and research practices so basic that they seem to evade all generalizing labels. These stories never succeed in being "about" Tujia, Achang, Yao, or Lisu medicines, and they keep spilling beyond the taken-for-granted domain of medicine. They fail even to preserve localness. The lives of the actors themselves are highly mobile, as they climb mountains, seek out storied practitioners in other districts, register for short courses, host government work teams or itinerant herbalists, and carry medicinal plants to the city to help a relative. The drugs themselves are in active circulation, as a visit to any periodic vegetable market shows. If we just confine our attention to the matters of concern we have taken up here, Tujia plants and "*tima* culture," Achang "theoretical" medicine, the Yao pharmacopoeia as it is standardized, and the herbal knowledge taught in health schools are all important and consequential for more than a few people. But with these encounter stories we perhaps have succeeded only in showing how difficult it is to hold such matters of concern, and their allied earth and heavens, "firmly in place."

This observation is consistent with a worry that is often expressed: precious indigenous knowledge around the world is under threat and disappearing. Other worlds of healing experience and unique forms of social solidarity are falling into obscurity behind the glare of scientific rationality and state production and regulation of knowledge. Certainly, most of the local nationality medicine experts we met were quite elderly, and few of them had transmitted their skills to disciples or younger relatives. Some techniques recognized to be "not superstitious, but rather, effective" (recall Dr. Brilliance Zhang's remarks at the beginning of the chapter) could not even be acknowledged in the world of textbooks, official drugs lists, and standardized tests. And health insurance does not pay for folk medical treatments.

As we tracked the salvaging and sorting, synthesizing and elevating projects of nationality medicine activists and their elderly teachers, however, we witnessed two sides of an emergent medical pluralism: certainly, the enframing and regulating state was hard at work articulating drugs, techniques, diseases, and health care workers so that a "medicine" could be held firmly in place. But at the same time, local experts of all kinds, women, men, young, old, Miao, Tujia, Achang, Lisu, Yao, Han, educated, "illiterate," continued to gather medicines in the mountains—or along the roadside, or among the tea bushes, or in kitchen gardens—lay them out in the sun or hang them from the ceiling to dry, add them to soups, mix them with honey, mash them into a plaster for a wound, and combine them in weighed proportions into "secret formulas."

Perhaps the most interesting aspect of the national salvaging and sorting moment that occasioned our diverse field encounters is that these two

currents of activity are swerving together—scientists and health administrators are talking with herbalists, bone-setters, diviners, forest ramblers,
ritualists, and even anthropologists. And these local experts are proving
willing to share some of their world with outsiders. Whatever the trajectory
of this broad movement, we cannot believe that its only direction in China
is decline.

Conclusions, and Then Some . . .

Yes, minority nationality medicines are a thing. Some of the *shaoshuminzu yiyao* (少数民族医药) that have appeared in the pages of this book are quite formally *instituted*, boasting rich stores of systematized *knowledge* that is expressed and made effective in the *embodied practice* of skilled doctors, and confirmed in the *bodily experiences* of sufferers. Minority nationality medicines depend on the powers of natural products—like the *wild plants* collected by "drug farmers" (*yaonong* 药农) and nomad herbalists (*lao caoyi* 老草医)—and they flexibly address particular situations (according to the time, the person, and the place) with trusted drugs, techniques, healing hands, mutual teaching, and assistance from the yin side. And then some.

The officially recognized nationality medicines we have explored in *Gathering Medicines* are creatures of particular times and places, assembled by actors who learn from collective past experience and work with local re-sources to craft new medical sciences that can be distinguished from the biomedical and traditional Chinese medical (TCM) services that are widely available in China. Twenty-first-century nationality culture and science are, as we have argued, more understandable as *local* phenomena than as ethnic or racial formations: modern Tujia medicine is different in Hubei and in Hunan, yet hard to distinguish from Miao nationality medicine anywhere. Qiang medicine in Mao County is different from Qiang medicine further west in Sichuan province, where it overlaps more with Tibetan traditions. The Yao medicine that can be accessed in Jinxiu's hospital does not offer some of the efficacies that can be had a few miles away in the private homes of Yao medicinal wine-makers, nor is it identical to what is on offer in the new Yao Hospital in Beijing. Most important, the "pattern discernment and therapy determination" reasoning held to be constitutive of the modern TCM Lili and Judith studied in the medical schools of China's big cities appears to be of very little interest to the theorists and methodologists of all nationality medicines. Diversity and heterogeneity notwithstanding, in the towns and cities we visited where nationality medical activists were at work, there was a strong sense of meaningful lived *place* growing up around the bodies and skills, tools and drugs, of some who identified as Zhuang or Qiang, Achang or Yao (and then some).

Some of the medical activities noted in this book have not yet, and may never, produce a locally influential system of nationality medicine. Lisu medical men appear more oriented toward learning directly from nature than engaging in "scholarly exchange" with other Lisu healers, and with those habits they may never achieve a textbook or a hospital. Li nationality residents of Hainan—an island province much taken over by plantations and mainland tourists—struggle to maintain a critical mass of nationality activists who could render local lore as transmissible formal knowledge beyond mere catalogs of botanicals. Academy Director Resolution Ma may never figure out the unique nature of the theoretical foundations underlying Achang medicine and distinguishing it from TCM.

Things like nationality medical systems are, then, heterogeneous and localized, but as we have shown here, they *gather* in a social process that can be observed and appreciated historically. We have traced the recent becoming of new traditional medicines—formidable achievements, in our view—through the writings, oral explanations, and ongoing practices of those activists who have taken up a challenge to development issuing from Beijing that started in the early 1980s. The gathering medicines process, however, has its discouraging side. National cultural policy may be turning away from nationality pluralism, and even in well-instituted areas there may not be enough knowledgeable experts to sustain present services and produce a coming medical community.

In the course of this work, we have been continually reminded of Zhuangzi's truism, "Human life is a gathering of qi: when it gathers, this is life; when it scatters, this is death."[1] Zhuangzi here points out the obvious against which creative activists and builders of heritage always struggle: it is folly to deny the inevitable tendency of all life—institutional life, human bodily life, plant and animal life, everyday social life—to scatter and come to an end. But, as the *Zhuangzi* corpus also reminds us, in an "outer chapter," the merest seeds, bugs, and worms end their lives-as-such in the "birth" of new forms—leopards, horses, humans! And who is to say that all that gathers into form does *not* eventually return, undifferentiated, rescattered, into "the unfathomable works"?[2]

The tendency of all things to fall apart, even those encouraged by ministries of health and a multicultural government, even those legally certified through carefully designed examinations, is a potential that is courageously battled by our friends in the nationality medicines movement. Formal knowledge—the textbooks and summaries that embody the nascent royal science taught to large classes of Zhuang and Yao interns, and still dreamed of by less fully instituted nationalities—is the secret weapon of those who would see the things of nationality medicines properly gathered. Those practitioners who know what drugs are powerful, where they can be found, how illness sufferers self-cure, what physiological flows need to be nudged, what local pathologies need to be controlled—these inspiring experts sometimes become disenchanted with institutional life and retire to the hills and forests to treat only family members and neighbors. Too often, local healers die without leaving disciples who could carry on their nomad science or help to build a new royal science. This sense of disappearing cultural and medical expertise may lie behind Laborjoy Wei's passion for continuing his hands-on (and shirt off) studies with old rural masters. At the same time, a sense of the inevitability of scatter may underlie his commitment to getting definitions and techniques for *sha* disease written down and published. Formal knowledge is a central weapon for energetic builders of nationality medicines like him, but it is not the only actor in play.

Like other ethnographies, this book has described forms of natural and cultural becoming that are specific to one region, southern and southwestern China, and especially those areas associated with minority nationality populations. This is a vast area, but it is not all of "China," nor does it tell us much about the rest of East or Southeast Asia. Perhaps there are no universally applicable lessons to be learned here.

Ethnographies are full of concrete things, some of them bounded material objects and some stabilized conceptual or ideological entities. All the things we have discussed, from large formations like hospitals, health departments, and mountain ranges, to minor actors like an egg marked with a mystic character or a table of contents in a Zhuang medicine textbook, are unique—they are concrete, recognized, relatively discrete, and located in time and space. We ethnographers can seldom explain the joy we take in each of these specific things. But, it bears repeating, all things that live are *gathered*. Rather than merely describe an entity—such as a brick-and-mortar clinic or a handful of fritillary bulbs—we turn as historians to the ongoing process of assembly that continues to construct viable nationality things. We have looked past the particular characteristics of the myriad local things to seek some generalities in the process of gathering itself. There has been a specific and instructive assembly process at work in China: salvaging and sorting, synthesizing and elevating minority medicines are social forms of work that are institutional, epistemological, bodily, and scientific. They discipline and intensify innovation, and they result from and express the seriousness and creativity of many actors in China. They are a version of gathering medicines from which other worlds can learn.

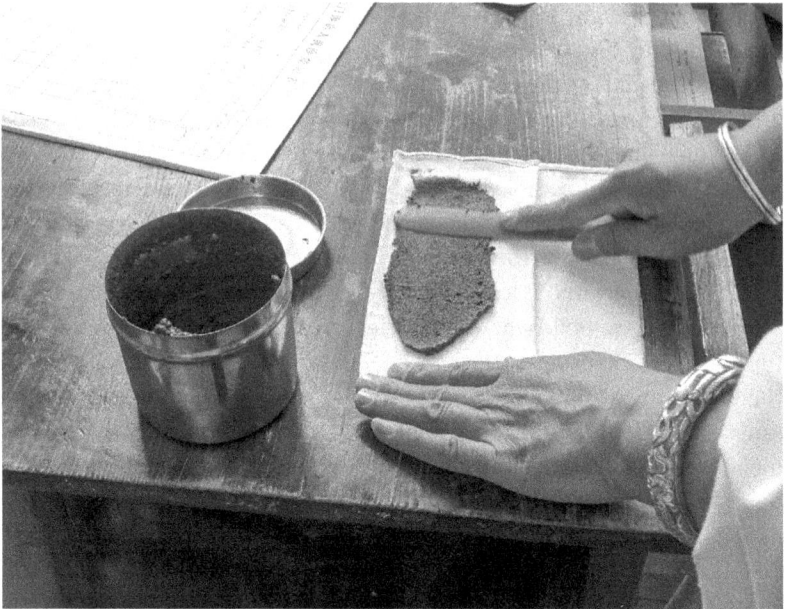

Figure 5. A Qiang nationality bone-setter prepares
an herbal plaster in his hospital clinic.

AND THEN SOME . . .

This ethnographic study set out to catch social becoming in the act. But
that is not a task that can be completed or concluded. The everyday activities of climbing the mountains to pluck medicines, attaching bamboo tubes
to draw out heat poison, laboring over a nomenclature chart in a tense conference room, checking daily blood pressures for elderly neighbors, writing
catalogs of symptoms and therapies, *and then some* — these practices continue to fascinate us, and yet all partially elude our analytical grasp. If there's
one thing that an ethnographer learns, it is that things themselves speak
anthropology and history better than scholars do.

So we close with a return to the concrete and the haptic: Consider the
herbal plaster. A folded gauze package of combined natural medicines
cooked and ground into a mash, damp and sometimes smelly, applied to
your ulcerated ankle, bound around your painful shoulder or wrist, held
against your aching lower back with bandaging, or taped to your bruised
ribs. You need to keep it pressed against your body for several days at least,
at times renewing the mixture of drugs gathered into the awkward package.
If you are a hospital inpatient with a painful chronic lesion, like Dr. Goldstamp Huang's lymphoma patient in the Jinxiu Yao Hospital, you might find

considerable comfort in a daily application of a warming, drying, and healing mash wrapped in soft gauze.[3] If you are an anthropological fieldworker walking a lot and traveling by bus between county towns (we're thinking of Judith's visit to Dr. Purity Chu's private clinic outside Jinxiu), you might find a thick plaster strapped around your knee quite inconvenient, even if it does ease your arthritis pain.

Plasters are ubiquitous across China's southern nationality areas, but they are not prominent in the national literature of traditional Chinese medicine. They appear only as minor technologies in TCM herbal pharmacy textbooks, and when they are noted in mainstream medical literature they are listed as part of the rather peripheral specialty of "external medicine" (*waike* 外科). External medicine in China tends to be left either to biomedical surgeons or to folk experts such as bone-setters and masseurs.[4] In the process of doing research across China's south and southwest, however, we saw many herbal plasters prepared and applied. Some "bone-setters," accustomed to treating injuries of many kinds, emphasized to us that the continuous hard work of southern mountain farmers puts them at risk for sprains, fractures, infected sores, and heatstroke. What is, thus, a minor and peripheral technology for urban and mainstream TCM becomes, in nationality hands, a valued form of what Laborjoy Wei called "microsurgery" working with the surfaces of porous southern bodies.

The herbal plaster renders concrete a wide scatter of natural-cultural relations. Have you got a disorder somewhere in your body? Put the powers of the forest up against the place and it will get better. But natural herbs and natural bodies are very mixed, local things, as we have shown throughout this study. The humble herbal plaster congeals in its down-to-earth obviousness a complex history of human and nonhuman actions spanning far-flung networks. It gathers knowledge, labor, efficacies, social relations, wild powers, institutional habits, affinities and antagonisms between things, and many specific processes of life and growth into a bundle that addresses your disordered body with direct contact, nudging your life toward healing.

Let us dwell for a moment on the nature of plasters, drawing first on the language of the TCM experts themselves. Plasters appear near the end of one mainstream herbal pharmacy textbook, defined in a way that would not be contested by nationality practitioners. In its small note on "external use drugs," the entry covers some of the salient characteristics and special powers of "pastes."[5]

> The term external use drugs refers to a part of the *materia medica* that is mainly for out-of-the-ordinary uses. . . . These drugs are variously effective to resolve poisons and reduce swelling, transform putrefaction and

draw out toxins, cause pus to discharge and pain to cease, enliven blood and stop bleeding. They are mainly used to treat ulcers and boils, scabies, external wounds, snake bites, burns, and disorders in the five senses. Locally smeared on, applied in a plaster, steamed/vaporized, used as eye, nose, or throat drops—these are the main modes of use. A few of these drugs are okay for internal use.

The list of discomforts addressed by this therapy is rather miscellaneous, and when you consider the complex dynamic whole that is the Chinese medical body, with its circulation tracks and interacting organ systems, these disorders are notably localized and superficial. From a TCM perspective, these are "out of the ordinary" utilities. External medicine pastes like this do not take up much space in textbooks, nor do patients with these problems often occupy the large wards of TCM hospitals. Indeed, after this definitional paragraph, there are only twelve drugs (of the thousands recorded in the same textbook) listed as usual for external application, eight of which "have *du*-poison [有毒]" in various degrees. This *Chinese Pharmacy* textbook thus leaves much to the imagination of the reader, who wonders how a practitioner would actually use, or localize, these listed medicines.[6] That is to say, the bulk of the knowledge is left to be taught on the job in practice supervised by relatively nomad knowers; these experts would need to be drawn from the peripheries of the royal science of TCM. And as our nationality medicine mentors have taught us, such peripheral agencies are often southern, often drawing their authority from gathering in the mountains.

The external medicines applied in plasters present unusual technical problems in a pharmacy field that, like TCM, mainly focuses on decoctions taken by mouth. Many of the drugs in use have a special relationship to the question of efficacy/toxicity (*du* 毒). The Chengdu pharmacy textbook does not fail to mention this issue, in the interest of promoting safe clinical usage:

> The majority of these drugs have some toxicity or are even poisonous. In external use of high-toxicity drugs the amounts used should be small, and the proportion of these drugs in a formula should not be great. The surface to which they are applied may not be too large lest it be easy through breathing to receive an overdose and be poisoned [*zhongdu* 中毒].

These modern technical warnings notwithstanding, everyone knows that those drugs classified as most toxin-bearing (*youdu* 有毒) are also the most effective against all manner of pathologies. Given the porousness and dynamic flows of the human body, plasters might be seen as a technology custom-designed for maximizing therapeutic value while controlling the dangers of powerful toxin-bearing drugs. Each plaster, in other words, containing a combination of natural drugs chosen for its appropriateness to the "particular illness condition,"[7] might act as a discriminating two-way filter, drawing specific toxins out of the body and sending in efficacies (forms of qi) that will have a wholesome and possibly systemic effect. The nationality medicine disorders we have listed elsewhere in the book add complexity: as we know, *du*-poisons are the main pathology in southern mountain China, so the power of plasters to "resolve poisons" and "draw out toxins" works in parallel with the high toxicity of external use drugs.

This gathering has yielded a powerful therapeutic agent. An herbal paste offering up its complex efficacies among the folds of sterile gauze is a gathered medicine *par excellence*. As such, it indexes—as metonym, a part representing an unknowable whole—many of the assemblages we have been exploring in *Gathering Medicines*. The questions raised and the large and small mysteries presented by the formulas and classifications found in both TCM and nationality medicine textbooks are not failures on the part of their clinician-editors.[8] Rather, such gaps are invitations to working healers and their disciples to craft locally sourced and locally serviceable medicines. A medicine may be a smelly and sticky mush folded in cloth and extending its qi toward the lurking pain of an arthritic knee, or it may be a salvaged and sorted, synthesized and elevated "medical system" recognized by the State Administration of Traditional Chinese Medicine in Beijing. Both senses of the term refer to something made, albeit not by one creator. These and the other medicines we have gathered in this book escape any comprehensive understanding. The thing itself escapes not because it is essentially unhistorical and nonlinguistic (we would argue that things properly understood are neither of these negatives) but because it is always too much to grasp, presenting an ontological excess.

Stories about plants, animals, and minerals; itinerant healers and gardening grandmothers; textbook writers and curriculum designers; Daoist mantras and transformed water; hands-on cooking and haptic therapeutics; ancient classics and modern toxicology; clinical trials and visiting regulators—these show us how ten thousand things collude to form an assemblage known as medicine (at any scale: the drugs, the techniques, the colleges, the profession, the archive). These are not accounts that can be "understood" or stories that can be completed. We can trace the itineraries of many kinds of related actors across far-flung networks of practice, witness as historians the material and powerful becoming of beneficent healing modalities, and analyze the large and small institutions that try to guarantee their goodness. We field researchers can ourselves be transformed in our mountain-climbing and computer-using lives as we encounter (often with pleasure, always with surprises) the diversities that are nationality-marked local medicines in China.

But we cannot claim to know the whole thing that is minority nationality medicine in China. Not only is it not one system, institution, sector, or subculture, it does not stand still to be described. As we have been watching the initiatives known as nationality medicine develop and change, with our activist friends we have been concerned for the future. We would hate to see the world forget how to prepare a healing herbal plaster in a farmhouse kitchen. And we still want to better understand the logic by which relatively poisonous drugs both apply toxic efficacy to an injury and draw out the "damp-heat" toxins that interfere with whole-body flow (*tong* 通). Some of this is written down for experts to consult. But writing leaves so many gaps! We hope the nationality healers of forest and clinic, hospital and storefront encountered in this book will long be able to compound their drugs and, with them, assemble viable futures for local knowledge.

Acknowledgments

We have elsewhere in this book acknowledged our many debts to the people and institutions that have been active in the emergence of minority nationality medicines, both as practical things-in-the-making and as scholarly subjects for anthropologists and historians. Collaboration and scholarly exchange are crucial for the development of new medicines in China, and these activities have also been indispensable to our work as anthropologists. The "Methodology, Collaboration" section of the introduction, in particular, has much to say about the specific contributions of a network of creative and energetic comrades who were recruited to this project along the way. Some of these researchers continue to study new medical developments across China. And our citations of other published authors, some of them working alongside us on minority nationality questions, have often been made with considerable gratitude for much inspiration. We have found teachers in so many unexpected places, and we have tried to respond by giving credit as often and early as possible. We hope none of our friends and comrades are being forgotten in this volume.

The State Administration of Traditional Chinese Medicine, a unit of the National Health Commission in Beijing, started us down this road with an invitation to Lili Lai to add anthropological methods to their nationality medicines development project. We relied heavily at first on Hou Fengfei of the SATCM to help us organize our field research and make the necessary contacts with local officials. Retired leader of the SATCM and long-time president of the China Medical Association of Minorities Zhu Guoben warmly encouraged us and gave us extremely useful books. And Professor Zheng Jin of the Yunnan Administration of TCM shared in the intellectual excitement of this research. Zhen Yan of the China Academy of Chinese Medical Sciences was a friend to our work from the beginning; she continues to kindly consult on issues that arise in minority medicine studies in China.

We are especially thankful for sustained help and challenges offered by the nationality medicine advocates we encountered in the course of our traveling field research. Our admiration and gratitude for these conscientious and creative experts should be clear in our storytelling throughout the book. But we especially want to thank Tan Laoxi in Nanning and environs and Ma Kejian in Yunnan for serving as true comrades and frequent interlocutors. Warm thanks are also due to Zhuang medicine scholars Huang Hanru and Huang Jinming, who solved many problems for us through their writings while finding time in their busy schedules to answer our questions in person. The lively curiosity and fieldwork companionship of Hou Jinian, chair of the local district Centers for Disease Control in Zhangjiajie, Hunan, were an unexpected and much appreciated gift.

At about the same time we were beginning to plan and engage in field research, in 2010, the University of Chicago established its center in Beijing near Renmin University of China. Over the ensuing years the center provided an excellent base for Judith Farquhar, and after 2016 both of us had offices there. We thank the entire staff of the center for allowing our conversations between rooms to dominate the faculty suite, and for tolerating our habit of making writing plans on classroom whiteboards. We are especially indebted to Liang Xueming and Beth Bader for their understanding and support of our work, and to Hannah Pickwell (when she was acting as a teaching assistant) for shouldering part of the burden of other responsibilities. The center very kindly hosted one of our research associate training sessions (during which the whole staff submitted cheerfully to being interviewed by trainees), and helped us entertain visitors, interviewees, and fellow researchers. We greatly benefited from the thoughtful assistance of University of Chicago interns Alex Ding, Sarah Friedman, Colin Garon, and Feng Ye; Lili's Peking University student Wei Wei helped us index medical books; and Sare Arecanli visited just in time to be recruited to a planning session with a whiteboard. The intelligent engagement of these friends with the book helped us avoid solipsism and remember the important questions.

Writing the book while based in Beijing meant that we could enjoy the company of stimulating interlocutors from several universities and disciplines. We thank Wang Min'an, Huang Yingying, Gong Haoqun, Fu Xiaoxing, Liu Liu, Liu Xueting, Liu Wennan, Su Chunyan, Xiao Suowei, Zhang Xu, Zhang Hui, and Kris Kardaszewicz for keeping the intellectual terrain there exciting and relevant for both of us. The support of Gao Bingzhong of the Anthropology Program at Peking University is much appreciated as well, and other anthropologists in China—Weng Naiqun, Zhang Wenyi, Tan Tongxue, Song Hongjuan, Zhou Yongming, and Li Ruohui especially— joined Professor Gao and his colleagues in Beijing as they helped us work out a non-Eurocentric contemporary anthropology. Colleagues not mentioned in the rest of this book—Duan Zhongyu, Li Chengwei, Qin Ana, and Liu Cheng—were valued companions in the process of thinking through medicine. Some who were passing through, or involved with us at a distance, also made anthropological contributions for which we are grateful (and which they might have forgotten): Mikkel Bunkenborg, Lorraine Daston, Bruce Doar, Eric Karchmer, Marshall Kramer, Vivienne Lo, Dale Martin, Carl Mitcham, Peter Redfield, and Gang Yue.

Lili Lai's colleagues and leaders in the School of Health Humanities of the Peking University Medical Center supported our anthropological approach to a history and sociology of medicine with sympathy and administrative help. We both thank Zhang Daqing, Zhou Cheng, Guo Liping, Wang Yifang, and especially Li Runhong for their generous support. We are also grateful to the publishers of some Chinese journals that accepted preliminary reports from our group. *Kaifang Shidai/Open Times* published our first Chinese research article; the *Guangxi Nationality University Report* produced a special issue on our research; and Chen Bin, editor of *Sixiang Zhanxian/Frontiers of Thought*, was especially welcoming of Lili Lai's theoretical writing.

In the course of the itinerant field research conducted for this study, we passed through a number of institutions as brief or longer-term guests. These included the Chongqing University Institute for Advanced Studies in the Humanities and Social Sciences; Hainan College of Traditional Chinese Medicine; Hospital of Traditional Chinese Medicine and Qiang Medicine in Mao County, Sichuan; Hospital of Yao Medicine in Jinxiu County, Guangxi; Hospital of Zhuang Medicine in Nanning, Guangxi; the College of Traditional Chinese Medicine in Hubei Minzu University, Enshi; the Institute of Minority Medicines in Xiangxi, Hunan; Yunnan Academy of Traditional Chinese Medicine, and the Yunnan University Department of Anthropology. We were always accorded the most gracious and sympathetic hospitality and assistance in these institutions.

In 2012 we received a generous research grant from the American Council of Learned Societies; this funding made it possible to monopolize the time of some of our field associates for a short but productive while, and also to free up some of Lili Lai's time, which she spent enjoyably in Chicago. Judith spent the 2015–16 academic year as a fellow of the National Humanities Center in North Carolina. The opportunity to present a preliminary account of nationality medicines to sophisticated audiences there and in universities and colleges around North and South Carolina was precious. But conversations with fellow fellows April Masten, Norman Kutcher, Bill Schwarz, and Janice Radway, in particular, were even more important.

Further research support over the years came from the Adolf and Marian

Lichtstern Fund of the Department of Anthropology and the Division of the Social Sciences at the University of Chicago. Judith Farquhar's colleagues and students at the University of Chicago have long modeled for us the kinds of activity that belong in a great research and teaching institution, so this research funding is only a small part of our debt. And finally, a research fund provided by the University of Chicago Global Engagement office and the Beijing Center supported some of the costs incurred in the writing process after 2016. We are humbly grateful for all this institutional support.

Priya Nelson and Karen Darling at the University of Chicago Press and the two anonymous reviewers they found were exemplary in their expeditious and intelligent processing of the book manuscript. Susan Tarcov did a wonderful job of copyediting, and Jenny Addison produced a map and a diagram for us with no muss and no fuss. We feel lucky to be read and helped by such discriminating professionals.

Our more personal debts are many. Judith Farquhar's thinking has been assisted through the Translating Vitalities project led by Volker Scheid (initially), Carla Nappi, and herself. There is not much about nationality medicines on the TV website (www.translatingvitalities.com), but our workshops over five or six years have considerably brightened the writing process for this book. In Chicago (and in North Carolina for the NHC year), James Hevia labored alongside this book, reminding us what good historiography is and nudging ours in more wholesome directions. In his readings of our drafts he always insists on sanity and clarity, and we thank him warmly for that.

Lili Lai has enjoyed the unflagging backing of her family in Shanghai as she has negotiated a career path in Beijing. She wishes to name her parents and sister here, even though inside the family, no one ever bothers to say thank you. Judith Farquhar thus presumes to thank Lai Guoquan, Tong Wuqin, and Lai Lilin, as well as Lili's dear and ever-supportive friend Nie Jianlan, for making our intercontinental and translingual collaboration on this book possible.

Most of all, we appreciate each other. As we have researched and written this book, our friendship has put down ever deeper roots, and our participation in new and old worlds has grown ever more joyful, as we have taught each other—we think!—how to be better anthropologists.

Appendix

The Emphasis on "Three Ways and Two Roads" in Zhuang Medicine and Pharmacy

Huang Hanru and Rong Xiaoxiang
This is a translation of an essay that appeared in
China News of Traditional Chinese Medicine, December 25, 2015.

INTRODUCTION

- Zhuang medicine (ZM) takes yinyang as the root, and the synchrony of the Three Qi, to be core theory. Within the relations of yinyang, ZM especially emphasizes the leading role of yang qi, such that emphasizing yang, regulating yang, strengthening yang, have become an important idea in ZM's prevention and treatment of disease. The human body is a small heaven and earth, the qi of the internal body's three parts (heaven, human, and earth) must circulate in synchrony, it must both restrict and transform generation if a healthy condition is to be protected.
- The "Three Ways" are the Grain Way, the Water Way, and the Qi Way. The Two Roads are the Dragon Road and the Fire Road. Though ZM has partly appropriated TCM's channels and collaterals theory (e.g., in channel sinews theory [*jingjin lilun* 经筋理论]), still, the Three Ways and Two Roads play a major and specifically [Zhuang] theoretical role. At the heart of the Three Ways and Two Roads is [the concept of] *tong* [通], or through-flow.
- Regulating qi, breaking down poisons, and supplementing depletion are not only Zhuang medical principles of treating diseases but also basic ideas used in Zhuang medicine to prevent disease and nurture health, having an important guiding significance in "treating the not yet ill."

Zhuang medicine is a nationality traditional medicine and pharmacy that has gradually formed and developed through the long process of struggle by Zhuang nationality people against hunger, disease, injury, and a hostile natural environment. Zhuang medicine and pharmacy is also an important component of traditional Zhuang nationality culture.

HISTORICAL EVOLUTION

The period during which experience of ZM diagnosis and therapy, techniques, formulas, and drugs accumulated stretches from the former Qin period [221-207 BCE] through to the early 1980s. Its [historical] periods can be divided into the two periods of the pre-Qin and the post-Qin periods. In the pre-Qin period needling and drugs were already in use, but this was a time of origins, so techniques and formulas were rather simple; the bronze needles dug up in old tombs are fairly short and could be used only for shallow needling, and the types of drug products unearthed are relatively few. After Emperor Qin Shi unified Lingnan [the South] the techniques and formulas used by Zhuang medicine became much more elaborate. Especially after the Tang and Song Dynasties [618-1279 CE], there was increased understanding of the diseases often seen in Lingnan, as well as of common diseases and their characteristics; not only did techniques mature, the drugs in use increased to more than 100 types. Medical books like *Formulas of the South* appeared, and especially after the Ming Dynasty records of eminent local doctors in many places began to appear in the gazetteers.

During the long period of accumulation of diagnostics, therapies, techniques, and formulas, although ZM developed comparatively slowly, still, by seeing as a whole the prevention and treatment needs of a vast territory's population, [the field] was able to achieve a certain level of development. Especially as regards needling therapies and the manufacture of metal needles; the knowledge and use of poison drugs and antidotes; and the rich experience of preventing and treating symptoms of *sha*-fevers, *zhang*-miasmas, *gu*-parasites, *du*-poison, wind, and damp diseases—with regard to all these, ZM developed the characteristic features of [medicine at] a high developmental level. At the Zhuang site of Yuanlong Village #101, Matou Town, Wuming County, a tomb of the Western Zhou [1050-770 BCE] yielded bronze needles for medical use, furnishing material proof of the passage in the *Inner Canon of the Yellow Emperor* that says, "the nine needles all come from the south." This remains the earliest find of bronze needles for medical use in China.

The period of the formation and rapid development of the theoretical system and medical education system of ZM dates from the First National Working Conference on Nationality Medicines held in 1984. In February 2002 the ZM theoretical system—incorporating the tenets of yinyang as the root, synchrony of Three Qi, the body composed of visceral systems, qi and blood, muscles, bones and flesh, emphasizing the disease causes of poison and depletion and the therapeutic principles of breaking down poison and supplementing depletion—was evaluated by the Guangxi Health Department and Science and Technology Department for the positive results of scientific research. At that time ZM received a second-place award for progress in Guangxi science and technology and a national TCM science and technology award. [Also by that time] many representative works of ZM theory and clinical specialties were being published as a series, e.g., *History of Zhuang Nationality Medicine, China's Zhuang Medicine, China's Zhuang Pharmacy, China's Zhuang Internal Medicine, China's Zhuang Acumoxa Medicine*, etc. The specialized work *History of Zhuang Nationality Medicine* received a first prize for Chinese nationality books and was nominated for a National Library award; it also received a third-place national science and technology progress award (for science and technology books) and was praised as a milestone of Zhuang medical history by medical historian Professor Cai Jingfeng. Formed on the basis of a ZM theoretical system, an ancient Zhuang medicine and pharmacy was elevated to become a discipline: Zhuang medicine.

A PARTICULAR MEDICAL REASONING
[*TESE YILI* 特色医理]

Yinyang as the root, synchrony of the Three Qi: the Zhuang nationality "sets great store by yin and yang" (chap. 17, Ming Dynasty Guangxi Gazetteer), so ZM takes yinyang to be the root and has the synchronization of the Three Qi as its core theory. ZM holds that every kind of normal and abnormal phenomenon of nature and the human body, and their changes, are a response to and result of the opposed, interrooted, waxing and waning, balancing, and intertransformative mutuality of yin and yang [qi]. In the yin and yang relationship, ZM especially emphasizes the guiding role of yang qi, holding that the traits of the lived body that have life are an expression of the existence and activity of yang qi. The human body's yang qi normally tends to scatter, so signs of yang depletion are often seen clinically. Increasing yang, regulating yang, and strengthening yang have become important ideas in ZM prevention and therapy. At the same time, ZM considers that yin and yang must normally stand in a state of relatively harmonious balance in order to maintain a certain stable equilibrium; if it is otherwise, no matter whether it is humans or the natural environment, disasters and illnesses will come about.

ZM calls qi "*xu*." Qi suffuses heaven and earth and the human body, being expressed as yang, motive power, energy, and as the life span that is the birth, growth, health, aging, and death of the human body; [this "*xu*"] depends on the qi of heaven and earth for its restraint and control. Human qi and the qi of heaven and earth intimately intermingle in their flow, they work in synchrony. Humans are the "magic" of the myriad things, they have a certain special agency in adapting to changes in the qi of heaven and earth. The human body is also a microcosm [*xiao tiandi* 小天地] such that the heaven, human, and earth qi sectors [called in ZM "the Three Qi"] inside the body must run in sync [*tongbu yunxing* 同步运行] and thereby mutually control the generation and transformation processes in the interest of maintaining a healthy condition. The significance of the "synchrony of the Three Qi" lies in "synchronizing," which means harmonizing movements and mutually controlling them in order to preserve a dynamic equilibrium between yin and yang.

Theory of Visceral Systems; Qi & Blood; Muscles, Skin, and Flesh; and the spirit-governing qiaowu: ZM holds that these are the basic structures of the body and the material basis of its various functions. Especially the *qiaowu* (brain), which is the central governing pivot that maintains the dynamic equilibrium of yin and yang.

In Yizhou, where many Zhuang people are concentrated, as early as the Northern Song period [960–1127 CE] there were records of human anatomy; moreover, [they] sketched out our nation's first human anatomy diagrams, the *Ou Xi Fan* [欧希范] *Pictures of the Five Viscera*. Most Zhuang nationality local folk still have the custom of "secondary burial," so ZM early on had an understanding of the human viscera and the bones, muscles, skin and flesh of the material body [*shiti* 实体] and their functions. ZM's knowledge of the material body and its functions, such as qi/blood/*jing*-essence/fluids and the *zang* yin organs and the *fu* yang organs—Heart, Liver, Lungs, Kidneys, Stomach, Intestines, and so forth—is basically the same as what has been recorded for TCM. But what needs to be particularly pointed out is that the Zhuang folk in dissecting and butchering animals repeatedly discovered that the spleen organ (in Zhuang language it is called the *weilong*) stored a lot of blood, and of course they had the expression that when people are angry they "vent their spleen" [*fa piqi* 发脾气], so they slowly came to understand that the spleen organ, in addition to the way TCM speaks of it as [governing] the movement-transformation function, is a qi and blood storage and regulation reservoir. Supplementing qi and blood and supplementing the spleen visceral system thus have a very close relationship.

The knowledge in ZM about the *qiaowu* (brain) has historically been rather exact, considering that the activities of the human spirit, language, and capacity for thought, as well as the regulation of the functions of the visceral systems and the sense organs, are all functions of the *qiaowu*; hence the formation of the theory that the *qiaowu* governs the spirit. The *qiaowu* is located in the upper part of the body (i.e., the heaven sector), its place is high and its powers are great, it lives up to its name as the guiding part of the human body. What is seen clinically is that, because of "*qiaowu* disorder" or "bad *qiaowu*" leading to mental dullness or mistakes, or producing disorder in every kind of function of the body, the three Qi are unable to be synchronized, yin and yang lose their regularity, and it's easy for diseases to come up.

Theory of the Three Ways and the Two Roads: The "Three Ways" are the Grain Way, the Water Way, and the Qi Way. The "Two Roads" are the Dragon Road and the Fire Road. Though TCM's channels and collaterals theory is partly accepted by ZM (as in channel sinew theory), the main and characteristic theory is still that of the Three Ways and Two Roads.

The Zhuang nationality and their precursors the Luoyue [骆越] people were one of the earliest groups in Chinese and world history to initiate irrigated agriculture, so they knew that irrigated grains are endowed with the qi of both heaven and earth to sprout and mature, they depend on the qi of heaven and earth to be harvested, and they receive the qi of heaven and earth to nourish the human body. So the through-channel that takes these into the body for digestion and assimilation is called the Grain Way (Zhuang: *tiaogen ai*), mainly indicating the gastric passage and the stomach and spleen, with the pivots of the transformations being the liver, gall bladder, pancreas, and spleen. Water is the source of life, so the body has the Water Way for taking in water and other liquids, and this occasions the most direct connection with nature. The Grain Way and the Water Way are the same going in but they differ coming out; after water and grain essences have been assimilated into nutrients, the Grain Way excretes fecal matter and the Water Way excretes sweat and urine, tears and saliva. The governing pivots of the Water Way are the kidneys and the urinary bladder. The Qi Way is the through passage that interchanges human body qi and the qi of nature to replenish body qi; qi enters the mouth and nose, and the pivotal visceral system of the Qi Way is the lungs. The characteristic of the "Three Ways" is that they mutually and directly flow through nature, and nature and the three material states of the body (the solid, the liquid, and the qi-gaseous) enter and exchange, realizing a metabolic through-flow. If the "Three Ways" are blocked or their regular flow is compromised, the synchrony of the Three Qi will be influenced and bring on disease.

The "Two Roads" are also ZM channels that allow the interior of the human body to maintain direct communication with nature, but both also maintain body mechanisms and they respond to two kinds of disease conditions that block extremely important circulation passages. Traditional Zhuang culture considers that the dragon governs water, so the Dragon Road in the body is the passage for blood, body fluids, and germinal essence; its function is mainly to transmit water and nutrient substances to the viscera and the muscles, bones, sinews, skin, and flesh. The Dragon Road has arteries and reticular collaterals spreading all over the interior of the body; its circulations come and go, and its pivot is the heart organ system. Fire is a thing that rises, its nature is quick (hence the expression, "like wildfire" [*huosu* 火速]). ZM holds that the Fire Road in the body interior is a route of transmission; in modern parlance it could be called the "information channel." It is more or less the same as modern medicine's nervous system. Like the Dragon Road, the Fire Road has arteries and collaterals, extending in all directions, making the normal body able to take in stimuli and information from the outside world, immediately, as an inner feeling. Managed through its central pivot of the *qiaowu*, [the "Fire Road" makes it possible to] quickly respond spontaneously to all the changes of the outside world, maintain a normal physiology, and realize the "synchrony of the Three Qi."

The relationship among the Three Ways and the Two Roads is very close. Their concrete functions are not identical; [rather, they] support and complete each other, and they similarly support the body's harmonious physiological functions. The core concept of the Three Ways and the Two Roads is the word *tong* 通, through-flow. The many diseases of the body, that is to say, its pathologies, are all made from obstacles to flow or even complete blockage in the passages. If you restore flow through the "Three Ways and Two Roads," you can prevent and treat numerous common and frequent diseases and even resolve puzzling and difficult acute disease symptoms.

Poison and Depletion Bring on Disease, and the Theory of Regulating Qi, Breaking Down Poisons, and Supplementing Depletion: ZM holds that one of the reasons *du*-poison brings on disease is that at root the propensity of poisons runs counter to that of normal qi; normal qi can expel pathogenic poisons, and pathogenic poisons can damage normal qi. The two engage in struggle, and if normal qi doesn't overcome *du*, this can influence the synchrony of the Three Qi and the harmony of yin and yang. A second reason is if some pathogenic *du* begins to clog up the "Three Ways and the Two Roads" (e.g., stasis *du*-poison), this directly affects the normal functions of the visceral systems and the bones, sinews, flesh, and skin. Depletion means that normal qi is depleted; this is both a very important cause of disease and a general response to a disease condition. With depletion, both the mechanisms of transmission-transformation and the defensive functions are reduced, and it is especially easy for external poisons to attack and for internal poisons to proliferate. Poison has both internal and external types, depletion can be congenital or post-natal, and clinically it's important to distinguish them.

ZM has targeted the poison and depletion causes of disease by systematically advancing the therapeutic principles of regulating qi, breaking down poisons, and supplementing depletion. The first involves working through body manipulations or drug formulas to recuperate the qi mechanisms that supplement depletions, improving and increasing the body's natural transmission-transformation functions and defensive capacities to meet the goal of fighting poisons and expelling poisons. The second is to use all manner of drugs with poison-attacking (or antidote) functions, working through the character and flavor of the drugs; after they have entered the body they can directly neutralize the poisons or work through the Three Ways to quickly expel the poison. Regulating qi, breaking down poisons, and supplementing depletions are not only ZM therapeutic principles for dealing with disease; at the same time they are also basic ideas of ZM for preventing and nurturing health; they have an important guiding role in curing the not yet ill.

SPECIFIC FORMULAS AND DRUGS

Guangxi's unique geographic and climatic environment richly produces Chinese herbal medicines. Cassia bark [肉桂], Pseudo-ginseng [田七], Job's tears [苡仁], Lohan Fruit, Honeysuckle [山银花], Bushy Sophora [山豆根], Chinese Holly [铁冬青], Niutali [牛大力], etc., are all Zhuang medicines in long use. The famous Tranquility County herbs market already has a thousand years of history. During the time that Zhuang medical experience was accumulating, a large number of specialized formulas and drugs were developed.

Pharmacy is divided into the two great types of "hen" and "cock" drugs: ZM drug qualities are divided into the five types of Cold, Hot, Warming, Cooling, and Neutral. The drug flavors are the eight types of sour, sweet, bitter, pungent, salty, numbing, bland, and astringent; these [characteristics] are classified under the hen and cock rubrics. The cock drugs are mostly warming, hot, filling, and supplementing drugs that regulate qi, such as Cassia bark [肉桂], raw Ginger, Purple Perilla [紫苏], Grains of Paradise [砂仁], Jingjie [荆芥], Milk Vetch [土黄芪], etc. The hen drugs are mostly correlated with cold, cooling, heat clearing, poison resolving, calming and guiding drugs, e.g., Chinese Holly [铁冬青], Ox Gall [青牛胆], Arrow-shaped Tinospora Root [地苦胆], Bushy Sophora [山豆根], Honeysuckle [山银花], Barberry [土黄连], etc. Hen and cock drugs counter yang syndromes and yin syndromes, respectively. The combining principles of ZM's classical formulas are very strong in assisting and guiding functions. The main drug targets the main disease and the main symptom, and the assisting drugs coordinate and strengthen the function of the main drug, or they assist in treating secondary symptoms, or they lessen the toxic functions of the main drug. Guiding drugs lead the various medicines to the site of the disease.

Preference for fresh drugs and singular formulas: These are important features of ZM. The plants and trees of the Zhuang region, green throughout all four seasons, provide the necessary environment and conditions for ZM's use of fresh herbs. There are more than 100 sorts of fresh medicinal herbs often used in ZM, e.g., Rohdia [罗裙带], Dandelion [蒲公英], Asiatic Pennywort [雷公根], fresh Aloe root [鲜芦根], Dendrobium [鲜石斛], Purple Perilla [鲜紫苏], etc. Among the orally administered fresh drugs, ZM selects those effective for moistening yin and clearing heat, and the fresh drugs relied on for external use mostly function to expel and break down poisons. The fresh animal-derived drugs, like red-spotted lizard, gecko, viper, and centipede, used alone or in combination with other Zhuang medicines, in clinical practice have demonstrated rather marked efficacy against many malignant tumors and various recalcitrant chronic diseases. In the treatment of broken bones and wounds, as well as snakebites, what is used is almost always fresh herbs, and most of these formulas are single-ingredients.

Preference for using poisonous and poison-dissolving drugs: This has to do with the Zhuang people's environment, which is rich in both poisons and antidotes. It is known that ZM uses nearly 100 types of poisonous and poison-countering drugs, and these are quite generally used internally and externally in all kinds of diseases, and in gynecology, pediatrics, dermatology, and other specialties. Examples are Datura [曼陀罗], Ericybe [丁公藤], Yellow Jessamyne [断肠草], Strophanthus [羊角扭], Schizocapsa [水田七], Four o'clock [紫茉莉], and Poke root [商陆], as well as mineral drugs like sulphur, pearl powder, and arsenic, and animal drugs like leeches, centipedes, blister beetles, and snake venom: though they have toxic properties, if used properly the effectiveness is quite marked.

SPECIFIC TECHNIQUES

ZM needling therapies: In *Illustrated Acupuncture Prescriptions for Sha Diseases* (manuscript edition), authored by renowned senior Zhuang doctor Luo Jia'an, twenty-plus needling and skin-pricking therapeutic techniques are recorded. ZM needle and pricking methods include multiple techniques, selected carefully for use as clinically needed: body, ear, palm, and sole needling; fire needling; skin-pricking; pricking for blood; gold needling; ceramic needling; etc. With the publication of Professors Huang Jinming, Lin Chen, et al.'s *China's Zhuang Medical Acumoxa* and *China's Zhuang Medical Needling*, and other books, a "Master Huang Zhuang medicine acumoxa current" has formed, and ZM acupuncture therapies have become more widely known and adopted.

ZM medicated thread touching moxibustion therapies: This therapy has come down to us from the Zhuang folk lineage of Master Long in Liujiang County, where it was kept secret and not shared with outsiders. But in 1986 Huang Jinming, Huang Hanru, and Huang Dingjian openly published their edited book *Zhuang Medicine Medicated Thread Touching Moxibustion Therapies*. This method can loosen up rheumatic stasis and pain, stop itching and expel winds, mobilize blood and transform qi, lessen swelling and loosen joints, etc., and it has clear efficacies in commonly seen or epidemic diseases. In 2011, medicated thread touching therapy attained to national-level status, being declared to be intangible cultural heritage.

ZM cupping therapy with medicated bamboo tubes: This therapeutic system was sorted out by renowned Zhuang doctor Chen Lizu. It uses [a bath of] various ZM medicines to sterilize special bamboo tubes with heat and then attaches the tubes by heat-induced suction to a therapeutic place on the surface of the patient's body. Working through the strength of the medicine, the heat, and the pressure of the suction, it facilitates the functions of expelling poisons and moving qi, dispelling cold and stopping pain, driving out winds and dampness, and enlivening blood and relaxing muscles. Presently this is one of the nation's major clinical techniques in those fields that emphasize treatment of rheumatic, or wind-damp, diseases.

ZM tuina massage therapy: This therapy takes the Three Ways and two sinews, and channel-sinew theory, as a guide, incorporating and synthesizing the rich experience in Zhuang nationality folk *tuina* and massage of rectifying musculature and setting bones. It has developed "stove inspection diagnosis" and "eliminating the stove and untying knots" disease treatments; these are characteristic *tuina* methods with marked effectiveness in many kinds of pain syndromes. At present, ZM *tuina* is deemed to be one of Guangxi Zhuang Medicine Hospital's nationally emphasized clinical specialties.

ZM herbal vaporizing, bathing, amulets, and pillows: Using various different Zhuang medicinals, singly or after combining them, treat the skin and flesh to reach therapeutic goals. These therapies are especially effective in children's diseases and chronic disorders.

PREPONDERANT DISEASE TYPES

The preponderant diseases of ZM are the disorders commonly seen in the southern parts of China, e.g., wind-damp and *sha/zhang/gu/du*-poison types of diseases [also see table 2.1]. In the list below, the Zhuang language names (italicized) are phonetically transcribed into standard Chinese characters. [Trans. note: We provide only the English translations here.] Specifically, ZM's main typical disease types are *sha* illness (subacute fevers), numbness/paralysis, asthma, stomachache, painful urination, watery edema, acute leukemia, stroke, hypertension, pain syndromes, dementia, diabetes, hemorrhoids, bone fracture, marrow inflammation, lower back pain, extruded disk disorder, cervical vertebra disorder, frozen shoulder, infertility, colds in children, asthma in children, urinary incontinence, mumps, acute conjunctivitis, runny nose, pharyngitis, etc.

DEVELOPMENT TRAJECTORY

In order to develop ZM and pass on its heritage, the Chinese Communist Party committee and the government of Guangxi Nationality Zhuang Autonomous Region, respectively, listed the "Decision on Speeding the Development of Chinese Medicine and Nationality Medicines" and other important documents and convened a regional convention on [Han] Chinese medicine, Zhuang medicine, and Yao medicine. The People's Congress of the Autonomous Region drew up and promulgated the "Guangxi Zhuang Autonomous Region ordinances/regulations to develop TCM and ZM" and organized enforcement and inspections.

In 2002 the Guangxi College of TCM decided to establish a Zhuang medicine department, organizing the editing of a series of twelve ZM textbooks and useful teaching materials, and also matriculating the first class of undergraduates majoring in TCM but with a ZM concentration. In 2011 the first class of students majoring in Zhuang medicine formally matriculated, thus creating a watershed in ZM undergraduate education. In August 2002, the Editing Committee of the Guangxi Regional Health Department decided to establish the Guangxi Zhuang Autonomous Region Hospital of Zhuang Medicine, based at the affiliated hospital of the Guangxi Nationality Medicines Research Institute (now the Guangxi Academy of Nationality Medicine Research). In 2009 this hospital was determined by the State Administration of TCM to be one of the top ten nationality medicine hospitals in China. Over the past thirty years, the Guangxi Nationality Medicines Research Institute, with the approval and support of the [National] Science Committee (now the Ministry of Science and Technology), undertook and completed more than three hundred programs of scientific research pertaining to ZM. Many of these research projects received provincial and higher awards for scientific progress, or book awards. ZM specialties in rheumatic (wind-damp) diseases and in tumor treatment, as well as ZM's ocular orbit examination, medicated thread touching moxibustion, and ZM's muscle and channel *tuina* techniques, have been cited by the State Administration of TCM as premier specialties that are needed to propagate the practical therapeutic technologies of nationality medicine. Of these, medicated thread touching moxibustion was declared to be a national intangible cultural heritage in 2011. The first and second volumes of *Guangxi Zhuang Autonomous Region Quality Standards for Zhuang Medicine*, incorporating 375 categories, were published respectively in 2008 and 2011.

Notes

1. Though most of our interviewees and associates in field sites were willing to be mentioned with their real names in this book, we still preserve research confidentiality herein by using pseudonyms. Our pseudonyms are constructed from a common Chinese surname (not usually the same as that of the research subject in question) and a translation of the forename that tries to preserve some of the meaning of the subject's (sometimes self-selected) given name.

2. Throughout this study we prefer the term "nationality" (which in common usage refers to a nationally recognized minority group) to "ethnicity." The introduction explains this decision more fully.

3. We took herbal baths ourselves at a Yao therapeutic spa on the edge of town; Judith found hers wonderfully restoring, but Lili had to give up early because the aromatic herbs made her dizzy This experience attests to the porousness of the body, as it is known to southerners, and also to the efficacies of herbal medicines; see chapters 3 and 4.

4. See Lai and Farquhar (2020) for more detail on this case.

5. Chinese anthropologist Fei Xiaotong had done fieldwork in the area decades before, as had many Chinese ethnologists over the ensuing decades. Ralph Litzinger worked for a long time in Jinxiu in the 1990s and produced an important book, *Other Chinas* (2000). This book, among its other accomplishments, demonstrates some of the historical reasons why "the Jinxiu Yao" are seen as a rather central emblem of ethnic traditionalism in China. In 2011 we quickly determined that the health department director who approved our anthropological research in the area had come to her post and to Jinxiu County only after Ralph was no longer personally active in the area. Apparently it was not a problem for her that we knew and asked after him.

6. Ralph Litzinger (2000) has extensively documented and analyzed the culture work that Jinxiu Yao activists have engaged in over the past few decades. Thanks to his assiduous historical anthropology, we had the luxury in 2011 of appreciating Yao local culture alongside our Yao medicine activist friends without having to critically evaluate the significance of this culture work for anthropological theory.

7. This is "Selena Huang," who also appears in chapter 4.

8. The bilingual text printed on inserts for these herbal bath kits emphasized the magic and mystery of the herbals found in the Great Yao Mountains.

9. See chapter 1, "Institution," for a consideration of the importance of "the wild" in the construction of minority medical authority and effectiveness. Also see Schein (1997)

for the relation of collective ethnic self-representations to Chinese (and global) imaginaries of exotic Miao nationality essences.

10. Thanks are due to Feng Ye for sharing insights from her 2017 fieldwork in the Beijing Yao Hospital with us.

11. See chapter 5 for an account of a nomenclature standardization meeting held at the Jinxiu Yao Hospital.

12. Between 2010 and 2013 we convened three five-day anthropology training sessions for the ten research associates who remained with us throughout the project. The first focused on participant observation methods, the second on interviewing (especially oral histories), and the third was devoted to the writing of ethnographic articles. See the *Journal of the Guangxi University for Nationalities* (广西民族大学学报) 36, no. 6 (2014) for some published results from the third workshop.

13. In Nujiang Prefecture, where we spent more than four weeks in 2014, Judith and Lili were accompanied part of the time by Gang Yue and Marshall Kramer. Our research assistant there was Sha Lina. We are grateful to all of them for many thoughtful exchanges and good companionship.

INTRODUCTION

1. On nomad science, see our discussion below and Deleuze and Guattari (1987); on hegemony and subalternity, see Guha (1997); Hardiman and Mukharji (2012); and on epistemological heterogeneity see Foucault (1996).

2. Popper (1972).

3. Farquhar and Lai (2014).

4. Smith (1988) has made us content to be relativists. For the usage of "statist" and "subaltern" medicines, see Hardiman and Mukharji (2012). These authors follow the pioneering work of Arnold (1993). On the pluralization of the abstract noun "knowledge," see Haraway (1988).

5. On styles of knowing in medicine, see Hsu (1999).

6. Farquhar (1987; 1994a); Lai (2017a).

7. Lai and Farquhar (2020).

8. Our translation. We have based our unconventional rendering on recent readings of Neo-Confucian commentators on the Great Learning.

9. See Harman (2010) for the distinction.

10. Ames (1983).

11. The language of "statist" (vs. subaltern or vernacular medicine) comes from the historical and ethnographic research on India's indigenous medicines of Arnold (1993); Lambert (2018); and Mukharji (2016). More recently than in the Chinese case, the "AYUSH" traditional medicines of India were integrated into the postcolonial public health system of India. AYUSH is short for "Ayurveda, Yoga, Unani, Siddha, Sowa Rigpa, and Homeopathy." A ministry of AYUSH medicines was established in 2014 in India. Mukharji and Lambert, among others, argue that these officially recognized traditional medicines exclude many more subaltern or vernacular experts, such as bone doctors and martial artists.

12. Scheid (2007).

13. Taylor (2005).

14. Deleuze and Guattari (1986, 17–40).

15. Deleuze and Guattari (1986, 28).

16. Deleuze and Guattari (1986, 28).

17. See, for example, Barker (1984); Foucault (1973); Jordanova (1989); Rabinbach (1990); Stengers (2003); K. Thomas (1983); Hacking (1983).

18. See Scheid (2002); Taylor (2005); Schmalzer (2008; 2016); Fa-ti Fan (2012); Andrews (2014); Fang (2014). On the historicity of notions of causation, see Farquhar (2020, appendix 1).

19. See Farquhar (1994a; 2020); Garon (2018); Lai (2004); Lu (2001); Zhang Dong (2016).

20. Karchmer (2005).

21. Anthropological considerations of medical pluralism in today's world have proposed all manner of complex relations between "medical systems." Leslie (1976); Hardiman and Mukharji (2012). And they have thrown interesting light on the "Complementary and Alternative Medicine" (CAM) world that has developed in the United States. We aim to show with this study that the analytical notions suitable to these other national situations—alternativeness, for example, or subalternity—are not quite right, or quite powerful enough, to describe fully the contemporary Chinese situation.

22. Foucault (1996, 199).

23. Lei (2014).

24. Lampton (1977).

25. Taylor (2005).

26. Anderson (2006).

27. See chapter 5 for a discussion of these survey techniques and their contemporary manifestations.

28. These are phrases ubiquitous in the mid-twentieth-century literature of Chinese medicine, serving as a legitimating premise for all that follows in just about any medical book.

29. Gordon (1988).

30. From the beginning of this research, Geoffrey Bowker's *Memory Practices in the Sciences* (2005) was a major inspiration for us. The tables of contents of medical books in Chinese, which have long interested us, are in their social and epistemological impacts quite like the database structures on which Bowker focuses.

31. In the course of field research we asked practicing doctors of local medicines what they read. None of the older practitioners appeared to use the new textbooks, relying instead on some ancient classic medical works, the Book of Changes, and especially various versions of local *bencao* (本草), or *materia medica* handbooks.

32. We could also translate this term *zongjie* as summing up or even systematizing. But we think synthesizing best captures the kind of activity undertaken by developers of nationality medicines.

33. Lai (2004).

34. Michael Dutton, in a forthcoming book that incorporates important readings of public representations in modern China (*The Book of Politics*), characterizes "the political" in China as advancing a telluric, or earth-bound, aesthetics and strategics. This quality of politics, we believe, is shared by contemporary ethnic and medical-cultural formations, especially since the most authoritative expertise tends to be that deemed to be the most wild and earthy (*tu* 土), or nomadic. This cultural tendency identified by Dutton helps us to see the form of emergence of minority nationality medicines as a specifically modern Chinese politics.

35. Also see Farquhar and Lai (2014).

36. Litzinger (2000).

37. Also in the preface we mention a TV documentary that considers Yao nationality medicine in the context of Yao nationality ritual, arts, and mystical connections to the Great Yao Mountains. Anthropologist Ralph Litzinger has reflected on these arenas of media-oriented traditionalism and cultural production among the Jinxiu Yao, sometimes working along with Yao intellectuals, in a series of rich articles and in his book *Other Chinas* (1995; 1998a; 1998b; 2000). In our study of medical-cultural production (especially the Yao parts of it) we see many parallels with the aims and anxieties he drew out in his engagement with local cultural experts. Most of his insights, however, date from fieldwork in the 1980s and 1990s, a time when (he argues) much collective representation and cultural performance expressed a critical perspective on a painfully remembered and relatively recent Maoist socialism. Times have changed in Jinxiu, however, and though the state is much involved in the production of nationality, minority, Yao-ness, culture, and locality, it is quite difficult to see state agendas as imposed from above, or to identify clear acts of resistance to "the state."

38. Thomas Mullaney's (2010, 103–6) study of the Yunnan ethnic classification project in the 1950s includes an account of how three quite disparate local groups were merged to become "the Achang."

39. For another example of rather strong ethnic commitment, recall the preface, in which we noted the discomfort a Zhuang colleague felt when she was asked to model the elaborate costume of a Yao woman. She wanted to oblige but felt there was something off about physically appropriating another person's national costume.

40. Joniak-Luthi (2013).

41. Like Mullaney's 1950s linguists, ethnologists, and historians, anthropologists have challenged the utility of every term in the Stalinist model of "nation." Indeed, any traveling anthropology of nationalities in today's China—at least in the south—tends to encounter nationality in fragments (Mullaney's "remainders") or, at best, as large or small construction projects led by activists.

42. Mullaney (2010, 103).

43. Mullaney (2010).

44. Hostetler (2001); Wang Hui (2016).

45. Wang Hui (2011) is not alone in noting that even as the national domestic sphere was being managed as multicultural under the Qing and in the early Republic, the proper boundaries and inclusions of "China" were also under debate.

46. Chatterjee (1993).

47. For non-East Asian examples of this situation see Steinmetz (1999).

48. "Folk" medicine and healing are still respected and studied in the PRC, but in minority nationality areas these nomad sciences are mostly being taken up, renamed, and incorporated within nationality medicine projects. For an important study of the modernity of folklore in Asia, see Ivy (1995). See also Li Hsiao-t'i (2001). On the biomedical eagerness to denounce nonbiomedical knowledges as charlatanism, see Isabelle Stengers (2003). On the mobile boundaries between, and the interdependences of, royal or state science and the nomad sciences, see Deleuze and Guattari (1986).

49. On social assemblage, see Latour (2005); Verran (2011).

50. Feld and Basso (1996). The Chinese word noted here, *tese* 特色, refers to "special characteristics" and is often used to talk about particular places and the local specificities. Its frequent invocation in southern mountain conversations reminded us again and again that nationality in China may be inseparable from locality, or place.

51. See Jackson (2005) on sincerity and racial/ethnic belonging.

52. See, for example, Zhu Guoben (2006).

53. We are not here referring to nationality territories, which in most of China (even in the Guangxi Zhuang Self-Governing Region) do not cohere as spaces that could be mapped and affiliated to a majority nationality.

54. Haraway (1988).

55. Roland Barthes in *Mythologies* (1972) shows how a power-suffused modernist ideology turns history into nature. In this book, chapter 3 on bodies and chapter 4 on plants especially explore the ways in which local knowledges and histories are embodied in things, and thus naturalized. We add "tools" to this list here, recalling a visit to a small museum of Zhuang medicine in Nanning, where we were shown some very ancient (Warring States period?) acupuncture needles that had been excavated in Guangxi. These needles were proof, we were told, that the original roots of Chinese traditional medicine are to be found in Zhuang territory, making TCM originally not Han at all, but Zhuang.

56. Heidegger and Tim Ingold, among others, have sought to better understand practices of dwelling in places, and our experiences in rural southern China have made this notion appealing to us. But we are wary of uncritically adopting this resonant metaphor of being in place, dwelling, for parts of East Asia where there has been so much travel by so many different kinds of people. Everywhere we went there were lots of people who showed no particular attachment to the life of the mountain forests that made up part of their environment. Heidegger (1971 [1954]); Ingold (2000).

57. All the groups we worked with for this study are thought of as "lacking written language" (mainly because they have no archive of classical texts like those that exist in Tibetan, Arabic and Turkish, Mongolian and Manchu, and Korean languages). This label holds even though some southern groups (e.g., Zhuang, Lisu, Qiang) have relatively recently invented and used, albeit somewhat spottily, alphabetic-phonetic languages. On the archiving of nationality medicines, see Zhen and Hu (2014).

58. We frequently refer to processes of development in this book. The commitment of the Chinese government to overall societal development cannot be overstated, so the notion of specific trajectories of *fazhan* (发展, or development) was often alive in the discourse of our interlocutors.

59. On "the wild," see Bennett (1994); on "nomad science," Deleuze and Guattari (1986). These terms are revisited in chapter 1.

60. The fieldwork also included assiduous collecting of published and unpublished writings on ethnic medicine projects in the southern mountains. The usefulness of this precious mini-library, stored in Beijing, will be evident in the citations of expert writing we make in the chapters that follow.

61. Scott (1998); Farquhar, Lai, and Kramer (2017). We must add that many healers we visited were incredibly generous with their insights, stories, notes, and herbs.

62. *Guangxi Minzu Daxue Xuebao* 广西民族大学学报 36, no. 6 (2014).

63. In chapter 5 we discuss a certain Maoist tradition of work-team-based rural survey research, a model that is enjoying an afterlife in public health research in contemporary China. Our reliance on health departments and local research units placed us in social research work teams in a way that was not entirely comfortable for two US-trained anthropologists. It was hard to get over the feeling that nine or ten researchers descending upon a farmhouse for an afternoon of interrogations was rather invasive, not likely to achieve anthropology's famous quality of "rapport." We were not always

in such large groups, and we enjoyed ourselves more when it was just the two of us and one very local host. But we also came to acknowledge that the work-team model offers a useful kind of collaboration consistent with our orientations in anthropology.

CHAPTER 1

1. Croizier (1968); Lampton (1977); Taylor (2005); Scheid (2007); Andrews (2014).

2. Following the lead of some of our nationality medicine colleagues in southern China, we will sometimes refer to TCM as Han Chinese medicine.

3. Samuel Weber (1987) has partly inspired this orientation on our part.

4. The mountains of western Yunnan have been traversed by itinerants of many sorts for hundreds of years, many of them spreading nomad sciences. See for example Scott (2009); Mueggler (2011).

5. Ethnicity—nationality on the Chinese side of the border—is a particularly complex and elusive issue for the Lisu, who are generally perceived to be relatively atomistic, transborder, and not ethnically organized. But Dr. Wang's Lisu self-governing county is surrounded by counties belonging to a Tibetan autonomous prefecture, so a certain contrastive identification process might be unusually important here.

6. Anyone functioning as a village doctor, however, would be the recipient of frequent health education memos, reports, and brochures from higher-level health agencies, all filled with information designed to improve and regulate village-level practice. Most of this information would rely on biomedical science and a standardized hygiene system. Dr. Wang impressed us as the kind of doctor who would conscientiously read and keep such communications.

7. Throughout this study we tend to refer to the medicinal substances that are gathered and used by minority nationality practitioners as "herbals." In addition to the plant drugs that are harvested in the south, there are also mineral substances and animal parts. But the Chinese words used to refer to natural drugs (*caoyao* 草药) and their expert users (*caoyi* 草医) make a clear reference to plants.

8. See the introduction for a more detailed discussion of the implications of "salvaging and sorting, systematizing and elevating" nationality medicines. See Lai and Zhen (forthcoming) for a historical account of the national level of instituting minority nationality medicines. This article emphasizes that one historical factor in generating relatively successful salvaging and sorting nationality medicine projects has been the support of local governments in autonomous nationality regions and districts. The scope and stability of the Zhuang institutions discussed below testify to the effectiveness of regional autonomy in respect of this kind of cultural production.

9. See chapter 5, "Encounters," for a discussion of some of these governmental practices.

10. "Preserving the essence and discarding the dross" of Chinese tradition is a slogan strongly associated with the history of salvaging and sorting TCM in the PRC.

11. Bowker and Star (1999).

12. The Chinese term, *zongjie* 总结, implies a kind of knotting together at a higher level of generalization, making, perhaps, a coherent assemblage (see Verran 2011; Latour 2005). In this chapter "system" generally refers to this modern Chinese idea of actively made coherence, knottedness, even synthesis.

13. Anthony Giddens's (1984) approach to institutionalization, in his development of the idea of structuration, emphasizes not only that "rules" of practice construct

institutions but also that "resources" are needed. Such resources are a lot more than money and information, of course, and in our research we found that some nationalities seemed to have much richer available resources than others did for gathering together minority medical systems. We like to think of this difference in terms of co-construction of institutions through the collaboration of both human and nonhuman actors/actants.

14. Latour (1990). This observation invokes the cosmopolitical process, or the human-nonhuman co-construction that we emphasize more in chapter 4, "Plants." Latour (2005 and elsewhere) argues that human societies need to make alliances with many nonhuman actors if there is to be any stability, if, in other words, there is to be any instituting.

15. Giddens (1984, xxii). We like this image of social practices "biting into space and time" mainly because it resembles our adopted metaphysical language in which we envision things emerging, as such, as they are gathered from the endless flow of the Dao into some particular form of existence. But we would not want to imply that "space and time" preexist the gathering process, or that social practices can "bite" from a place external to the great spontaneous Way called the Dao.

16. Giddens (1984) returns frequently in his discussion to a reasoned rejection of Emile Durkheim's influential argument that "society is sui generis."

17. Laclau (1983).

18. Also see Mitchell (1991).

19. Nancy Munn (1986) has made Melanesian ethnography into a comparative metaphysics by insisting, first, that space and time are inseparable from each other as co-varying specificities, and second, spacetime is always a particular qualitative configuration, like the ontological work of culture.

20. The close relationship between ruling power and excellent calligraphy has long been noted in Chinese studies. See, for example, Kraus (1991) and Zito (1997).

21. Keane (1997); Markell (2009).

22. Mullaney (2010).

23. Farquhar and Zhang (2005).

24. In China, a country with many regional dialects and mutually unintelligible languages, writing tends to be national and use Han Chinese (Mandarin, or "the common tongue" [*Putonghua* 普通话]) written characters. The exceptions to this rule that we encountered in our research were few: some commercial signs in Nanning supply the relatively young Zhuang language script alongside Chinese, but many locals cannot even read it; a rural village doctor in Nujiang Prefecture had kept his 1960s health school notes in Lisu writing; and a project to standardize the Yao names of drugs was frustrated by the need to translate Yao speech phonetically into Chinese ideographic characters (see chapter 5).

25. Dr. Zhao had more formal schooling than many of the healers we visited. He had received barefoot doctor training and had also attended an early formal academy at Baise that combined Zhuang medicine and TCM. This history, in addition to his study with his father and grandfather and his continuing service as a teacher, helped legitimate his claims to a leadership position.

26. On "the wild," see Bennett (2010); Casey (1996).

27. The herbal medicine academy at Baise, where Wonderfont Zhao had studied, was an even earlier and equally unusual contribution to the extension of Zhuang medicine institution into the future.

28. This is a phrase used by Stephan Feuchtwang to gloss the kind of charisma

he sees at work in Chinese folk religion. See Feuchtwang and Wang (2001, 172). This important study also makes the point that the determination of positive social change in rural China has more to do with leaders' personalities and idiosyncratic histories than with more systemic factors. In our consideration of the importance of historian Huang Hanru and ZM doctor Huang Jinming below, we tend to concur.

29. See Jane Bennett's (2010) usage of this term.

30. While working in Zhuang areas of Guangxi we were privileged to spend field-work and scholarly exchange time with Dr. Laborjoy Wei as he visited rural healers and sought to learn, as a clinician, their special techniques and favored local drugs. Dr. Wei's enthusiasms and practices will reappear in chapters 3, 4, and 5.

31. See Farquhar (2015) for a parallel exploration of ontological issues in modern TCM.

32. There are other key figures in the development of Zhuang medicine, some of whom will appear in this chapter and others of whom will surface in other chapters.

33. There was no fully elaborated Zhuang written language until PRC linguists began to develop a standardized and partially Romanized transcription of one dialect from northern Guangxi in the early 1950s. This writing system was not very functional for this large, diverse, and "Han-ized" (thus, Mandarin-using) nationality region; it was reformed in the early 1980s to become a fully Romanized system based on oral language. There is still very little publishing in Zhuang language, however.

34. Anagnost (1997). In the course of his career Huang showed that he had a well-rounded vision of the salvaging and sorting project, successfully laying foundations for research (including compiling historical records), education (all levels of training and higher education, and publishing textbooks), standardization (for both clinical practices and the pharmaceutical industry), and legal regulation (certification exams approved by the state medical examination center). But in our conversations with him it was not this administrative work that most animated him; rather, it was Zhuang medical history.

35. Perhaps he first encountered Wonderfont Zhao there at that time, and he certainly was aware of the early Zhuang medicine teaching going on in the Baise Academy nearby.

36. Huang Hanru et al. (1998, 616–17).

37. This is obviously consistent with national policy. In 1981, the National Planning Group on Editing and Publishing Classic Literatures was established; in 1984, the National Leading Planning Group on Editing and Publishing Nationalities Classic Literatures was established, and work on an overall plan for the national development of nationalities classic literatures was begun in its collaborative development phase. The 1984 "Hohhot meeting" made it clear that "to salvage and sort the heritage of nationality medicines," it would be necessary to accomplish "the publication project of classic nationality medicine literatures from 1985 to 1990," during the seventh five-year plan. See Lai and Zhen (forthcoming).

38. Huang Jinming is widely thought of as the foremost clinical specialist of Zhuang medicine. He is also a theorist, and a sketch he made for us of the body according to Zhuang medicine will appear in chapter 3.

39. Wang Bocan, Huang Hanru's first MA-level graduate student, is now the executive director (*bangongshi zhuren* 办公室主任) of the Guangxi Nationality Medicines Research Institute.

40. The May 7 Cadre Schools were agricultural farms where cadres and intellectuals were sent to "transform their thought." The name comes from the letter Mao Zedong

wrote to Lin Biao on May 7, 1966, in which he approved Lin's recommendation that, as the army had been participating in agriculture production, this educational activity could be extended to all cadres. But the May 7 Cadre Schools didn't become popular until 1968, when Heilongjiang started one that was praised by Mao. The schools were officially suspended in 1979. http://news.163.com/05/0525/18/1KK9NCRS00011247 .html

41. Huang Hanru and Huang Jinming (1986).

42. Body-surface therapies like acupuncture, moxibustion, acumoxa cupping, and medicinal thread cautery, however, are almost impossible to study as randomized controlled clinical trials. The perennial question is, how would you design a control or "placebo" practice?

43. See Huang Hanru et al. (1998, 593). More details on the "theoretical system of Zhuang medicine" can be found on this page as well.

44. As early as 1985 the Guangxi College of CM offered a master's degree in Zhuang medical history. Huang Hanru hoped from the beginning to enroll undergraduate students in Zhuang medicine; this early master's program aimed at producing teachers for the College of Zhuang Medicine.

45. The examination includes 40 percent Chinese medicine content, 20 percent Zhuang medicine, and 20 percent Western medicine. According to Huang Hanru, there have been around four hundred applicants but the passing success rate has been only 30 percent. As we indicate elsewhere, tensions surround this kind of standardized test and its legal implications. In respect of Zhuang medicine, Huang said they are considering making special arrangements for experienced senior doctors.

46. There is also no space here to detail the many national and international Zhuang medicine training institutes run from Huang Hanru's base in Nanning (but see Huang Hanru et al. 1998, 609) and the extensive academic exchange that has been taking place throughout the region, in which Zhuang medicine is a leading exemplar. It is important to note, however, that when we talked with him, Huang Hanru wanted us to particularly acknowledge these far-flung and cosmopolitan activities.

47. Before the reform and opening up policies of 1978, all traditional medicines were put into the one category of "herbal medicine" (caoyi 草医). See Lai and Zhen (forthcoming).

48. This is a vision that seems to take the necessity of modernist progress and development for granted. But it should be borne in mind that Huang Hanru is also a teacher, and like anyone in any academic setting, he would like to see jobs for his graduated students continue to open up. If scientistic biomedical critics were to succeed in delegitimizing nationality traditional medical practice, a great many people would be out of a job, and (as any clinician would point out) a number of effective techniques for the treatment of stubborn disorders would become unavailable to sufferers.

49. Hospital Director Bao explained the timing of this institution's establishment. In the late 1980s a provincial commission visited Maoxian seeking to learn about Qiang medicine. The head of the county health bureau at that time was of Qiang ethnicity, so it was easy to garner his support for the new institute after he and Bao had witnessed the interest of those higher up.

50. The direct supervision of a Qiang salvaging and sorting process by a national agency stands in contrast to the provincial-level management of Zhuang medicine by public health and nationality authorities in the Guangxi Autonomous Region. Perhaps the relative autonomy in Guangxi, and support from state agencies responsible for

ethnic group development, are responsible for the greater (but not perfect) institutional stability achieved by Huang Hanru and his collaborators.

51. Zhang Yi and Zhong Guoyue (2005).

52. Chapter 2, "Knowledge," discusses the contents of this book and its theories more fully.

53. Earth beings is Marisol de la Cadena's term (2015). Though earth beings and their human allies in the Andes, about whom she writes, are quite different from those that disrupted northwestern Sichuan in 2008, any study of "Qiang religion" would raise similar issues. For accounts of Qiang culture and religion, see Wang Kang et al. (1992); Wang Mingke (2008); Zhou Yuhua (2010); Ruan Baodi (2011).

54. This Qiang style of domestic architecture looked a little invented to us, owing more to generalized southwestern ethnic traditions than to the distinctive Sichuan buildings that have been well documented in other sources (Wang Mingke 2008). Qiang homesteads and villages were usually built from stone on slopes above the valleys. The new housing was wood, concrete, and stucco and took the form of consolidated villages clustered in the (more easily administered) valleys.

55. There is even a small museum of Qiang medicine, built since 2008.

56. Local therapies in most of southern China are often developed and offered by bone-setters. Bone-setting is a traditional healing modality that includes a great many ways to treat injuries, speeding natural healing and preventing permanent disability. See also chapter 3.

57. Director Bao praises Dr. Li's clinical abilities and depth of understanding, including him in his short list of those truly authoritative Qiang healers who remain active in the county. But he too has been frustrated about the licensing issue. When we asked him about this problem in 2013, he saw no legal way to recognize Virtuefont Li as a Qiang nationality doctor in the eyes of the government.

58. Zhang Dan (2016).

59. Lili's notes on the research reports of the 2012 meeting remind us that participants talked openly about *shibi* (释比), the Qiang ritual experts who seem to enjoy high social status. In a previous interview with Bao, he talked about the importance of the local *shibi*, saying that these healers tended to be masters of most Qiang medicine knowledge. Bao even said that Qiang medicine would be incomplete if it didn't include *shibi* practice. This attitude seems rather inconsistent with mainstream salvaging and sorting values.

60. Zhang Dan (2016).

61. We have frequently referred to nationality medicine *activists* in this chapter partly because they are a minority even among herbalists and healers. There are plenty of local medicine practitioners in southern ethnic China who are uninterested in the state's minority nationality medicine development projects; though most healers told us they had plans for building a future for their skill, e.g., through taking disciples, quite a few of these doctors were not actively engaged in instituting. As the case of Zhuang medicine shows particularly well, however, a few activists can successfully establish a rather impressive group of agencies devoted to a minority medicine.

CHAPTER 2

1. Judith Farquhar (1994a) developed this idea at length in her study of the clinical encounter of traditional Chinese medicine, based on field research in Guangzhou,

China, in the early 1980s. Many other writers have insisted on the same point; see, for example, Bachelard (1984); Mao (1967 [1937]); James (1920 [1907]); Citton (2017); Weber (1987); and the much earlier Chinese philosophers Xunzi and Wang Yangming, who are known for their insistence that knowing and going gather as one (*zhi xing he yi* 知行合一). Lili Lai and Farquhar (2020) have discussed the unity of knowledge and practice in Chinese contexts.

2. See Bowker (2005) for more on information in the modern sciences.

3. There is plenty of scientific evidence to be had supporting TCM safety and efficacy, after several generations of biochemical and clinical research in the field. Farquhar (1994a) reports at length, however, that Chinese medical doctors and scholars, and the books they were writing in the early 1980s, emphasized "experience" (*jingyan* 经验) and "practice" as the foundations of their knowledge. Lei (2014) has described the rise of an emphasis on "experience" in the field of Chinese medicine in the twentieth century as a response to attacks from scientific modernizers and their carefully synthesized evidence.

4. Hsu *(1999)*; Zhan (2009).

5. This critical anxiety is especially pervasive in some quarters of TCM pedagogy and practice. A global evidence-based medicine movement has been influential in TCM institutions, leading to disciplined clinical trials and many standardized protocols. But patients and medical professionals often express their preference for, and their greater trust in, the flexibility and virtuoso skills of senior, experienced, and traditionally trained doctors. Such cultural preferences are evident in the genre of publishing that collects the "experience" of "renowned senior doctors." See, e.g., Zhou et al. (1981–85).

6. Hardiman and Mukharji (2012). Other historians have excelled at showing how medical facts can be crafted as tools of colonial domination. See Arnold (1993); Langford (2002); Vaughan (1991). But the political situations that have configured medical knowledge in India, Africa, and China differ with consequences for the forms that knowledge takes.

7. Foucault (1984).

8. Spivak (1988).

9. We see this situation as different from the struggles over "indigenous knowledge" that have been so important in (at least) Latin America (Blaser 2010; Kohn 2013; Hayden 2003), Africa (Green and Levine 2012), and Australia (Verran 1998; Povinelli 2016). But the histories of such struggles raise important issues for the history of medicine anywhere.

10. This group of medicine developers includes national-level academics, staff at the State Administration of Traditional Chinese Medicine (SATCM) in Beijing, and some people responsible for medical education and licensing in the Ministry of Education. In this chapter, though, we pay more attention to the sorting and systematizing work of regional and local experts.

11. In this chapter we mainly draw on textbooks that were produced for medical education. But we also mean "textbook" in the broader sense of conventional and consensual knowledge.

12. Angela Zito's (1997) study of Qing (Chinese) imperial ritual usefully explores the power/knowledge nexus under the heading of text editing, seen as a dimension of the performance of imperial power.

13. As we noted in chapter 1, Zhuang nationality medicine has Wonderfont Zhao's textbook pamphlets and his annual academy helping to construct a future for the field.

More important in the long run are Zhuang medicine's larger institutions: a Zhuang medical school and hospital in Nanning (Guangxi); an impressive library of textbooks and academic research reports available online, in journals, and as books; and for the past few years, licensing examinations that have staffed many clinics and transformed the legal regulatory environment for the practice of this "folk" medicine.

14. Though we are treating this essay written by the founder of modern Zhuang medicine as authoritative and objective, it does have a somewhat polemical cast. The title, for example, "The Emphasis on 'Three Ways and Two Roads' in Zhuang Medicine and Pharmacy," would be challenged by some other leaders in the field, who prefer to place an emphasis on the Three Qi (heaven, earth, and the human) at the center of the field. Or by others, like Laborjoy Wei (see chapter 3), who are developing noncanonical models of the ZM body.

15. See also chapter 5, for a different approach to Director Ma's research in Yunnan.

16. We suspect that Director Ma had begun to seek a "deeper" level of knowledge especially actively after initial contacts with our anthropological project. Perhaps he saw in anthropology and its methods a way of dignifying and conserving the culture and knowledge of one of China's smallest minority populations, the Achang.

17. Lei (2014); Scheid (2007); Taylor (2005); Lampton (1977); Croizier (1968); Andrews (2014).

18. Are these terms especially suitable for a medicine that has drawn so deliberately on East Asian nomad sciences? See the appendix.

19. Chinese medicine historian Liao Yuqun (2006) locates the first appearance of the "medicine is reasoning" idea in the Latter Han period (the *Hou Han Shu* 《后汉书》, c. 940–50 CE), though he believes that *yi* (意) in that context meant attentiveness rather than reasoning. Because (he argues) acupuncture was a more important therapeutic mode during the earlier period, "attentiveness" was a particularly valued medical skill. When, after the Song (960–1279), herbal pharmacy became important, *yi* in this frequently repeated phrase referred more to the thinking involved in designing herbal formulas and adopting therapeutic strategies. This medical reasoning, in turn, was acknowledged by Neo-Confucian "pattern studies" (*lixue* 理学) philosophers as a form of resonance with the rhythms of the universe, in other words, much more than cognition or calculation. In addition, Jane Geaney (personal communication) reports from her research on pre-Han Confucian writings that the *yi* we are translating as reasoning (for modern purposes) was more like speculation or guesswork for the first Confucians (Geaney, forthcoming). The contemporary doctors and scholars who invoke the phrase "medicine is reasoning" may know nothing of classical or early modern philosophy, but they like the idea that the knowing practice of medicine is thoughtful, philosophical, and reasoned. See also Lai and Farquhar (2020); and Farquhar (2020).

20. We have met primary care doctors, for example, who insist, in their daily practice, which is almost completely devoted to the dispensing of biomedical drugs and treatments, on using TCM reasoning to diagnose syndromes and in that way determine the most rational (biomedical) therapies. State Follower Wang in Lisu nationality Yunnan was especially articulate on this point, explaining it to us as we inspected his little-used herbal medicine pharmacy. Colin Garon (2018) has shown in detail how the logic of TCM and that of biomedicine can "integrate" in clinical practice.

21. The parts of this project centering on the drugs themselves were quite important from the point of view of the funding agency, the SATCM. National researchers emphasized very concrete "data collection"—drug sampling and video recording of tech-

niques—in preference to the more interpretive and holistic methods Director Ma was also teaching his team to adopt.

22. These herbal medicine surveys were remembered with respect by a number of the healers and researchers we interviewed. We know of no historical study of this state-led "local *materia medica*" movement, but it can be thought of in parallel with other forms of mass science initiated in Maoist China. See chapter 5; also see Fa-ti Fan (2012) on seismology and Sigrid Schmalzer (2008; 2016) on paleontology and entomology.

23. We also persuaded him that anthropological analysis, if it is to "go deep," needs to rely on the results of long periods of participant observation in the places where people live and work. Director Ma saw the importance of this method, but as far as we know he has not found the resources to support longer-term ethnographic research on nationality medicines in Yunnan.

24. Scheid (2007).

25. See Barry Allen's (2015) argument contrasting the "onto-theological" biases of Western epistemology with a classical Chinese approach to what knowledge is and how it works. Allen's insights are very resonant with some approaches to knowledge we describe in this book, and there is a definite genealogy that could be traced from the classical times he studies through the Neo-Confucians, the *kaozheng* (evidential scholarship) philosophers, Wang Yangming, some modernizing pragmatists (maybe even John Dewey!), to Mao Zedong and the theorists of modern TCM. But for most of this chapter we are reading and presenting a particularly modernist and even transnational structuring of medical information, as it appears, cut-and-dried, in textbooks.

26. Latour (1993).

27. Our Achang hosts, when pressed about the "theory" underlying their clinical strategies, and perhaps with a certain exasperation at our ignorance, tended to repeat the theoretical terms of TCM. Unlike Director Ma, they were not troubled by the apparent absence of a specifically Achang theory of "medicine" or way of thinking (*silu* 思路).

28. This deeper level may be inarticulately felt to be necessary for good medical practice because "theory" allows for flexible, responsive, and creative medical management of diseases. Medicine *is* reasoning, after all. Many biomedical doctors resist the protocol-driven practice of the evidence-based-medicine movement. But TCM and ZM have the advantage of sharing underlying principles like "taking yin and yang to be the basis" (*yi yinyang wei ben* 以阴阳为本) and "struggle between normal and pathogenic qi" (*zhengxie douzheng* 正邪斗争) to help practitioners think on their feet.

29. Leading Group (2013, 3). The list of important texts that follows this observation about the recent origins of systematic Zhuang medicine includes one "early" text, published in 1959, and twenty-three general and specialized works that began to appear in print in the early 1980s.

30. Leading Group (2013, 3).

31. Croizier (1968; 1976); Taylor (2005); Yang (2009); Zhao Hongjun (1983).

32. Scheid, (2007); Hanson (2011).

33. See Weber (1987) and Bachelard (1984) for extended discussions of how knowledge institution relies on the epistemological and ethical-political task of distinguishing same from different, excluding and including matters of concern in spheres of attention.

34. Textbooks for use in medical school courses include guidelines on writing proper case records in hospital and clinic settings. These medical records are structured almost identically to both TCM cases and to those of biomedicine, following forms of medical record-keeping that were developed in the United States and Europe in the twenti-

eth century. The recording technique works like a kind of paperwork infrastructure of knowledge that grounds all forms of medicine in a single imaginary of the human body, disease, and natural causes in physiology and pathology. We still argue here that Zhuang medicine (among other sorts) works with some unique entities that are missed, or mistranslated, in the written record.

35. The assembly of a body of knowledge and language of medicine for the Zhuang nationality has taken place under conditions of considerable diversity. This large minority population speaks numerous local languages and occupies territories far beyond southern Guangxi. The development of ZM propagated mostly in "the common speech" of Han Chinese can thus be seen as a method of ethnic consolidation and even identity formation.

36. Dai (2006).

37. *History of Zhuang Nationality Medicine* also credits a number of other Zhuang medicine experts with the work of salvaging and sorting the system, and it notes the several academic and government agencies supporting editing projects and collaborative workshops from the early 1990s forward.

38. Dai (2006, 88).

39. When asked, many ZM practitioners will say that they don't really think with the Three Ways and the Two Roads, but they do not deny the existence of these pathways. In their daily practice they probably also presume the existence and functionality of the yin and yang organs in the ZM body.

40. We cannot dwell on these fascinating metaphysical issues here, all of which lurk in (Han) TCM discourses. There are rich discussions of writings surviving from the Zhou, Warring States, and Han periods (770 BCE–220 CE) that appreciate the depth and diversity of the assumptions built into the language and worldview of classical medicines (e.g., Needham 1956; Graham 1989; Jullien 2007).

41. Farquhar (2015).

42. In the literature of Zhuang medicine, for example, an uneasy compromise between the subsystems of the "Three Qi" (heaven, earth, the human) and the "Three Ways and Two Roads" is evident. The logical and mechanical connection between these two subsystems is not theorized in the textbooks we have read, partly because they are arguably incompatible and advocated as "core essences" by different experts.

43. Leading Group Bureau (2013).

44. See our discussion of the problem of things in chapter 4. Also Farquhar (2015), in which Lu Guangxin's use of the relational term *duixiang* 对象 for "object" is discussed (Lu 2001).

45. Bowker and Star (1999, 10).

46. Later in this chapter we mention that Laborjoy Wei's father has a way of "sending qi" that says involves a kind of "information exchange." The term he uses for "information" (*xinxi* 信息) is a modern compound not associated with classical terminologies of qi; perhaps it is a way for the senior Dr. Wei to explain to scientific visitors what is going on when he works with a local sense of qi.

47. Farquhar (1994a).

48. Hanson (2011).

49. It is interesting to note that Dai Ming's *Zhuang Medical History* seldom mentions a Zhuang nationality claim without at the same time stating a local identity. This habit persists in spite of the fact that everyone knows that nationality groups in the south of China very seldom map cleanly over territory (cf. Huang 2001, 435–36).

50. Yanhua Zhang (2007).

51. Michel Foucault, "Introduction" in Georges Canguilhem, *The Normal and the Pathological*, 1989; Smith (1988).

52. Law and Mol (2002); Stengers (2003).

53. Dai (2006, 104).

54. As will be seen in the next chapter, on bodies, Zhuang synthesizers have accepted the yinyang-patterned body as foundational to both ZM and TCM, but like a significant number of critical TCM practitioners they are much less interested in five phases relationships of generation and constraint among the five great organs, or visceral systems.

55. Some Zhuang medicine experts use a language of "expelling" poisons (*paidu* 排毒) with ZM techniques rather than "breaking them down" to make the Ways and Roads flow (*jiedu* 解毒). Choices that have been made between these images and terminologies, in the editing projects of ZM over the past several decades, exemplify the contestation legible just below the bland surface of textbooks. Cf. Ya (2009).

56. Scheid (2002).

57. Huang (2001, 422–36); Dai (2006, 102–13).

58. Bruno Latour uses the concept of "settlement" as a kind of temporary political compromise in ontological struggles in *We Have Never Been Modern* (1993).

59. This famous idea, which we are paraphrasing from Thomas's original argument, is taken from W. I. Thomas and D. Thomas (1929, 572).

60. Kuriyama (1999).

61. Huang (2001, 432–36).

62. Dai (2006, 109), italics added.

63. Near the end of his comparative section, after considerable discussion of the similarities among the nationality medical systems, Dai (2006) says that, given their local and historical divergences, these various systems are like "many roads returning to the same place" (110).

64. Hu (2011, 58).

65. Stated in more sociolinguistic terms, these "keywords" and the names of the bodily targets of medical action are performative: they bring the entity they name into existence as a lasting mode of participation in the world. This kind of linguistic performativity is particularly *medical*: there is a lot at stake in acknowledging the material reality of a functional process, or a Way, or a Road.

66. See also chapter 3, "Bodies."

67. As was noted in chapter 1, Dr. Wei's parents are both village doctors in Guangxi, and in their long careers they developed styles of practice that are nowadays seen as Zhuang medicine. Laborjoy first trained with them, then joined a two-year "integrated Chinese and Western medicine" training course, graduating with a certificate in 1994.

68. *Sha* in ordinary language could also be glossed as sunstroke or heatstroke, but it is interesting that the editors of contemporary ZM seem to avoid invoking one commonsense referent for the term. Here and in chapter 3 ("Bodies") we follow their lead in perceiving many types of *sha* and inquiring about the several modes of diagnosis and treatment known to specialists like Laborjoy Wei.

69. But see chapter 3, in which Laborjoy Wei characterizes *sha* as an often self-limiting disease that is seen in clinics in only a minority of cases.

70. Zhu Hongmei et al. (2014, 43–44).

71. As a stubborn recurring condition known for its uneven symptomatic expressions

and vague complaints, *sha* poisoning is the kind of illness that might be scoffed at or dismissed in a biomedical clinic. Dr. Wei's diagnostic techniques thus combat a certain professional skepticism about the reality of *sha* by recording its concrete bodily signs. Also see the appendix, where, in his long list of "preponderant disease types," Huang Hanru lists *sha* first but then follows it up with disease names that are mostly biomedical. The *zhang*-miasmas and *gu*-worms, also ontologically problematic, are neglected, and very few of Huang's listed diseases are labeled as *du*-poisons. Further, it is worth noting that the process in which Wei (and others) assemble *sha* disease is logically parallel with the story of syphilis recounted by Ludwik Fleck (1979), a classic case of medical ontology or thing-gathering (see Heidegger, 1971 [1951]).

72. Dr. Fan listed eight types of *sha* for us, using names that were in part derived from diagnostics and in part (we think) from symptomatic experiences: woolly *sha*, gut-twisting *sha*, Yellow River *sha*, white down (hair) *sha*, black down *sha*, red down *sha*, tangled thread *sha* (a pain syndrome), and ordinary *sha* (involving headaches and dizziness). This was a somewhat idiosyncratic list, but probably on its way to becoming a component of formal ZM by way of the relationship Dr. Fan had with Laborjoy Wei.

73. Classical images of the itinerant healer, who was both an herbalist and Daoist ritualist, generally included his two-lobed *hulu* (bottle gourd) containing secret medicines.

74. He said the man had a disorder of the Stomach Channel and made him up some medicine, five days' worth. The Weis use a lot of powdered medicines, which they dry and grind up at their "research base"; see below. Dr. Wei senior said that his little packets of combined medicinal powders should be steamed with pork and eaten as food.

CHAPTER 3

1. *Tu*, earth or earthy, is a polysemic term often used to indicate localness or indigeneity, but it also, in urban usage, suggests crudeness or lack of sophistication.

2. We don't know whether this riverside practitioner, like other *baguanr* experts, chose the position of tubes with reference to acupoints. In any case, Zhuang medicine circulation tracks and acupoints are different from those well known in Chinese medicine, and there is, further, no reason to presume that the points used by this Donglan cupping practitioner were similar to those systematized and published by ZM experts in Nanning.

3. This practitioner supplemented her *baguanr* treatment with some needling, which let a few drops of blood from the sites where the tubes were placed. She cleaned the resulting small wounds with alcohol.

4. The bamboo tube method was also introduced to us by Yao practitioners in the main herbals market in Nanning, and there, as in Donglan, the technique was supplemented with a local form of strong needling.

5. Vice Director Wei tended to refer to the folk practitioners he didn't respect as "village grannies." He referred to the widely practiced surface scraping technique of *guasha* (刮痧) as a charlatan's practice, and he said the "old peasant women" won't use the hospital because they have "no culture, no licensing, no training . . . indeed, they're untrainable." Obviously, we couldn't agree.

6. In the course of field research we often saw medical treatments of patients from outside a nationality area. Lili herself was the occasional beneficiary of a massage or

acupuncture treatment; Judith's arthritic feet were treated with "transformed water" by a Tujia healer, and her knee with a Yao medicinal plaster (which kept slipping off); our colleague Luo Jie was happy to help a *zhentiao* expert in a Zhuang hospital demonstrate the method of treating her shoulder stiffness; and Dr. Goldstamp Huang of the Yao nationality hospital in northern Guangxi was sometimes visited by Beijingers, who would drive ten hours by car to get a Yao medicine workup with him.

7. One could go on and on, remarking on "the" [modern] body as best known through dissection, as consisting of relatively discrete organ subsystems, as having five senses, containing circulations, supporting an ontologically distinct "mental" existence, etc., etc. It is not the aim of this chapter to critique the very complex knowledge developed in the history of biomedicine that has taught the world so much about human bodily activity. Nor do we lack interest in the recent new models of bodily function developed through bioscientific research (Landecker 2013; Scheid 2014). Rather, our purpose here is to pluralize the lives of bodies, in the tradition of philosophical pragmatism. And then to ask how practical translation among ontological pluralities might work.

8. This medical and epistemological modernism and universalism does not prevent nationality medicine activists from multiplying real entities in their emergent systems. When we realize that our bodies too have Three Ways and Two Roads, not to mention the Four Pillars of Dai medicine and the Life Gate of TCM, we begin to feel that we are truly in the realm of "the ten thousand [emergent and gathered] things" making up China's many developing nationality medicines.

9. Lai (2017b).

10. Zhang Wenyi (2020).

11. Kuriyama (1999, 8).

12. Kuriyama (1999, 8).

13. Kuriyama (1999, 12).

14. Wang and Cheng discuss the classical origins of Chinese medicine's adjustments of its therapies according to the time, the place, and the person, citing as illustration only some of the many passages in the *Plain Questions* and *Divine Pivot* where this idea is advanced. See Wang Xinqi and Cheng Xiankuan (2010).

15. Lock (1993). Also see Lock and Nguyen (2010, 90–92).

16. Hanson (2011).

17. Zhao Jinghua (2005, 11).

18. Zhao Jinghua (2005, 11).

19. Sivin, and Farquhar after him, among others, have translated the heart, kidneys, liver, and other organs of traditional Chinese medicine as "visceral systems of function" precisely to highlight their holistic dynamism in a body of patterned flows. Some very important visceral systems of TCM—the spleen system, the triple burner—are not mentioned by Zhao Jinghua, while "brain" appears in the Tujia list but not the TCM list. Textbook TCM and Tujia medicine really do look different if we confine our attention to this "rather simple anatomy." Yet we also have observed a certain reliance on the holistic or processually patterned logic of TCM at work in clinics where Tujia practitioners practice.

20. Zhao Jinghua (2005, 13).

21. Zhao Jinghua (2005, 13). This account of the body includes nothing about the senses apart from the function of the eyes to see and the mouth to taste. Nor is the skin treated as an organ.

22. Zhang Yi and Zhong Guoyue (2005).

23. Zhang Yi and Zhong Guoyue (2005, 39–43). But we will later suggest that there are some external body structures perceived and used by practitioners of manual therapeutics that do not make it into these published lists.

24. Zhang Yi and Zhong Guoyue (2005, 39).

25. The kidneys, for example, are described as ruling the genesis and release of germinal essence, in a way familiar in TCM and closely connected with the reproductive organs, and as ruling the separation of clear from turbid fluids and promoting the flow of urine. The spleen, rather than functioning as a rather passive filter (as in biomedicine), is an assertive manager of digestive processes. Both of these organs look quite a lot like their TCM counterparts, though in Qiang medicine the heart and brain organize bodily activity rather differently from the way "heart-mind" (*xin* 心) does in Chinese medicine. Even more fundamentally, it is semiotically important that while canonical TCM has five *zang* and six *fu*, and these two lists correlate with a number of analytical systems that go by fives and sixes, Qiang medicine prefers to list six *zang* and eight *fu*. The system role of any given organ seemingly shared by these two systems would have to be counted as different in practice. In other words, a TCM heart is not the same thing as a Qiang heart.

26. Zhang Yi and Zhong Guoyue (2005, 38).

27. A slightly more adventurous comment in the last chapter of the book leads us closer to Qiang specificity, however: "Although Qiang medicine at present is not equipped with a complete system of medical theory, still in its understanding of factors leading to illness it has its own special character. Qiang medicine holds that wind, qi, water, fire, rain, and stone are the six great causes of illness. Unique among them, the idea that rain causes illness arises from the fact that people work outside on rainy days; and stone as a disease factor amounts to receiving a punishment for offending supernatural forces (e.g., gods and ghosts)." Zhang Yi and Zhong Guoyue (2005, 325–26). This paragraph goes on to point out some other differences from TCM, finally arguing that Qiang medicine has its own "self theory" that makes it different from either TCM or Tibetan medicine.

28. See Farquhar (1994a) for explanations of how a classificatory science like Chinese medicine sorts the conventional correlations of all manner of things (sensory data, symptoms, drugs, bodily structures, etc.) under rubrics (not unlike "the Three Ways and the Two Roads") and in so doing places things into relation in a complex life dynamic. Entities sorted into pigeonholes interact, for good or ill, in ways that become predictable once a sorting process has been achieved. Most nationality medicines, as they salvage and sort "folk" knowledge, are emerging as correlational systems of this kind.

29. We have relied upon the well-written and thoughtful characterizations of ZM to be found in this essay by Huang Hanru and Rong Xiaoxiang because Huang in particular is a very authoritative founder of modern ZM; because the essay is short and can be read in the appendix in its (translated) entirety; and because its content is quite consistent with the standard knowledge now being taught in ZM colleges and academies.

30. Scheid (2018). Yanhua Zhang has also emphasized *tong* through-flow in her study of TCM's management of emotional disorders.

31. Diagnostic correlations possible at microcosmic sites on the body are another topic altogether. Eyes, palms, physiognomy, tongue, and, of course, pulse convey whole-body information to the experienced examiner.

32. Farquhar (1994b).

33. Mol (2002).

34. This was probably a *zhentiao* treatment. *Zhentiao* is a needling method that inserts and then removes strong needles deeply enough to pull out a bit of dermal tissue. It is thought of as breaking some of the tiny threads that weave over the surface of the body. It sometimes produces a drop of blood, but it should not be thought of as bloodletting per se. *Zhentiao* was explained and demonstrated to us by Dr. Wei and other Zhuang and Yao doctors on other occasions, but we did not discuss it on this, our first visit to Dr. Wei's hospital clinic.

35. Wei contrasts this list of eight with the thirty-six or seventy-two types of *sha* detailed in Zhuang medicine textbooks. He says his grassroots authorities have seen only eight types in many years of practice, and the longer lists in textbook are worked up logically rather than in experience.

36. *Tuina* (push and pull) massage is a body manipulation known and used in many parts of East Asia.

37. But also see the appendix, where authors Huang and Rong say that it is "information" that especially flows along the "Fire Road."

38. Deleuze (1993).

39. Marisol de la Cadena's (2015) phrasing.

40. Patriot Sun was a convivial constant presence in his large clinic, which was stuffed with gurneys, electro-acupuncture machines, an X-ray viewing light box, and physical therapy equipment. There were always a few patients visiting for their regular treatments, and emergency cases—like a dislocated shoulder we saw reseated—would interrupt the rather mundane everyday life of an evolving community of patients and practitioners. There was a drawing of a Buddhist-inspired hand on one wall, labeled "magic hands." Dr. Sun told us what he most enjoyed about his work was the daily life of joking and laughing with patients. So though Trooper Guo was angry about his accident (and the delayed compensation he was due) and anxious about recovery, our visit with him was not really sad; he was part of a shifting and convivial clinic community centering on the wounded but magical body of Patriot Sun.

CHAPTER 4

1. Translation by Judith Farquhar.

2. Foucault (1996, 199).

3. Koerner (1999).

4. See Nappi (2009) for a richly suggestive study of Li Shizhen's *Compendium*.

5. We are indebted to Marilyn Strathern for first drawing our attention to Maria Sybilla Merian, in a conference presentation.

6. See Bennett (1994). Even more interesting, chapter 17 of Thoreau's *Walden* (1961) includes a rhapsody on natural intertransformation quite similar to Zhuangzi's playful natural history that begins this chapter. Thanks to Joy Kasson for pointing this out to us.

7. Mueggler (2011).

8. Raj (2005).

9. There is a growing rural industry developing to supply the vast market in traditional herbals with plantation-produced drugs. These projects face many difficulties: first, it is difficult to find suitable tracts of land, cleared and legally available to be consolidated into factory farms, where plant drugs can be grown in bulk and where large

processing facilities can be maintained nearby. Second, only a few medicinal plants (numbering, perhaps, in the dozens) have been shown to thrive under plantation conditions; forest plants are famously fussy about who their neighbors are. And finally, most potential customers for herbal drugs much prefer to use wild plants selectively gathered by herbalists, healers, and other nomads. Wild plants processed with natural methods (sun-dried not heat-processed, for example) are the only ones considered to be trustworthy and of high quality.

10. This notion of "nearing" comes from Martin Heidegger's essay "The Thing" (1971 [1951]), and it recalls his discussion of "the age of the world picture" (1977). Timothy Mitchell has developed the critique of world-picture representation as a profound history of colonialism and the modernization of politics, even of being itself, in *Colonising Egypt* (1988). The medicine-gathering itinerants we spoke with, read in the light of Heidegger's critique of modernity, are as much moderns as the townspeople who come to them for treatments and the researchers like us who visit in search of folklore; they are no strangers to a modernist alienation of objects from subjects.

11. On meshwork as opposed to network, see Ingold (2011, 5–6).

12. See Heidegger (1971 [1951]). François Jullien (1995) has shown the central, but seldom theorized, importance of a notion of propensity in medieval Chinese aesthetics. The word he traces through a number of literatures is *shi* 势. The way this term congeals the tendencies, intentions, configurations, dispositions, efficacies, and powers of things of all kinds (certainly far beyond the merely human) is completely consistent with the argument of this chapter, and has partly inspired it. It is interesting, however, that Jullien takes up neither classical Chinese medicine (healing) nor premodern geography (locality), domains in which we think he could have found even more illuminating propensities to appreciate.

13. Lu (2001).

14. Heidegger (1971 [1951]).

15. Harman (2010, 22–43).

16. Heidegger (1977).

17. Heidegger (1977, 164).

18. Butler (1993, 7).

19. This is the "analytico-referential" practice that Timothy Reiss (1982) has shown unevenly developing within the "patterning" discourses of early modern scientific and philosophical writing. Structuralist and deconstructive critiques notwithstanding, in our everyday usages we have not progressed much beyond Jeremy Bentham's utilitarianism of language and logic, or the discursive empiricisms of nineteenth-century science. Further, as science studies scholars following Latour and Woolgar (1979) have argued, the sciences tend to perform a "splitting and inversion" that produces an entity in a (nominalizing) discursive-material practice and then posits it as simplistically always already having existed.

20. Chudakova (2013), especially chapter 3 on making Tibetan medicines, has much influenced our thinking in this respect.

21. Heidegger (1971 [1951], 172–75). In this he is echoed by Bruno Latour and Peter Weibel (2005) in an important discussion of things as collectives, and thus thoroughly social, political, and hybrid natural-cultural.

22. The essay has an elaborate discussion of the simultaneous oneness of being and "fourness" (or "fouring") of things. Thus what the jug gathers for Heidegger is a fourfold relation between heaven and earth, mortals and immortals. This vision impresses us as

leading away from the metaphysical assumptions informing the gathering work of our interlocutors in China, so we do not consider it here.

23. TCM doctors, especially in the philosophically active 1980s, often spoke of their field's flexibility and adeptness as *linghuo* 灵活 (Farquhar 1994a).

24. Nappi (2009, 57).

25. The things that interest us are also understandable as actants in actor-networks (Latour *2005*). But we are so persuaded by the concepts of agency and relationality developed in actor-network theory that we tend to let this fact go without saying, in the main text at least.

26. In May 2008 Mao, Wenchuan, and Beichuan Counties were at the epicenter of an earthquake measuring 8.0 on the Richter magnitude scale. The massive loss of life, destruction of buildings, and damage to agricultural and forest environments (landslides are still frequent everywhere) have left an indelible mark on the area in every respect.

27. Zhang Dan (2014). For most of his career Dr. Li had practiced medicine at home in the mountains, but after the 2008 earthquake that caused so much suffering and drew so much government funding into health services in the area, he was persuaded by his son and the local Qiang medicine leader, County Hospital Director Bao, to come "down" to the county town to "serve more people" and help to develop Qiang medicine. See also chapter 1, "Institution."

28. Zhang Jing received her PhD in Chinese medicinal pharmacy from the Chengdu University of Chinese Medicine, Sichuan.

29. Zhang Jing (2013).

30. An "herb farmer" (*yaonong*) is as much a collector as he is a cultivator; the term is not usually used for people who set up large plantations to produce commodity drugs in bulk.

31. Heidegger (1977).

32. Frustrated with the legal limitations placed on his practice as an unlicensed herbalist, a few years ago Dr. Li and his sons left the county hospital and opened a private clinic in an apartment building in the town. The family is also still pursuing the establishment of an "herbals medicines base" in the land around their ruined family home.

33. Feuchtwang 1992; 2010).

34. Later she became a schoolteacher, and then the party secretary of her village. From that position she was promoted to the county bureau of discipline and inspection. Here it is impossible to adequately explore the important role of the 1960s and 1970s program of appointing, training, and supporting barefoot doctors in rural areas all over China. The majority of the nationality healers we have met, or their parents, had some experience as barefoot doctors (Fang 2012 and see chapter 5).

35. Dr. Huang and her relatives liked to point out to us that lineage and residence among the Pan Yao subgroup to which they belong is quite often matrifocal, with daughters often taking the names of their mothers rather than their fathers.

36. In the preface and in chapter 5 we describe some of the forms of Yao medicine and pharmacy that are being deployed and developed in the Yao Medicine Hospital in a town near where Drs. Huang and Feng lived. Informed by many conversations with Dr. Yang Jian, who was a member of our research team, we tend to agree that this hospital cannot maintain the ethnic and herbal purities that interested Huang. But we nevertheless feel that this institution, and others like it, do cultivate a healing charisma of local powers beyond the state-regulated rationalities of public health and formal medicine.

37. For Huang and Feng, this concept and practice of "tasting" had relatively little to do with the canonical TCM method of classifying drugs according to "the five flavors" (*wuwei* 五味). Speaking of new approaches to systematizing local drugs and Yao nationality medical knowledge, Dr. Feng said that many Yao experts have difficulty figuring out which of the five flavor categories an herbal might belong to, even though they know how it tastes perfectly well.

38. Yellow jessamine, also known as *dachayao* or poison hemlock, is often used to treat rheumatic disorders, but, Huang and Feng emphasize, it requires proper technique to use it; otherwise things could go terribly wrong.

39. Sun Simiao was a medical man who died in 682 CE. He famously authored the *Qian Jin Fan* [千金方, Essential Formulas Worth a Thousand in Gold] and is commonly thought of as "the Medicine King." He also receives offerings and prayers in temples and at shrines like Dr. Su's throughout China.

40. He was actually not very comfortable speaking in standard Chinese, and his nephew translated most of the interview as we went along. His everyday language was a local Lisu language.

41. Actually there was some ambiguity in the interview about which senior family member it was who visited in dreams.

42. Actually, he was dismissive about the idea that women could be fated to learn medical work. This strong bias toward male specialists may be rather particular to Lisu communities; in some other areas we found healers were willing to consider taking female junior relatives as disciples. Everywhere except in "matrifocal" Yao country and in the Li communities of Hainan Island, however, there was a clear bias toward transmitting healing skill to males.

43. Su Lao's "literacy" was not in question; noting some common mistakes in word choice—the sort of thing any of us might slip into—on his pink satin medicine pockets, we believed that the names, labels, and classifications in use in his pharmacy were written by him.

44. Butler (1993).

45. Porkert (1974); Graham (1989); Granet (1975); Farquhar, Lai, and Kramer (2017).

46. Harman (2010).

47. Farquhar (1994a, 217–20).

48. McLuhan and Powers (1989); Harvey (1989; 2007); Hardt and Negri (2000).

49. Equal to about $100 at the time.

50. This event is described and some background on Wang Jie's work as an herbalist is given in an online newspaper article, Dong (2012).

51. Zhu Guoben (2006, 472–86).

52. Liu (2003). Both of the Yang sisters were on the editing committee of this volume, and they are generally credited with being the chief authors of its content.

53. In our visits to Hainan we learned about the island's long history of plantation agriculture. We presume that the socialist collectives were organized plantation style in Hainan, and very likely to exclude agricultural workers who were of the "bad classes."

54. "Characteristics" is the conventional English translation of *xingneng*; and *xingwei* according to Wiseman and Feng (1998) is "nature and flavor." In keeping with the argument of this chapter, however, we would be inclined, following Jullien, to translate *xing* as propensities. Joseph Needham (1956, 51 et passim) translates the term for ancient Chinese science as "inherent nature," in a context where he emphasizes the propensities (*shi* 势) of each of the myriad things to seek out a certain place and show affinities and

antipathies with certain things. This is a vision of the active specificity of all things that Needham draws on (and extends into his own vision of "organicism") from his reading of Zhuangzi and his contemporaries, the "Daoist school" (*Tao Chia*). Further, A. C. Graham (1986, 14) in a discussion of the word *xing* (*hsing*) as it appears in the same early sources ends up translating the word as "nature." From the Zhuangzi, he defines it as "the course of life (*sheng* 生) proper to a thing."

55. Dong (2012).

56. Sister Wang expressed some frustration with the limits to her career as a doctor stemming from her poor education. She may feel that her history, national attention notwithstanding, has made it impossible for her to sustain a wider fame and a bigger practice.

57. *Yaofang* become objects with their own integrity: the very fact that proprietary formulas (*mifang* 秘方) can be kept secret even as researchers are welcomed to examine them (see chapter 5) suggests that as drugs "thing" and become "objects" of attention and use, they stabilize for a time into secrets that withdraw in part from knowledge (Harman 2010, 19); they do not openly declare their properties, and not everyone can perceive their qualities.

CHAPTER 5

1. Latour and Weibel (2005, 246).

2. 人之生, 氣之聚, 聚則為, 散則為死 (《知北游》1). Latour and Weibel (2005) expand on the nature of "the thing" as a gathering of multiple agencies at some length, in a rather Heideggerian mode. Their approaches to gathering are argued through an etymological riff on an old Saxon word, *das Ding*, which means both an object and a convocation. Zhuangzi's image of the gathering of vital Qi is advanced as part of one of his many relativizing pronouncements about life and death; because in the chapter cited he goes on to talk of how the beauty and wonder of gathered life transforms into the corruption and putridness of a dispersed death, he is not just speaking of human life.

3. Sapir (1995); Lai and Farquhar (2020).

4. Samuel Weber (1987, 3–17) in his reading of Saussurian semiotics argues that signification itself is always an encounter with otherness. We agree, and though we are uncomfortable with the classical "self-other divide" in modern anthropology, we still see difference and some sense of an other as fundamental to anthropology.

5. The reader is asked to bear in mind that when we use the word "social" in this book we are referring to relations embracing both human and (all manner of) nonhuman actors. Also, we should note that in contexts like this, when we speak of "experience" we are using it in a pragmatist sense derived from both William James (2003 [1904]) and the writings approaching philosophy of science from a Chinese medicine perspective. Not, in other words, a secret individual possession like the commonsense notion critiqued by Jay (2005).

6. We are indebted to Anna Tsing (2011) for this useful notion.

7. Lei (1999). Our chapter 1, "Institution," is our extended effort to replace a state-people divide.

8. See Callon and Latour (1981) for a (non)distinction between micro-actors and macro-actors that informs our perception of the state in action. For them, macro-actors are constantly made with "translations" that link and transform the actors involved in any matter of concern. Here we focus on encounter with the understanding that trans-

lations in this sense are a form of encounter, though the latter term is more agnostic about communication. Also see Lai (2016) for a critique of the sociology that presumes China's fabled urban-rural divide.

9. We have found Louis Althusser's (2006 [1993]) essay "The Underground Current of the Materialism of the Encounter" a thought-provoking interlocutor in this connection. Gilles Deleuze's (1993) book *The Fold: Leibniz and the Baroque* is suggestive in this respect too.

10. In "The Underground Current of the Philosophy of the Encounter," Louis Althusser 2006 [1993] discussed the atomic metaphysics of Epicurus, who saw the origin of specific being as resulting from a swerve in the smooth flow (or "rain") of atoms. The notion of encounter as swerve or uncaused event, which Althusser develops in other ways in this late essay, helps us to think of our field research as salient outside a predictive or determinist social science framework.

11. Mullaney (2010).

12. In this signboard structuration of available services, the type of disease would seem to trump the nationality character of the cures on offer. Most traditional medical systems in the southern mountains claim a special expertise in treating rheumatic diseases (*fengshi bing* 风湿病).

13. But note that Dr. Tian too has published on both Miao and Tujia medicine, and thus frequently encounters local mixtures of nationality traditions. Here we want to express our warm thanks to Dr. Tian and his health research associates in Xiangxi for their hospitality and creative collaboration in nationality medicines research.

14. We want to leave behind the "doctor-patient relationship," the "Self-Other encounter," and a lot of sociolinguistic and ethnomethodological reductions that presume the modern individual as a basic unit.

15. We could even grow quite metaphysical on the subject of these contingencies: Following Epicurus, and then Marx, and then Althusser, we are noting only a particular series of swerves in the rain of unconnected atoms. Or, following the cosmogonic writings of China's Warring States period, we witnessed just a particular phasing or configuration of the flow of qi from the source. These are nondeterminist and nonreductionist ways of understanding "the underground current" of emergence and event (Althusser 2006 [1993]).

16. *Earthbound China* is the interesting translation of the title of a classic anthropological study by Fei Hsiao-Tung, 《云南三村》 (or "Three Villages in Yunnan"), 1945.

17. *Diaocha* is a term with a relatively deep history in modern China. It tends to refer to both survey research and field investigation. The modern history of state-led *diaocha* began, we think, with Mao Zedong's (1967 [1927]) essay "Report on an Investigation"; Farquhar (2012) discusses the history of *diaocha*.

18. Director Ma was also conducting surveys in the Dehong area, further to the west, where a somewhat better-documented variant of Achang medicine had been found to be active.

19. In 2011 the team consisted of Director Resolution Ma, senior staff members Cloudscape Zhao and Cosmic Gift Lu, two younger members of the research staff, a reporter named Energy Chen, and Director Ma's pharmacy student son, who had brought along a professional field video kit. And Lili and Judith.

20. At one point Dr. Zhu suggested that his approach to therapeutics was a "localization" (*bentuhua* 本土化) of traditional Chinese medicine. But he also insisted that the records in his notebook belonged to "Achang medicine."

21. In one conversation with Director Ma, Judith described to him some of her experience in researching traditional Chinese medicine in Guangzhou in the early 1980s. She tried to persuade him that she had found very few clinicians who could hand over their "theory" on an epistemological silver platter. Normally the researcher himself would have to reason out the principles of a medical system—to find its systematicity, as it were—through a long-standing engagement with practice.

22. Stephan Feuchtwang (2013) defines and discusses the mass line and its legacies in post-Mao China.

23. He was too tactful to say so, but there was little evidence in the Caojian area of nationality "culture" of any other kind. The research team had gathered evidence that this nationality had long had a presence in the Southwest and an importance in regional history (for example as contract warriors, horsemen, and carters). But in today's ways of salvaging and sorting China's minority nationalities, they take up little cultural space. Not much for folk dancing, and known for simple clothing, they could not compare to the exotic Others consumed by tourists all around them in Yunnan province.

24. In the academic world of ethnology and anthropology in China, where these fields are growing, similar critical debates have been lively for several decades.

25. The five tigers listed in the draft catalog, which we discuss below, were the names of five Yao herbals: "Entering Mountains Tiger," "Climbing Mountains Tiger," "Descending Mountains Tiger," "Furry Tiger," and "Fierce Tiger."

26. Prof. Dai is based at a pharmacy research institute in Nanning, and Dr. Li (who also practices Yao medicine) heads a Yao medicine research center in that city.

27. Anthropologist Ralph Litzinger lived and conducted fieldwork in Jinxiu in the early 1990s. See Litzinger (2000) for a sensitive ethnographic account of Yao ethnicity politics and local place-making.

28. See Bowker and Star (1999).

29. Around Jinxiu we were told that the Yao nationality (in Guangxi, at least) is composed of five subgroups: Pan Yao 盘瑶, Chashan Yao 茶山瑶, Ao Yao 坳瑶, Guoshan Yao 过山瑶, and Hualan Yao 花篮瑶. The nationality medicine leaders we worked with seemed to hold that Yao medical authority rested mainly with those in the Pan Yao group. We even noted during the meeting that considerable prior work on the pharmacopoeia done by an Ao Yao herbalist was disvalued, ostensibly on nationality grounds. And though he was local, he was not invited to this meeting.

30. Yao medicine was thriving in the entirely private sector. Dr. Purity Chu, a senior relative of Hospital Director Liang, had established a successful private clinic (modernized from his long-standing village practice) and opened several allied businesses in a nearby township. In the town of Jinxiu we met other private practitioners (some of them retired from the health department) who had opened businesses supplying herbals and medicinal wines. Because Jinxiu was a tourist destination (known to be cooler than Nanning in the summer), and because the Great Yao Mountains have a commercially attractive reputation as a source of magical healing powers, it seemed that many local experts had no need of an institutional framework in which to practice Yao medicine. Maybe this is one reason the three old doctors at the meeting could retreat to a "more or less" or "whatever" kind of attitude. Perhaps they felt they could leave the constraints of legal institutional medicine behind if all the regulation became too onerous.

31. See chapter 4 for reasons why this was not a comfortable process.

32. Like hospitals in the United States, Director Liang's organization was forced to engage in entrepreneurial profit-seeking. With declining support from local and central

government, and incompletely effective insurance schemes, hospitals and clinics have little choice in this matter. In 2013 we toured a new outpatient facility for "boutique" Yao medicine services, which had been built alongside the main building; and we heard plans from Director Liang to develop a Yao *materia medica* base (i.e., an herbal medicine plantation) on hospital land. He also was planning a spa-hotel near a new manmade lake on the edge of town, hoping to attract medical tourists.

33. In most of the clinical institutions of the minority nationality medical groups we studied, senior practitioners with formal appointments had not been required to pass licensing exams. Many of them had some formal medical training. But it was clear that without their local and uncertified expertise, there would be no "nationality medicine." Their authority had to be grandfathered in.

34. A reader who is unpersuaded by the idea of nonhuman agents being active in a supremely social event like the standardization meeting might object that "the list" was far from being a naturally occurring or internally coherent agent: it was assembled by human actors. But who among us human writers and readers was not assembled, and indeed, what agents are not still and always under construction?

35. Bowker (2005).

36. We note that *zuan* 钻 is a phonetic transcription into a Chinese character (it means drill or bore) of a Yao language name.

37. Hathaway (2013); Harwood (2014); Giersch (2006). The most spectacular and historically interesting (if somewhat unreliable) account of this "wild" region is Winnington (1959).

38. See our discussion of a former county town in this area, Bijiang, in which we trace the shifting relationship between strong state socialism and a place thought to be mostly wild or anarchic: Farquhar, Lai, and Kramer (2017); Scott (2009).

39. Sha Lina was then an anthropology student at Yunnan University. She kindly assisted us in Nujiang, her home area, and was especially generous in connecting us with healers and experts she knew.

40. Shortly after Dr. Hu retired, in the 1990s, new regulations were put in place requiring that medical practitioners hold one of several kinds of licenses. Because Benefits Hu was not a medical school graduate, he was required to forgo his medical license at that time, though he was still allowed to sell herbal drugs from his pharmacy in Pihe. We are sure, however, that his regular patients still often sought him out for herbal prescriptions. See Farquhar, Lai, and Kramer (2017) for a description of his pharmacy.

41. The public health importance of the barefoot doctor program that formally began in the late 1960s cannot be overstated. See Xiaoping Fang's (2012) history of the program in one area near Shanghai; see also Fang (2014).

42. The Liuku training seems to have been an early and local form of the nationwide programs to train barefoot doctors. The well-known "Barefoot Doctors' Manual," which reflects a systematic curriculum in both Chinese and "Western" medicine, was first properly published in 1970. Shanghai and Zhejiang Colleges of TCM (1970).

43. We are grateful to Mr. Zhou Yuanchuan, whose book, 《怒江流域民族医药》, was our first access to Nujiang Lisu medicine and who assisted us with introductions for part of our time working in the prefecture.

44. Market days, which operate on variable schedules in different areas of rural China, are times when people gather to buy, sell, and make use of services in the county town or township, in Nujiang sometimes traveling long distances from their houses scattered along the narrow valley.

45. Bone-setting (*zhenggu* 正骨) is a time-honored specialty among "folk" practitioners in East Asia. The skills of a bone-setter include treating not only broken bones but also sprains, wounds, and a variety of aches and pains. They are perhaps comparable to barber surgeons in the nineteenth-century United States.

46. Dr. Zhang was not optimistic about being able to help her, though he tried. A few days later we saw this patient on the street and asked her how she was doing, and she said the arm was still not properly set; obviously in great discomfort, she told us she was on her way to the hospital to accept and pay for their treatment. Dr. Zhang charged little or nothing for his services on market days, by contrast.

47. Farquhar, Lai, and Kramer (2017).

48. See Fang (2014).

49. Rifkin (1972).

50. Fang (2014).

51. See any translation of the *Dao De Jing* by Laozi for this famous first line.

CONCLUSIONS, AND THEN SOME

1. 人之生, 氣之聚也, 聚則為生, 散則為死 (*Zhuangzi* 22《知北游》Knowing Wanders North 1).

2. *Zhuangzi* Chapter 18:《至乐》Happiness Attained 7.

3. We have discussed at greater length Dr. Huang's use of a rare herbal medicine to treat a lymphoma-associated lesion in Lai and Farquhar (2020).

4. Acupuncture and moxibustion, important parts of the modern TCM canon, are not usually taught as *waike* "external medicine" practices, though they do work on the body surface. *Tuina* massage is often offered in acupuncture departments of TCM, but *tuina* and other haptic treatments are also strongly associated with the bone-setters and professional massage services that operate outside of the major TCM institutions. We have also noted that most masseurs in China have studied some medicine and frequently advise their clients on therapies. There is also a commoditized home-remedy form of herbal plaster: this is a medicinal adhesive patch, usually infused with aromatic and warming herbs, that should be applied to the skin near the site of deep or superficial discomfort. There are many varieties and lots of homely advice for care associated with these commercial products. But doctors do not consider them to be as effective as the hand-prepared herbal plaster discussed here.

5. From Chengdu College of TCM (1978, 334).

6. There is, however, a marvelously detailed protocol for the home production of herbal plasters, along with several fascinating classic examples of external use herbal formulas, in Editing Committee (1987). That encyclopedia entry specifies more disorders treatable with herbal plasters than the Chengdu College textbook we discuss here, and more of these illnesses are of the body interior, not just surface injuries.

7. Editing Committee (1987, 265).

8. The first editor of the *Encyclopedia of Chinese Medicine* was historian Xie Guan, who founded this massive project in the 1940s after writing the first modern history of medicine in China; Xie (1935). The *Encyclopedia* now appears in many subdisciplinary volumes. Its descriptive definitions usefully reflect the ongoing work of a huge profession in achieving consensus about the nature of the many things, abstract and concrete, that are kept in play in the large and very popular field of TCM.

Bibliography

Allen, Barry. 2015. *Vanishing into Things: Knowledge in Chinese Tradition*. Cambridge, MA: Harvard University Press.

Althusser, Louis. 2006 [1993]. The Underground Current of the Materialism of the Encounter. In *Philosophy of the Encounter, Later Writings 1978–87*. London: Verso.

Ames, Roger T. 1983. *The Art of Rulership: A Study in Ancient Chinese Political Thought*. Honolulu: University of Hawai'i Press.

Anagnost, Ann. 1997. *National Past-Times: Narrative, Representation, and Power in Modern China*. Durham, NC: Duke University Press.

Anderson, Benedict. 2006 [1983]. *Imagined Communities: Reflections on the Origin and Spread of Nationalism*. London: Verso.

Andrews, Bridie. 2014. *The Making of Modern Chinese Medicine, 1850–1960*. Vancouver: University of British Columbia Press.

Arnold, David. 1993. *Colonizing the Body: State Medicine and Epidemic Disease in 19th Century India*. Berkeley: University of California Press.

Bachelard, Gaston. 1984. *The New Scientific Spirit*. Boston: Beacon Press.

Barker, Francis. 1984. *The Tremulous Private Body: Essays in Subjection*. London: Methuen.

Barthes, Roland. 1972. *Mythologies*. New York: Hill and Wang.

Bennett, Jane. 1994. *Thoreau's Nature: Ethics, Politics, and the Wild*. Thousand Oaks, CA: Sage.

———. 2010. *Vibrant Matter: A Political Ecology of Things*. Durham, NC: Duke University Press.

Blaser, Mario. 2010. *Storytelling Globalization from the Chaco and Beyond*. Durham, NC: Duke University Press.

Bowker, Geoffrey. 2005. *Memory Practices in the Sciences*. Cambridge, MA: MIT Press.

Bowker, Geoffrey, and Susan Leigh Star. 1999. *Sorting Things Out: Classification and Its Consequences*. Inside Technology. Cambridge, MA: MIT Press.

Butler, Judith. 1993. *Bodies That Matter: On the Discursive Limits of "Sex."* New York: Routledge.

Cadena, Marisol de la. 2015. *Earth Beings: Ecologies of Practice across Andean Worlds*. Durham, NC: Duke University Press.

Callon, Michel, and Bruno Latour. 1981. *Unscrewing the Big Leviathan; Or, How Actors Macrostructure Reality, and How Sociologists Help Them to Do So?* In A. V. Cicourel and K. Knorr-Cetina, eds., *Advances in Social Theory and Methodology: Toward an*

Integration of Macro and Microsociologies, 277–303. Boston: Routledge and Kegan Paul.

Canguilhem, Georges. 1989. *The Normal and the Pathological*. New York: Zone Books.

Casey, Edward S. 1996. How to Get from Space to Place in a Fairly Short Period of Time. In Steven Feld et al., eds., *Senses of Place*, 13–52. Santa Fe: SAR Press.

Chatterjee, Partha. 1993. *The Nation and Its Fragments: Colonial and Postcolonial Histories*. Princeton: Princeton University Press.

Chengdu College of Traditional Chinese Medicine, eds. 1978. 《中药学》 [TCM Pharmacy]. Shanghai: Shanghai Science and Technology Press.

Chudakova, Tatiana. 2013. *Recovering Health: Tibetan Medicine and Biocosmopolitics in Russia*. PhD diss., Department of Anthropology, University of Chicago.

Citton, Gaston. 2017. *The Ecology of Attention*. Malden, MA: Polity Press.

Croizier, Ralph C. 1968. *Traditional Medicine in Modern China: Science, Nationalism, and the Tensions of Cultural Change*. Harvard East Asia series 34. Cambridge, MA: Harvard University Press.

———. 1976. The Ideology of Medical Revivalism in Modern China. In C. Leslie, ed., *Asian Medical Systems: A Comparative Study, 341–55. Berkeley: University of California Press.*

Dai Ming 戴铭. 2006. *Zhuangzu Yixue Shi* 壮族医学史 [Zhuang Medical History]. Nanning: Guangxi Nationalities Press.

Deleuze, Gilles. 1993. *The Fold: Leibniz and the Baroque*. Minneapolis: University of Minnesota Press.

Deleuze, Gilles, and Felix Guattari. 1986. *Nomadology: The War Machine*. Trans. Brian Massumi. New York: Semiotexte.

———. 1987. *A Thousand Plateaus: Capitalism and Schizophrenia*. Trans. Brian Massumi. Minneapolis: University of Minnesota Press.

Dong Yaling, 董亚玲. 2012. 朱镕基总理慰问那位五指山黎医 [How President Zhu Rongji Expresses His Care for a Wuzhishan Li Healer]. http://lizu.baike.com/article-310124 .html.

Editing Committee of the 《中医大辞典》. 1987. 《中医大辞典, 外科骨伤五官科分册》. Beijing: People's Health Press, 1987.

Fan, Fa-ti. 2012. Collective Monitoring, Collective Defense: Science, Earthquakes, and Politics in Communist China. *Science in Context* 25: 127–54.

Fang Xiaoping. 2012. *Barefoot Doctors and Western Medicine in China*. Rochester, NY: University of Rochester Press.

———. 2014. Barefoot Doctors and the Provision of Rural Health Care. In Bridie Andrews and Mary Brown Bullock, eds., *Medical Transitions in 20th Century China*. Bloomington: Indiana University Press.

Farquhar, Judith. 1987. Problems of Knowledge in Contemporary Chinese Medical Discourse. *Social Science and Medicine* 24, no.12): 1013–1021.

———. 1991. Objects, Processes, and Female Infertility in Chinese Medicine. *Medical Anthropology Quarterly*, n.s., 5, no. 4 (December): 370–99.

———. 1992. Time and Text: Approaching Contemporary Chinese Medicine through Analysis of a Case. In Charles Leslie and Allan Young, eds., *Paths to Asian Medical Knowledge*. Berkeley: University of California Press.

———. 1994a. *Knowing Practice: The Clinical Encounter of Chinese Medicine*. Boulder, CO: Westview Press.

———. 1994b. Multiplicity, Point of View, and Responsibility in Traditional Chinese

Medicine. In Angela Zito and Tani E. Barlow, eds., *Body, Subject, and Power in China*, 78-99. Chicago: University of Chicago Press.

———. 2012a. Afterlives of the Field Survey: Several Modern Moments in Chinese State Knowledge Production. Keynote address, Soyuz conference, Ann Arbor, MI, March 23.

———. 2012b. Knowledge in Translation: Global Science, Local Things. In Lesley Green and Susan Levine, eds. *Medicine and the Politics of Knowledge*, 153-70. Cape Town: Human Sciences Research Council Press.

———. 2015. Metaphysics at the Bedside. In Howard Chiang, ed., *Historical Epistemology and the Making of Modern Chinese Medicine*, 219-36. Manchester: Manchester University Press.

———. 2020. *A Way of Life: Things, Thought, and Action in Chinese Medicine*. New Haven: Yale University Press.

Farquhar, Judith, and Lai Lili. 2014 Information and Its Practical Other: Crafting Zhuang Nationality Medicine. *East Asian Science and Technology Studies* 8: 417-37.

Farquhar, Judith, Lili Lai, and Marshall Kramer. 2017. A Place at the End of a Road: A Yinyang Geography. *Anthropologica* 59, no. 2: 216-27.

Farquhar, Judith, and Qicheng Zhang. 2005. Biopolitical Beijing: Pleasure, Sovereignty, and Self-Cultivation in China's Capital. *Cultural Anthropology* 20, no. 3: 303-27.

Fei Hsiao-tung. 1945. *Earthbound China: A Study of Rural Economy in Yunnan*. Chicago: University of Chicago Press.

Feld, Steven, and Keith H. Basso, eds. 1996. *Senses of Place*. Santa Fe: SAR Press.

Feuchtwang, Stephan. 1992. *The Imperial Metaphor: Popular Religion in China*. London: Routledge.

———. 2010. *Anthropology of Religion, Charisma, and Ghosts: Chinese Lessons for Adequate Theory*. Berlin: de Gruyter.

———. 2013. Political History, Past Suffering, and Present Sources of Moral Judgment in the People's Republic of China. In Charles Stafford, ed., *Ordinary Ethics in China*. London: Bloomsbury Academic.

Feuchtwang, Stephan, and Mingming Wang. 2001. *Grassroots Charisma: Four Local Leaders in China*. London: Routledge.

Fleck, Ludwik. 1979. *Genesis and Development of a Scientific Fact*. Chicago: University of Chicago Press.

Foucault, Michel. 1970. *The Order of Things: An Archaeology of the Human Sciences*. New York: Pantheon.

———. 1973. *The Birth of the Clinic: An Archaeology of Medical Perception*. New York: Pantheon.

———. 1977. *Discipline and Punish: The Birth of the Prison*. New York: Vintage Books.

———. 1978. *The History of Sexuality*. New York: Pantheon.

———. 1984. Right of Death and Power over Life. In Paul Rabinow, ed., *The Foucault Reader*, 258-72. New York: Pantheon.

———. 1996. The Masked Philosopher. In Sylvere Lotringer, ed., *Foucault Live: Interviews, 1961-1984*, 193-202. New York: Semiotexte.

Garon, Colin. 2018. Clinical Concrescences: Integration in Contemporary Chinese Medicine Gynecology. BA Thesis, Program in History, Philosophy, and Sociology of Science, University of Chicago.

Geaney, Jane. In press. *The Emergence of Word Meaning in Early China*. Albany: SUNY Press.

Geertz, Clifford. 1993. *Local Knowledge: Further Essays in Interpretive Anthropology*. London: Fontana Press.

Giddens, Anthony. 1984. *The Constitution of Society: Outline of the Theory of Structuration*. Cambridge: Polity Press.

Giersch, C. Patterson. 2006. *Asian Borderlands: The Transformation of Qing China's Yunnan Frontier*. Cambridge, MA: Harvard University Press.

Gordon, Deborah R. 1988. Tenacious Assumptions in Western Medicine. In Margaret Lock and Deborah R. Gordon, eds., *Biomedicine Examined*. Dordrecht: Kluwer Academic.

Graham, A. C. 1986. *Studies in Chinese Philosophy and Philosophical Literature*. Singapore: NUS Institute of East Asian Philosophies.

———. 1989. *Disputers of the Tao: Philosophical Argument in Ancient China*. Lasalle, IL: Open Court.

Granet, Marcel. 1975. *La Pensée Chinoise*. New York: Arno Press.

Green, Lesley, and Susan Levine, eds. 2012. *Medicine and the Politics of Knowledge*. Cape Town: Human Sciences Research Council Press.

Guha, Ranajit, ed. 1997. *A Subaltern Studies Reader, 1986–1995*. Minneapolis: University of Minnesota Press.

Hacking, Ian. 1983. *Representing and Intervening: Introductory Topics in the Philosophy of Natural Science*. Cambridge: Cambridge University Press.

Hanson, Marta E. 2011. *Speaking of Epidemics in Chinese Medicine: Disease and the Geographic Imagination in Late Imperial China*. Needham Research Institute series. Milton Park, Abingdon, Oxon: Routledge.

Haraway, Donna. 1988. Situated Knowledges: The Science Question in Feminism and the Privilege of Partial Perspective. *Feminist Studies* 14, no. 3: 575–99.

Hardiman, David, and Projit Bihari Mukharji, eds. 2012. *Medical Marginality in South Asia*. London: Routledge.

Hardt, Michael, and Antonion Negri. 2000. *Empire*. Cambridge, MA: Harvard University Press.

Harman, Graham. 2010. The Theory of Objects in Heidegger and Whitehead (1997). In *Towards Speculative Realism: Essays and Lectures*, 22–43. Winchester, UK: Zero Books.

Harvey, David. 1989. *The Condition of Post-Modernity: An Enquiry into the Origins of Cultural Change*. Oxford: Blackwell.

———. 2007. *A Brief History of Neoliberalism*. Oxford: Oxford University Press.

Harwood, Russell. 2014. *China's New Socialist Countryside: Modernity Arrives in the Nu River Valley*. Seattle: University of Washington Press.

Hathaway, Michael. 2013. *Environmental Winds: Making the Global in Southwest China*. Berkeley: University of California Press.

Hayden, Cori. 2003. *When Nature Goes Public: The Making and Unmaking of Bioprospecting in Mexico*. Princeton: Princeton University Press.

Heidegger, Martin. 1971 [1951]. The Thing. In Albert Hofstadter, ed./trans., *Poetry, Language, Thought*, 161–84. New York: Harper and Row.

———. 1971 [1954]. Building Dwelling Thinking. In Albert Hofstadter, ed./trans., *Poetry, Language, Thought*, 141–60. New York: Harper and Row.

———. 1977. The Age of the World Picture. In William Lovitt, trans., *The Question concerning Technology and Other Essays*, 115–54. New York: Harper and Row.

Hostetler, Laura. 2001. *Qing Colonial Enterprise: Ethnography and Cartography in Early Modern China*. Chicago: University of Chicago Press.

Hsu, Elisabeth. 1999. *The Transmission of Chinese Medicine*. Cambridge: Cambridge University Press.

Hu Hui 胡惠. 2011. *Guipai Ming Laozhongyi: Zhuanji juan, Huang Jinming* 桂派名老中医•传记卷:黄瑾明 [A Renowned Senior Chinese Doctor of the Guangxi School: Biography of Huang Jinming]. Beijing: China Chinese Medicine Press. 北京: 中国中医药出版社.

Huang Hanru 黄汉儒. 2001. *Zhongguo Zhuang Yixue* 中国壮医学 [China's Zhuang Medicine]. Nanning: Guangxi Nationalities Press.

Huang Hanru 黄汉儒, Huang Jingxian 黄景贤, and Duan Zhaohong 段昭红, eds. 1998. 壮族医学史 [Zhuang Medical History]. Nanning: Guangxi Science and Technology Press.

Huang Hanru 黄汉儒 and Huang Jinming 黄瑾明. 1986. 广西靖西壮族民间医药情况考察报告 [Report on a Survey of the Situation of Zhuang Folk Medicine and Pharmacy in Tranquility County, Guangxi]. *Guangxi Chinese Medicine and Pharmacy*, no. 6.

Huang Hanru 黄汉儒 and Rong Xiaoxiang 容晓翔. 2015. 重'三道两路'理论的妆医药 [The Emphasis on "Three Ways and Two Roads" in Zhuang Medicine and Pharmacy]. *China News of Traditional Chinese Medicine* [中国中医药报], December 2, 2012, no. 4.

Ingold, Tim. 2000. *The Perception of the Environment: Essays on Livelihood, Dwelling, and Skill*. London: Routledge.

———. 2011. *Redrawing Anthropology: Materials, Movements, Lines*. Burlington, VT: Ashgate.

Ivy, Marilyn. 1995. *Discourses of the Vanishing: Modernity, Phantasm, Japan*. Chicago: University of Chicago Press.

Jackson, John L., Jr. 2005. *Real Black: Adventures in Racial Sincerity*. Chicago: University of Chicago Press.

James, William. 1920 [1907]. *A Pluralistic Universe*. New York: Longmans Green.

———. 2003 [1904]. A World of Pure Experience. In *Essays in Radical Empiricism*, 21–47. New York: Dover Press.

Jay, Martin. 2005. *Songs of Experience: Modern American and European Variations on a Universal Theme*. Berkeley: University of California Press.

Joniak-Luthi, Agnieszka. 2013. The Han Minzu, Fragmented Identities, and Ethnicity. *Journal of Asian Studies* 72, no. 4: 849–71.

Jordanova, Ludmila. 1989. *Sexual Visions: Images of Gender in Science and Medicine between the Eighteenth and Twentieth Centuries*. New York: Harvester Wheatsheaf.

Jullien, François. 1995. *The Propensity of Things: Toward a History of Efficacy in China*. New York: Zone Books.

———. 2007. *Vital Nourishment: Departing from Happiness*. New York: Zone Books.

Karchmer, Eric I. 2005. *Orientalizing the Body: Post-colonial Transformations in Chinese Medicine*. PhD diss., University of North Carolina–Chapel Hill, Department of Anthropology.

Kasoff, Ira E. 1984. *The Thought of Chang Tsai (1020–1077)*. Cambridge Studies in Chinese History, Literature, and Institutions. Cambridge: Cambridge University Press.

Keane, Webb. 1997. *Signs of Recognition: Powers and Hazards of Representation in an Indonesian Society*. Berkeley: University of California Press.

Koerner, Lisbet. 1999. *Linnaeus: Nature and Nation.* Cambridge, MA: Harvard University Press.

Kohn, Eduardo. 2013. *How Forests Think: Toward an Anthropology beyond the Human.* Berkeley: University of California Press.

Kraus, Richard. 1991. *Brushes with Power: Modern Politics and the Chinese Art of Calligraphy.* Berkeley: University of California Press.

Kuriyama, Shigehisa. 1999. *The Expressiveness of the Body and the Divergence of Greek and Chinese Medicine.* New York: Zone Books.

Laclau, Ernesto. 1983. The Impossibility of Society. *Canadian Journal of Political and Social Theory* 7, nos. 1, 2: 89-92.

Lai Lili. 2004. Irresistible Scientization: The Rhetoric of Science in Institutional Chinese Medicine. MA thesis, Department of Anthropology, University of North Carolina.

———. 2016. *Hygiene, Sociality, and Culture in Contemporary Rural China: The Uncanny New Village.* Amsterdam: University of Amsterdam Press.

———. 2017a. 生殖焦虑与实践理性: 试管婴儿技术的人类学 [Reproductive Anxiety and Practical Reasoning: An Anthropological Observation of IVF-ET]. *Journal of Southwest Minzu University* 9: 21-28.

———. 2017b. 日常生活再出发: 身体, 体现, 体验 [Resetting Everyday Life: Body, Embodiment, Experience]. Conference paper for Research Forum on Everyday Life, Renmin University of China, October 28-29.

Lai, Lili, and Judith Farquhar. 2015. Nationality Medicines in China: Institutional Rationality and Healing Charisma. *Comparative Studies in Society and History* 57, no. 2: 381-406.

———. 2020. Toward Knowing: Engaging Chinese Medical Worlds. In John Law and Annemarie Mol, eds., *On Other Terms.* Sociological Review Monographs.

Lai, Lili, and Yan Zhen. Forthcoming. Minority Medicine: Institutionalization and State Policy. in *The Routledge Handbook of Chinese Medicine.*

Lambert, Helen. 2018. Indian Therapeutic Hierarchies and the Politics of Recognition. *Asian Medicine 13*: 115-33.

Lampton, David M. 1977. *The Politics of Medicine in China.* Boulder: Westview Press, 1977.

Landecker, Hannah. 2013. Metabolism, Reproduction, and the Aftermath of Categories. *Feminist & Scholar Online* 11, no. 3.

Langford, Jean. 2002. *Fluent Bodies: Ayurvedic Remedies for Post-colonial Imbalance.* Durham, NC: Duke University Press.

Latour, Bruno. 1990. Drawing Things Together. In Michael Lynch and Steven Woolgar, eds., *Representation in Scientific Practice*, 19-68. Cambridge, MA: MIT Press.

———. 1993. *We Have Never Been Modern.* Cambridge, MA: Harvard University Press.

———. 2005. *Reassembling the Social: An Introduction to Actor-Network-Theory.* Oxford: Oxford University Press.

Latour, Bruno, and Peter Weibel, eds. 2005. *Making Things Public: Atmospheres of Democracy.* Cambridge, MA: MIT Press.

Latour, Bruno, and Steve Woolgar. 1979. *Laboratory Life: The Social Construction of Scientific Facts.* Beverly Hills: Sage Publications.

Law, John, and Annemarie Mol, eds. 2002. *Complexities: Social Studies of Knowledge Practices.* Durham, NC: Duke University Press.

Leading Group Bureau for the Medical Professional Qualifying Exams in Chinese Medi-

cal Specialties (Zhuang Medicine) 中医类别中医 (壮医) 医师资格考试领导小组办
公室. 2013. *Zhuang Yixue* 壮医学. 上册 [Zhuang Medicine, vol. 1]. Nanning: Guangxi
College of Traditional Chinese Medicine (internal publication).

Lei, Hsiang-Lin. 1999. *When Chinese Medicine Encountered the State, 1910–1949*. PhD
diss., Committee on Conceptual Foundations of Science, University of Chicago.

———. 2014. *Neither Donkey nor Horse: Medicine in the Struggle over China's Modernity*.
Studies of the Weatherhead East Asian Institute, Columbia University. Chicago: University of Chicago Press.

Leslie, Charles, ed. 1976. *Asian Medical Systems: A Comparative Study*. Berkeley: University of California Press.

Levi-Strauss, Claude. 1966. *The Savage Mind*. Chicago: University of Chicago Press.

Li Hsiao-t'i. 2001. Making a Name and a Culture for the Masses in China. *Positions* 9,
no. 1: 29–68.

Liao Yuqun 廖育群. 2006. *Guanyu Zhongguo Chuantong Yixuede Yige Chuantong Guan-
nian: Yizhe Yi ye* 关于中国传统医学的一个传统观念——医者意也 [On a Traditional
Concept in China's Traditional Medicine: Medicine Is Reasoning]. http://www1
.ihns.ac.cn/members/liaoyq/yzyy.htm, accessed April 5, 2016.

Litzinger, Ralph. 1995. Making Histories: Contending Conceptions of the Yao Past. In
Stevan Harrell, ed., *Cultural Encounters on China's Ethnic Frontiers*, 117–39. Seattle:
University of Washington Press.

———. 1998a. Memory Work: Reconstituting the Ethnic in Post-Mao China. *Cultural
Anthropology* 13, no. 2: 224–55.

———. 1998b. Reimagining the State in Post-Mao China. In Jutta Weldes et al., eds.,
Cultures of Insecurity: States, Communities, and the Production of Danger, 293–318.
Minneapolis: University of Minnesota Press.

———. 2000. *Other Chinas: The Yao and the Politics of National Belonging*. Durham:
Duke University Press.

Liu Mingzhe, chief ed. 2003. 《黎族民间草药集锦》. Haikou: Hainan Nationalities Religious Affairs Department 海南省民族宗教厅.

Lock, Margaret. 1993. *Encounters with Aging: Mythologies of Menopause in Japan and
North America*. Berkeley: University of California Press.

Lock, Margaret, and Vinh-kim Nguyen. 2010. *An Anthropology of Biomedicine*. Malden,
MA: Wiley Blackwell.

Lu Guangxin 陆广莘. 2001. *Zhongyixue zhi Dao: Lu Guangxin lun yi ji* 中医学之道: 陆广
莘论医集 [The Way of Chinese Medicine: Collected Medical Works of Lu Guang-
xin]. Beijing: Renmin Weisheng Chubanshe.

McLuhan, Marshall, and Bruce R. Powers. 1989. *The Global Village: Transformations in
World Life and Media in the 21st Century*. New York: Oxford University Press.

Mao Zedong. 1967 [1927]. Report on an Investigation of the Peasant Movement in
Hunan. In *Selected Works of Mao Tse-Tung*, 1: 23–59. Beijing: Foreign Languages
Press.

———. 1967 [1937]. On Practice. In *Selected Works of Mao Tse-Tung*, 1: 295–309. Chi-
nese publication: 实践论: 论认识和实践的关系—知和行的关系 [On Practice: On the
Relation between Knowledge and Practice, on the Relation between Knowing and
Going]. 毛泽东选集第一卷 [Selected Works of Mao Zedong, vol. 1]. Beijing: People's
Press, 1951.

Markell, Patchen. 2009. *Bound by Recognition*. Princeton: Princeton University Press.

Mitchell, Timothy. 1988. *Colonising Egypt*. Berkeley: University of California Press.

———. 1991. The Limits of the State: Beyond Statist Approaches and Their Critics. *American Political Science Review* 85, no. 1: 77–96.

Mol, Annemarie. 2002. *The Body Multiple: Ontology in Medical Practice*. Durham, NC: Duke University Press.

Mueggler, Erik. 2011. *The Paper Road: Archive and Experience in the Botanical Exploration of West China and Tibet*. Berkeley: University of California Press.

Mukharji, Projit Bihari. 2016. *Doctoring Tradition: Ayurveda, Small Technologies, and Braided Sciences*. Chicago: University of Chicago Press.

Mullaney, Thomas. 2010. *Coming to Terms with the Nation: Ethnic Classification in Modern China*. Berkeley: University of California Press.

Munn, Nancy. 1986. *The Fame of Gawa: A Symbolic Study of Value Transformation in a Massim (Papua New Guinea) Society*. New York: Cambridge University Press.

Nappi, Carla. 2009. *The Monkey and the Ink-Pot: Natural History and Its Transformations in Early Modern China*. Cambridge, MA: Harvard University Press.

Needham, Joseph. 1956. *Science and Civilisation in China*. Vol. 2. Cambridge: Cambridge University Press.

Popper, Karl R. 1972. *Objective Knowledge: An Evolutionary Approach*. Oxford: Clarendon Press.

Porkert, Manfred. 1974. *The Theoretical Foundations of Chinese Medicine: Systems of Correspondence*. Cambridge, MA: MIT Press.

Povinelli, Elizabeth. 2016. Can Rocks Die? Life and Finitude outside Biontology. Chap. 1 of *Geontologies: A Requiem to Late Liberalism*. Durham, NC: Duke University Press, 2016.

Rabinbach, Anson. 1990. *The Human Motor: Energy, Fatigue, and the Origins of Modernity*. New York: Basic Books.

Raj, Kapil. 2005. Surgeons, Fakirs, Merchants, and Craftspeople: Making *L'Empereur's Jardin* in Early Modern South Asia. In Londa Schiebinger et al., eds., *Colonial Botany: Science, Commerce, and Politics in the Early Modern World*. Philadelphia: University of Pennsylvania Press.

Reiss, Timothy. 1982. *The Discourse of Modernism*. Ithaca: Cornell University Press.

Rifkin, Susan B. 1972. Health Care for Rural Areas. In Quinn, Joseph R., *Medicine and Public Health in the People's Republic of China*. Washington, DC: US Department of Health.

Ruan Baodi. 2011. 羌族释比口述史 [Oral Histories of Qiang Shamanism]. Beijing: Nationalities Press.

Sapir, Edward. 1995. The Unconscious Patterning of Behavior in Society. In Ben G. Blount, ed., *Language, Culture, and Society: A Book of Readings*. Prospect Heights, IL: Waveland Press.

Scheid, Volker. 2002. *Chinese Medicine in Contemporary China: Plurality and Synthesis*. Durham, NC: Duke University Press.

———. 2007. *Currents of Tradition in Chinese Medicine, 1626–2006*. Seattle: Eastland Press.

———. 2014. Convergent Lines of Descent: Symptoms, Patterns, Constellations, and the Emergent Interface of Systems Biology and Chinese Medicine. *EASTS* 8, no. 1: 107–39.

———. 2018. Promoting Free Flow in the Networks: Reimagining the Body in Early Modern Suzhou. *History of Science* 56, no. 2: 131–67.

Schein, Louisa. 1997. Gender and Internal Orientalism in China. *Modern China* 23, no. 1: 69-98.

———. 2000. *Minority Rules: The Miao and the Feminine in China's Cultural Politics.* Durham, NC: Duke University Press.

Schmalzer, Sigrid. 2008. *The People's Peking Man: Popular science and human identity in 20th century China.* Chicago: University of Chicago Press.

———. 2016. *Red Revolution, Green Revolution: Scientific Farming in Socialist China.* Chicago: University of Chicago Press.

Scott, James C. 1998. *Seeing Like a State: How Certain Schemes to Improve the Human Condition Have Failed.* New Haven: Yale University Press.

———. 2009. *The Art of Not Being Governed: An Anarchist History of Upland Southeast Asia.* New Haven: Yale University Press.

Shanghai and Zhejiang Colleges of Traditional Chinese Medicine, eds. 1970. 《赤脚医生手册, 修订本》 [*Barefoot Doctors Manual, Revised Edition*]. Shanghai: Shanghai Revolutionary Publishing Group,

Shi Chih-yu. 2007. *Autonomy, Ethnicity, and Poverty in Southwestern China: The State Turned Upside Down.* London: Palgrave Macmillan.

Sivin, Nathan. 1987. *Traditional Medicine in Contemporary China.* Ann Arbor: University of Michigan Center for Chinese Studies.

Smith, Barbara Herrnstein. 1988. *Contingencies of Value: Alternative Perspectives for Critical Theory.* Cambridge, MA: Harvard University Press.

Spivak, Gayatri Chakravorty. 1988. Can the Subaltern Speak? In Cary Nelson and Lawrence Grossberg, eds., *Marxism and the Interpretation of Culture*, 271-313. Urbana: University of Illinois Press.

Steinmetz, George, ed. 1999. *State/Culture: State Formation after the Cultural Turn.* Ithaca: Cornell University Press.

Stengers, Isabelle. 2003. The Doctor and the Charlatan. *Cultural Studies Review* (Melbourne) (November): 11-36.

Taylor, Kim. 2005. *Chinese Medicine in Early Communist China, 1945-1963: A Medicine of Revolution.* New York: Routledge.

Thomas, Keith. 1983. *Man and the Natural World: A History of the Modern Sensibility.* New York: Pantheon.

Thomas, William I., and Dorothy Thomas. 1929. *The Child in America.* 2nd ed. New York: Alfred Knopf.

Thoreau, Henry David. 1961. *Walden.* New York: Crowell.

Tsing, Anna Lowenhaupt. 2011. *Friction: An Ethnography of Global Connection.* Princeton: Princeton University Press.

Vaughan, Meghan. 1991. *Curing Their Ills: Colonial Power and African Illness.* Cambridge, UK: Polity Press.

Verran, Helen. 1998. Re-imagining Land Ownership in Australia. *Postcolonial Studies* 1, no 2: 237-54.

———. 2011. On Assemblage: Indigenous Knowledge and Digital Media. In Tony Bennett and Chris Healy, eds., *Assembling Culture*, 163-76. London: Routledge.

Wang Hui. 2011. *The Politics of Imagining Asia.* Cambridge, MA: Harvard University Press.

———. 2016. *China's Twentieth Century: Revolution, Retreat, and the Road to Equality.* Ed. Saul Thomas. London: Verso.

Wang Kang, Li Jianzong, and Wang Qingbao. 1992. 神秘的白石崇拜: 羌族的信仰与礼俗 [The Mystical White Stone Worship: Qiang Ritual and Belief]. Chengdu: Sichuan Nationalities Press.

Wang Mingke. 2008. 羌在汉藏之间:四川羌族的历史人类学研究 [The Qiang between Tibet and the Han: Historical Anthropology of Sichuan's Qiang Nationality]. Beijing: China Book Company.

Wang Xinqi and Cheng Xiankuan. 2010. 浅谈《内径》中的三因制宜思想 [Discussion of *Inner Canon* Thought on Adapting to the Three Causes]. *Reports of the Yunnan College of TCM* 33, no. 3: 16–17.

Weber, Samuel. 1987. *Institution and Interpretation*. Minneapolis: University of Minnesota Press.

Winnington, Alan. 1959. *The Slaves of the Cool Mountains: The Ancient Social Conditions and Changes Now in Progress on the Remote South-Western Borders of China*. London: Lawrence and Wishart. Rpt. 2008 as *The Slaves of the Cool Mountains: Travels among Head Hunters and Slave Owners in South-West China*. London: Birlinn.

Wiseman, Nigel, and Feng Ye. 1998. *A Practical Dictionary of Chinese Medicine*. Brookline, MA: Paradigm Publications.

Xie Guan (Xie Li). 1935. 《中国医学源流论》 [Origin and Development of China's Medicine]. Fuzhou: Fujien Science and Technology Press, 1935.

Ya Yanyi 牙延艺. 2009. *Zhuang Medicine Guasha Poison-Expelling Therapeutics* [壮医刮痧排毒疗法]. Nanning: Guangxi People's Press.

Yang Nianqun 杨念群. 2009. 再造"病人":中西医冲突下的空间政治 1832–1985 [Remaking "Patients": The Politics of Space in the Conflict between Chinese and Western Medicine, 1832–1985]. Beijing: Renmin University of China Press.

Zhan, Mei. 2009. *Other-Worldly: Making Chinese Medicine through Transnational Frames*. Durham, NC: Duke University Press.

Zhang Dan. 2014. 民族民间医疗的规范化新探—以老羌医的被规范化为例 [Analysis of the Standardization of Ethnic and Folk Medicine: A Case Study of an Old Qiang Doctor Being Standardized]. *Journal of Guangxi University for Nationalities (Philosophy and Social Science Edition)*, 36, no. 6: 17–20.

———. 2016. 新时期少数民族传统医药传承和发展困局探析 [Preliminary Discussion of a Dilemma Encountered in Inheriting and Developing Minority Nationality Traditional Medicines in the New Era: Taking Qiang Medicine as an Example]. Paper presented at the Fourth Forum on China Nationalities Medical Education, Annual Meeting of the China Nationalities Medical Association, and the "One Region, One Road" Summit Meeting on Nationalities Medicine and Culture of the Qiang, Tibetan, and Yi Corridor. Chengdu, January 6–8.

Zhang Dong 张东. 2016. 元气神机: 先秦中医之道 [Original Qi, Vital Machine: The Way of Pre-Qin Chinese Medicine]. Xi'an: World Book Publishers.

Zhang Jing. 2013. 从医者需要对草药付出多少情感和关注? [How Much Affection and Attention Is a Medical Practitioner Required to Put In?]. Conference paper presented at the Southwest Anthropological Forum, Chongqing, China, 西南人类学论坛.

Zhang Wenyi. Forthcoming. Interview with Judith Farquhar. *China Anthropologist*.

Zhang Yanhua. 2007. *Transforming Emotions with Chinese Medicine: An Ethnographic Account from Contemporary China*. Albany: State University of New York Press.

Zhang Yi 张艺 and Zhong Guoyue 钟国跃. 2005. 羌族医药 [Qiang Nationality Medicine]. Beijing: Chinese Literature and History Press.

Zhao Hongjun 赵洪钧. 1983. 近代中西医争论史 [History of the Struggle between Chinese and Western Medicines]. Hefei: Anhui Science and Technology Press.

Zhao Jinghua 赵景华, ed. 2005. 土家族医药学概论 [Outline of Tujia Medicine and Pharmacy]. Beijing: Chinese Medicine Ancient Literature Press.

Zhen Yan and Hu Yingchong. 2014. The Collection of Early Texts and the Establishment of Databases for Chinese Nationality Medicines. *East Asian Science, Technology, and Society* 8, no. 4: 461-78.

Zhou Fengwu et al., eds. 1981-85. 名老中医之路 [Paths of Renowned Senior Chinese Doctors]. 3 vols. Jinan: Shandong Science and Technology Press.

Zhou Yuhua. 2010. 白石, 释比与羌族 [White Stones, *Shibi*, and the Qiang]. Beijing: China Wenlian Press.

Zhu Guoben. 2006. 中国民族医药散论 [Essays on China's Nationality Medicines]. Beijing: China Medical Science and Technology Press.

Zhu Hongmei 朱红梅 and Tan Laoxi 谭劳喜. 2014. *Zhuangyi qianci cisha jifade wajue he zhengli* 壮医浅刺治痧技法的挖掘和整理 [Unearthing and Sorting Zhuang Medicine's Shallow Pricking Technique for the Treatment of *Sha* Disease]. China Journal of Nationality Medicines 2014, no. 7: 43-44.

Zito, Angela R., 1997. *Of Body and Brush: Grand Sacrifice as Text/Performance in Eighteenth-Century China*. Chicago: University of Chicago Press.

Index

www.ingramcontent.com/pod-product-compliance
Lightning Source LLC
Chambersburg PA
CBHW060029030426
42334CB00019B/2241